The Breast Cancer Prevention and Recovery Diet

Suzannah Olivier is a qualified nutritionist and is herself a breast cancer survivor. She is a lecturer with the Institute for Optimum Nutrition and a committed campaigner for women with breast cancer. Her first book, *What Shall I Feed My Baby?*, was published in 1998. She lives in Norfolk

The Breast Cancer Prevention and Recovery Diet

Suzannah Olivier

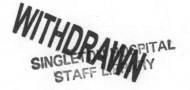

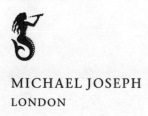

MICHAEL JOSEPH
LONDON

MICHAEL JOSEPH

Published by the Penguin Group
Penguin Books Ltd, 27 Wrights Lane, London W8 5TZ, England
Penguin Putnam Inc., 375 Hudson Street, New York, New York 10014, USA
Penguin Books Australia Ltd, Ringwood, Victoria, Australia
Penguin Books Canada Ltd, 10 Alcorn Avenue, Toronto, Ontario, Canada M4V 3B2
Penguin Books (NZ) Ltd, Private Bag 102902, NSMC, Auckland, New Zealand

Penguin Books Ltd, Registered Offices: Harmondsworth, Middlesex, England

First published 1999
10 9 8 7 6 5 4 3 2 1

Set in 10/14pt Stone Serif
Typeset by Rowland Phototypesetting Limited, Bury St Edmunds, Suffolk
Printed in Great Britain by Clays

A CIP catalogue record for this book is available from the British Library

ISBN 0-718-14395-7

Disclaimer

The contents of this book are not intended as an alternative to conventional medicine and you must take professional medical advice on all aspects dealing with cancer. The information in this book is intended for use for preventive measures, or as an adjunct to conventional treatment with the knowledge of your medical doctor. If you currently have cancer, it is recommended that you also consult a suitably qualified nutritionist or herbalist, with your doctor's knowledge, before embarking on an extensive programme. None of the advice in this book is appropriate for children.

Thanks to . . .

My husband **Laurence** for his patience while home life took second place to producing this manuscript, and for being a fierce and eagle-eyed editor; **Mr Mike Hudson**, breast cancer surgeon at Queen Elizabeth Hospital, for giving me invaluable advice on all things medical; **Marjorie Green** for encouraging, and haranguing, me throughout my career as a nutritionist and without whom this book probably would not have had its genesis; **Fiona Jenkins** for her commitment to finding every last statistic and piece of research I needed and working way beyond the call of duty; **Mr Dudley Sinnett** and **The Royal Marsden Hospital** for giving me back one of my nine lives ten years ago; my parents **Mo and Cy Endfield** and my sister **Eden Endfield** for being there when I needed them most.

Contents

Contents

Foreword

by Mike Hudson, Consultant Surgeon, Queen Elizabeth Hospital, King's Lynn

Here is a book for all women to read, particularly those who have had breast cancer, and those who wish to reduce their risks of developing it. Suzannah Olivier is an expert in the field of nutrition and has researched her subject thoroughly. Throughout the book her infectious enthusiasm bubbles through, and practical advice and help are to be found throughout. It is not the whole answer, as she is the first to admit, but it makes sense. It offers a means of taking control of one's body, of adopting a positive approach and saying, 'This is what I can do to help myself.'

I met Suzannah Olivier when, typically, she was hosting a dinner in aid of a breast cancer charity. She herself had developed breast cancer at an early age. She took a positive approach to her illness and during her treatment decided that her diet and lifestyle were wrong and set about changing them. She is now, over ten years later, a picture of health and a testimony to her convictions. Many people would be content with just that but Suzannah felt that her experience needed to be passed on to others. As a nutritionist she started advising women with breast cancer, and now with this book she is able to reach an even wider audience. She is at pains to point out that attention to diet is and must be complementary to conventional medical treatment and I obviously endorse this.

Diet has been known to be a factor in the development of some cancers for a long time. There are many other factors, of course, but sufficient heed has not been taken of diet, and advice, when given, frequently falls on deaf ears. Eating is a habit after all which, like many other habits, may at first seem hard to change.

As a surgeon specializing in the treatment of breast diseases I have, all too frequently, to utter those fateful words, 'You have breast cancer.' For the patient a period of anxious waiting has ended and life will never be quite the same again. It is then my task, together with my dedicated team, to treat that patient. The emphasis here is the word 'patient' – not just the cancer, but the whole patient.

Over twenty-five years ago I spent my research year in America working on the immune response to breast cancer and I have always been aware of the need to preserve this immune response. The body has its own natural defence mechanism against cancer cells – the immune system. Antibodies to breast cancer cells are produced in the same way as they are to infections. These antibodies attach themselves to the cancer cells and inhibit their ability to divide. Treatment therefore needs to be directed towards eradicating the tumour by conventional means – surgery, radiotherapy, chemotherapy or hormonal manipulation – and restoring the balance in favour of the immune system. Surgery, radiotherapy and chemotherapy will themselves cause temporary immunosuppression, but the overall benefits in destroying the tumour are of greater value, and the adverse effect on the immune system is a temporary one.

One of the first things to do is to build a positive approach which involves being outgoing and looking forward. Saying, 'What can I do to help myself?' Improving one's general health and level of fitness will boost the body's immune system, and here diet, exercise and stress-reduction play an important part.

The past fifty years have seen a dramatic increase in the incidence of breast cancer. Is it just coincidence that our diet has changed along with this? We look with dismay at the food our teenagers are eating, ready-prepared foods abound on supermarket shelves, sugar and salt are added to canned foods, and so-called fresh fruit and vegetables have withstood the onslaught of chemicals and pesticides. The pace of life has increased and food too has become 'fast'. We expect and demand more and more, yet stress levels rise and we remain discontented. Nor should we ignore the other changes in our lifestyle. The majority of breast cancers are hormone dependent, that is to say they are stimulated by the body's oestrogen. Nowadays, we can test the cancer cells for oestrogen receptors as a means of predicting whether they will respond to hormone manipulation using, for example, the drug Tamoxifen. Suzannah discusses the changes in our lifestyle that have changed women's hormone balance – the move towards having smaller families later in life, the contraceptive pill and HRT.

Suzannah is the ideal person to write this book and will, I'm sure, inspire her readers with her common sense and advice. **Read on. . . .**

Introduction

Moving Towards Health

As I write this, I am ten years post-diagnosis for breast cancer and I am going to do everything in my power to give other women with breast cancer the tools to make this, and more, a very real possibility for them. Eighty per cent of breast lumps and irregularities turn out not to be breast cancer, and there is much that can be done to prevent this disease. For the 20 per cent of women for whom the diagnosis does turn out to be cancer, there are many ways in which they can give themselves the best chance of recovery. Breast cancer is not a disease against which we are helpless. It is the result of a series of biological and environmental imbalances, and we are all able to take action to adjust these conditions.

My story

At the time I was diagnosed, I was thirty years old – a very young statistic – and found that the cancer had spread to half of my lymph glands. Whilst apportioning 'blame' for the development of cancer is probably ill-advised, I decided in later years, if there was a walking example of a woman most likely to get breast cancer I was probably her (genetics aside). I had not had any pregnancies; I had started my periods early in life; I had been put on the contraceptive pill as a young teenager to 'regulate' my periods and had stayed on it for many years; my diet was based on what was speedy and easy rather than nourishing and healthy; my food was certainly not organic; my stress levels were fantastically high; I had stopped doing any appreciable amounts of exercise, and so on.

After the initial shock of the discovery of the lump I set to work. The first item on my agenda was to find expert help. I asked around and found the most wonderful breast surgeon at a specialized National Health Service cancer centre. I had learnt that being operated on by a specialist, rather than a general surgeon, was likely to improve my chances of survival. He was sensitive to the fact that I was going

3

through a divorce and felt extremely vulnerable, and was happy to do a lumpectomy and lymph gland clearance instead of a mastectomy. It was only as the 1980s were clicking over to the 1990s that this became an option, and I have since spoken to many women with much smaller cancers who endured far more radical surgery only a few years previously.

Then I learned an interesting thing. The incidence of breast cancer had been rising steadily, and significantly, since the Second World War. It was startlingly obvious to me that there must be something that we were doing, as a nation, for this to be so.

Providence then came into play. A friend, and nutritionist, Marjorie Green, started putting packets of vitamin C through my letter-box, along with books to read. She was reduced to using my letter-box as I was feeling so low, emotionally and physically, that I would frequently avoid answering the door-bell. I was very depressed at this stage and it is hard to motivate yourself when you are feeling low and are on your own. I was having a bad reaction to my chemotherapy and feeling very unwell. Then I finally did as I was advised and started taking the vitamin C (I had slowly started to address my diet earlier). The vitamin C helped me turn the corner and the remaining three months of chemotherapy had nothing like the same negative impact.

Making changes

Subsequent to this I started to address other areas of my life that needed changing, always with a view to improving my chances of survival. I did not become a 'martyr to the cause' but made changes at a steady pace as and when I was able. First on my hit list was improving my diet further. I became fascinated with the subject of nutrition and it is, of course, the one area where we have the most control. Along the way I cleared up a number of other health issues that had plagued me in previous years – they would make good reading for a hypochondriac: an underactive thyroid, digestive problems, pre-menstrual swings, yeast infections and others. I believe that addressing all my health issues is what really made the difference, because these are not isolated processes that have no bearing on each other. By addressing the whole I am sure I was putting myself in the best possible position to avoid succumbing to breast cancer again, either with the original cancer spreading (if any microscopic amounts were left after hospital treatment) or new cancers having the opportunity to develop. I also addressed other key areas which I believe made a difference. I learned all about stress, its impact on the body and ways to make changes, some of which were quite radical. And I am still evolving. After fits and starts, I have been much better about taking regular exercise in the last two years and since remarrying and becoming pregnant with our son, he has been the catalyst I needed to get really serious about ensuring that most of our food comes from organic sources. In the first half of my forties, I feel physically much better than in the second half of my twenties.

Knowledge is power

As I researched this book, I hoped to include personal stories from long-term breast cancer survivors – and to my delight women came out of the woodwork in their droves, all of them wonderful, warm and keen to let other women know that life goes on. I often heard repeated from these women similar stories about how they coped at the time, how breast cancer has changed their view of life, and if they could have their time again how they would have wanted more information. As late as the mid-1980s breast cancer was not a widely discussed subject, but it has come out of the closet and women are prepared to share their experiences with others. Knowledge is power, and all these women feel that they have learnt from their experience and applied the information gained for the benefit of themselves and their families. Rarely did I encounter women who did not radically change their attitudes to life, living more for the moment and savouring precious times. The majority of them felt empowered by learning and changing their lifestyles and diets and were happy that they had become more aware of their health. And when I say the majority, these were not a carefully selected group of nutritionally paranoid women, but women that I met at breast cancer support groups who came from all walks of life. The one thing that is assured these days, if you are unfortunate enough to have just been diagnosed with breast cancer, is that you have a wealth of opportunities to meet other women who have been through a similar experience and who are willing to listen or provide information, as needed.

Loading the dice

I have a major question which I have been asking ever since my own encounter with cancer: *If some survive and some don't, what can we learn from the survivors and what can we do to load the dice in our favour?* The bald truth is that it is up to us to do what we can to help ourselves. Our families and friends can encourage and support us, but doing what it takes to give ourselves the best opportunity to thrive must come from within. Nobody gets it right all the time, but as long as we are making educated choices for ourselves we know that we are giving it our best shot.

Prevention is best

Today I practise as a nutritionist specializing in the care of women with breast cancer and I find myself becoming frustrated that insufficient attention is paid to prevention of this disease. It must be obvious to most people that it is a better strategy to avoid such a problem than to pick up the pieces afterwards. 'Reliable evidence shows that what we eat and drink is crucial in determining our risk of cancer,' stated Professor Philip James when launching the World Cancer Research Fund report in 1998. 'The evidence linking diet to cancer is now as compelling as the evidence on diet and heart disease,' added Professor Walter Willett of Harvard University, one of the world's leading nutritional epidemiologists.

Why do more people not concern themselves with prevention when the information is out there? Cancer is a difficult subject for most people. It is feared far more than cardiovascular disease even though, statistically, heart attacks and strokes outnumber cancer as killers. Breast cancer in particular is very threatening to women – it attacks their sense of attractiveness as well as forcing them to deal with the issue of mortality. The fear of death, the fear of losing a breast to surgery, of hair loss during chemotherapy, of tiredness and sickness during treatment are huge issues. And many of us are ostriches. If we don't think about it or address the problem, then maybe it will not happen. Even those who do think about it don't know how far to take preventive measures – there is a mass of information, much of it conflicting, so it is often easier just to ignore it all. And then there is a feeling of helplessness. If, as it seems, environmental factors are so important, and chemicals in our diet, and in the water we drink and the air we breathe contribute to breast cancer, what do we do – stop breathing? It can all seem quite complex. Others are simply unaware that diet, environment and lifestyle may have an impact – until they have no choice but to face the issues.

Ideally this is a book that will be used for prevention. This is, without a doubt, the area where the most significant changes to women's health can be made. In the last thirty years the incidence of breast cancer has increased by a massive 50 per cent. If these cases could have been prevented, we would have avoided untold heartache and saved millions of pounds.

Though prevention is the ideal, women who have already been diagnosed with breast cancer can benefit enormously from nutritional intervention. It is these women who are most likely to heed such advice – and these are the women who will bring the message to others. Every woman with breast cancer touches the lives of others and, whether she realizes it or not, is a bearer of information about this disease. It is my hope that this book will be read by the female relatives and friends of breast cancer patients for their own benefit. Their male relatives and friends may also take an interest – breast cancer affects the whole family. **This book is about choices, opportunities and hope.**

What can nutrition offer those with breast cancer?

Quite a lot, as it happens. You should be able to improve your quantity and quality of life and your chances for remission, without any conflict with your existing treatment and with no downsides – an insurance policy without significant cost.

A tumour is not a disease. A tumour is a consequence of a disease state. A disease state is, fundamentally, a metabolic disorder, and while surgery, chemotherapy and radiation will deal with the immediate crisis they do nothing to change the original factors, the metabolic imbalances or disorders, which allowed the condition to develop. By changing these imbalances you can create an environment where the cancer finds it difficult to survive.

There is a lot of information – several thousand research papers – to support the use of nutrition in the return to health of breast cancer patients, but doubters will always be looking for more research before recommending such measures. It must be stated plainly that the area of nutrition and cancer is controversial, and is regarded with scepticism by some members of the medical profession. Nevertheless hundreds of women have asked me for information about how to support themselves nutritionally after a diagnosis of breast cancer, and I have no doubt as to the need for, and the value of, this advice.

Costly research is a luxury that many people do not have the time for, and the wait could be fatal for some. Common sense dictates that, with the amount of data already available, those who want to adopt nutritional and lifestyle changes have clear incentives to act now.

How far, how fast?

We are all different. There is no one approach that is right for everybody, with nutrition as with anything else. We know from studies that the right sorts of fat in the diet, less overall fat, more vegetarian sources of protein, more fruit and veg, more oily fish, less alcohol, more soya, will decrease the risk of developing breast cancer. And yet, for some, the reforms required to lead a nutritionally exemplary life would be so tiresome, or even stressful, that they are not feasible – at the moment.

This book outlines the information needed to make personal choices for a way forward and sets out the most widely accepted nutritional and lifestyle factors in managing breast cancer. You may not want to follow all the advice, and even if you want to do as much as you can, you don't have to do it all in one go. Establishing new habits takes time, and these should be viewed as habits for life – not just for the weekend.

You may be reading this book while only half-way through treatment and may not have time, as suggested, to 'prepare' for surgery or chemotherapy, or you may feel that the mental stamina needed to change your diet is more than you have strength for at this time. I set before you the information; it is up to you to decide how far you want to take it.

An active role in your return to health

For some women the mental tonic of taking charge and doing something positive is a tremendous boost. If you are lucky, you will have a partner, family or friends to support you – though do not expect them to want to do as you do. Remember, there is nothing worse than a preaching convert!

Find your own place within this framework, and go at the speed you find acceptable. Don't let anyone dissuade you with 'It's not proven' or 'You are wasting your time'. If it feels right, do it. The power of the mind in the healing process is not the domain of this book, but never under-estimate its impact. Don't measure yourself against other people who may be doing more or less – it's not a race! This is a time, more than any other, when you are probably taking stock and becoming body-aware – maybe more than you want to. As with any other health regime, you will quickly become aware of what makes you feel good and what doesn't – listen to this inner wisdom. The seriousness of breast cancer does not detract from that, and probably gives an extra incentive which may have been lacking in the past. If I could patent the feel-good factor (FGF) of nutrition I would be rich! Take some of the FGF for yourself and make it your own.

Does Diet Really Influence Breast Cancer?

In the past, those who drew a link between breast cancer and diet endured a degree of ridicule from the establishment. However, it appears that the climate is now changing, with many important studies backing up the claims that diet and breast cancer do have strong links. Evidence shows that food choices can make a significant difference to the risk of developing the disease and this is now almost becoming received wisdom. The National Cancer Institute of Canada made the prediction that dietary modifications (in particular increasing fruits, vegetables, vitamin C and reducing saturated fats) could reduce breast cancer statistics by 24 per cent in post-menopausal women and by 14 per cent in pre-menopausal women.[1] If dietary changes are likely to make this much difference, and you then incorporate other influencing factors such as hormone balance, exercise and reduced exposure to environmental chemicals, you begin to see how you can make a really dramatic impact on a disease which affects so many women.

The body cures cancer daily

Cancer doesn't just 'happen'. Breast cancer takes an average of ten years to develop from the point where damage is done to a cell, until it has replicated itself to the point where a cancerous mass can be found.

Cell damage occurs daily, but we have many ways of dealing with this development. We can stop the damage happening in the first place, or at least dramatically reduce the chances of it developing. We can repair damage to DNA or cell membranes. We can get rid of, or detoxify, carcinogens. We can recognize cells that have mutated, and even started to proliferate, and eliminate them. We can encourage cells to live out their pre-programmed healthy lifespan, instead of going on to become cancer cells which do not die. There are several stages along the way in the development of cancer, and the healthy body can interrupt the process at most stages.

It is only when we are overwhelmed by cancer-causing or cancer-promoting factors, or when our defence mechanisms are not sufficiently able to deal with the abuses and imbalances, that cancer – in this case, breast cancer – gets a hold. Prevention of breast cancer makes sense because, if you can enhance your natural mechanisms which deal with early cancer, you may be able to avoid the traumatic experience of medical intervention.

A significant number of women, if they apply the principles in this book, may avoid the initiation of breast cancer. Or if they are in the very early stages of breast cancer which are as yet undetectable they may help to reverse the process. Even more astounding is the potential for women who have a genetic predisposition to breast cancer possibly to avoid their fate by applying these measures. Diet and lifestyle appear to be more significant influences on the development of breast cancer than is a genetic susceptibility. Women are likely to be able, literally, to reprogramme their genes.

Beyond a basic eating plan, we all have individual health issues that predispose us to an increased risk of breast cancer. For some it may be a question of hormone balance, for others their immune system may not be as effective as is ideal, and others still may not have the 'cast-iron' digestive systems that allow them to get away with dietary discrepancies. Taking a very personal approach, and working out which are the most important issues for you, can significantly raise your level of health and energy, enabling your defence mechanisms to work to maximum efficiency. Balance, or homeostasis, is what the body is always seeking to achieve, and if you allow this natural state to happen you are better disposed to deal with the threat of breast cancer.

Preventing recurrence

Whilst it is widely accepted that nutrition plays an important part in breast cancer prevention, the corollary that nutrition can be involved in reducing the recurrence of this disease is sometimes still viewed as novel. Research into this area is still at an early stage, and is looking promising,[2] but it will probably not be confirmed until well into the twenty-first century that we can help to prevent recurrence with dietary measures. The closest we come to anything that resembles evidence are Japanese women, whose low incidence of breast cancer is linked to their diet, and who also have a much better chance of their breast cancer not returning. Why? Probably because they are carrying on doing what they have been doing all along, eating a diet which is protective against breast cancer.[3] So this is where you have to apply some logic to the situation and decide for yourself if the link between nutrition and breast cancer prevention is likely or not. The truth is that when all the evidence is in, sorted and made sense of, you will probably have died of old age anyway. Why wait? Given that dietary manipulation doesn't do any harm, and you believe that you may be loading the dice in your favour, why not go with your instincts? It really is a no-lose situation. A key principle of the Hippocratic Oath, to which all doctors owe allegiance, is 'First Do No Harm'. Nutrition, when used wisely, at the very least does no harm and, at most, can make all the difference in the world. Supporting the body's defence mechanism and giving it the raw materials that it needs to function optimally can do a massive amount to help thousands of women to live many years beyond their initial diagnosis of breast cancer.

Members of the medical profession cannot relish being at the sharp end when watching patients decline. In fairness to most doctors they can only use the procedures at their command. Hospitals have limited resources and, for the most part, have to rely upon treatments which are based upon years of research. It must be added that few doctors have formal training on the effects of diet, and supplements, on breast cancer.

In all other fields the advice given for secondary treatment – in other words, prevention of recurrence – is the same as that which is given for initial prevention. This is the rule, not the exception. If you have a heart attack you will be told to reduce salt, reduce saturated fat, take exercise and avoid smoking – the same strategies that are suggested for avoiding heart disease in the first place. If you have osteoporosis you will be advised to take calcium and do exercise, as will a person who wants to prevent the disease. If you have kidney stones you will be asked to drink a lot of water, as this is known to prevent them in the first place.

And, it may not be just nutrition that works – the knock-on effect of doing something positive which may be helpful can bring into play the little-understood matter of the power of the mind in the healing process. A woman who is actively participating in her return to health will probably have the edge.

There is another exciting way in which nutrition can be used, to improve not only a woman's chance of surviving the cancer, but her recovery from the treatment she undergoes to deal with the disease. The treatment may have worked, but for some women may not have been 100 per cent successful in the long term. Nutrition can create the right environment for the immune system to operate optimally, mop up any residual cancer, recover from surgery and other treatments, and create an environment which is hostile to the development of new cancers.

What is good for prevention *must* be good for promoting recovery and preventing recurrence.

Nutrition and research

The 'gold standard' of research is the Randomized Double-Blind Cross-Over Placebo-Controlled Trial. This means that a substance is tested on people (or animals) who do not know if they are receiving the substance in question. It is all controlled by sealed, numbered doses, and at some point in the trial the participants are 'crossed over' from the substance being tested to the placebo, or vice versa. This method is fine if you are testing a drug, but if you are examining the merits of a vitamin or a food it has severe limitations.

Nutrition does not lend itself well to studies and trials and in years to come trials may need to be redesigned in order to obtain meaningful data from this whole area. To quote one researcher, 'The tools being applied are generally blunt instruments that are simple for the scientist to administer and analyse.'[4] Furthermore, most experiments are not funded for more than a few months (at best), while the effect of nutrition, though it can sometimes be speedy, takes longer in most cases and depends on long-term lifestyle changes.

Researchers at the International Agency for Research on Cancer put it succinctly when they said, 'Understanding the multi-dimensional nature of diet and of its relationship with different cancers is a major scientific challenge.'[5] To put it another way: with nutrition, the whole is greater than the parts.

There is now a significant body of research building up, with thousands of papers available examining the influences of nutrition on cancer. Evidence is accumulating that points firmly towards a useful therapy with no side-effects.

Magic bullets?

The search has been on for many years now to find magic bullets which are effective as the 'cure' for breast cancer and other diseases. None has yet been found, despite billions of dollars spent on research looking for what are termed 'biological response modifiers'. Attempts to 'bottle' the substances we make in our bodies which play a part in fighting cancer, such as interferon, tumour-derived activator killer cells and interleukin, have all been disappointing, expensive and have had traumatic side-effects for patients.

But suppose that drugs being developed as biological response modifiers had shown successful results, without any side-effects at all. You can imagine the blaze of excitement which would have been generated by such 'miracle drugs' and the huge effort which the drug companies would devote to having them patented, licensed and publicized.

Well, guess what? Such substances have been found. Foods are now being described by scientists as 'chemopreventive' and it is acknowledged that certain foods have a pharmacological effect – items such as broccoli, soya, oriental mushrooms, garlic and live yoghurt. These foods have been shown to:

- support the immune system
- balance hormones and block their effect on breast tissue
- improve the liver's handling of carcinogens
- block cancer-promoting growth hormones
- stop damage to DNA and the excessive cell growth that leads to cancer

Powerful stuff indeed. The problem is that these foods and nutrients can't be patented and there is no money to be had in researching them, meaning that any research is motivated by academic interest rather than profit. Nevertheless, the fact that trials are taking place at all, with the considerable funding that is required, is a strong indication of how seriously the role of nutrition in the prevention and treatment of breast cancer is being taken. Money is not thrown around for such research, and reputations are at stake; results which are meaningful are sought.

Throughout this book we will look at ways in which foods in our diet can lower the risk of, and promote recovery from, breast cancer by maximizing these pharmacological effects.

The best strategy

Certain concepts of holistic health care are alien to the medical profession as a whole. One is 'cleansing' the body of toxins, another is the idea of a 'healing crisis' where symptoms get worse before they get better. Whilst both can have value in the right context it is vital to differentiate between healing phenomena and the symptoms of serious disease, such as cancer.

It is the experience of many clinicians (and I have read this in every single orthodox book on the subject of cancer) that occasionally patients will come to them saying they noticed an abnormality a while ago, but had been told that it was the result of toxins in the body, or had been given some other explanation. This is a dangerous situation as early diagnosis is a life-saver. I must stress that if any lump or other untoward symptom is encountered, medical advice must be sought to rule out cancer. Professor Baum said in 1995 that he saw one person a month who delayed treatment while they tried other therapies, and that the other 3,000 consultant surgeons around the country probably had similar experiences.

Cancer is an area where alternative programmes and remedies abound. Some alternative therapies advocate rigorous dietary regimes, consisting of exclusively vegan, macrobiotic or fruit- and vegetable-based diets encompassing juices and enemas. Whilst these may have had merit for some individuals, there is insufficient evidence that they can stand alone as successful therapies for the majority of people. And by far the majority of people who can be helped with nutrition are not going to entertain such strict regimes, let alone disciplines which might advocate not using conventional treatments.

If cancer has been diagnosed, the optimum way forward for the majority of people, with our current state of knowledge, is to use the best that conventional medicine can offer and the best that nutritional therapy can offer, along with a smattering of 'what makes you feel good' therapies.

Nutrition – the adventure

Many people avoid the subject of diet and other lifestyle changes because they are worried about what they are going to be asked to give up. Food is a great pleasure for most of us and I prefer to think of changes in a more positive framework. It helps if you are a 'foodie' and enjoy different cuisines, the preparation of food and planning menus – and, of course, if you have the energy and time to devote to this issue. It is also helpful if you have a supportive family, especially if you are feeling unwell. But healthy eating can also be made simple and doesn't have to take up a lot of time. I would urge you to find ways to enjoy healthy food and good nutrition – this is meant to be a positive experience. For those who are not so hot in the kitchen, I have put in my own simple recipes. Rather than featuring lists of ingredients that need to be carefully weighed out, these are more the sort of recipe that reads 'a handful of this, and a pinch of that'. They are meant to be guides rather than 'the law'. The recipes are all short on preparation time and long on taste, enjoyment and healthy ingredients.

How to use this book

This book will take you through the facts about breast cancer, including its development, diagnosis and medical treatment. We will look at risk factors and how to use this information to help prevent the disease developing. The main thrust is to examine dietary, lifestyle and environmental impacts on breast cancer.

In **Your Basic Nutrition and Supplement Plan** (page 197), the measures covered are appropriate for all of us, whether we already have a diagnosis of breast cancer or are interested in preventing the disease. **Your Basic Nutrition and Supplement Plan** will offer ways of changing habits and providing the tools to optimize the fight against breast cancer.

But we are not all clones of each other and the influences of body chemistry are different in every individual. To give you the best of all chances in avoiding or recovering from breast cancer **The Five Pillars of Health** (page 235) provide measures to individualize your plan to suit your personal body chemistry and optimize your prevention or recovery goals. The check-lists at the front of the book will guide you to the areas which are most important for you to address.

Finally, for those who are undergoing, or about to undergo, medical treatment for breast cancer, **Supporting Your Medical Treatment Choices with Nutrition** (page 301) will provide measures to reduce side-effects that may be encountered.

Some people are browsers, some are readers, some are hoppers and skippers and some just want to get straight to the point. It would be great if you were to read this book from cover to cover, and then make a plan which is right for you. Those who do not wish to do that, or who do not have the time, could go straight to the **Basic Nutrition Plan** (page 202). Here guidelines are outlined for changes to get on with straight away, providing the basics of using nutrition to fight breast cancer for both prevention and recovery. You can then go on to the more 'advanced' information outlined in **The Five Pillars of Health** for measures which are specific to you, to rebalance your body chemistry. However, I would strongly urge you at some point to read the other chapters giving you the background to what you are doing and why. Educate yourself on the reasons behind the plan and you will be more effective at making informed choices at all stages.

Five Inspiring Stories

The following stories are from women who used nutrition as an intrinsic part of their healing process from the moment they were told of their diagnosis. Each has a touching and inspiring tale to tell:

Persephone Arbour's story

Extract from a letter sent by Persephone, a 'veteran' of breast cancer, to Mary, newly diagnosed with the disease.

'When I was diagnosed, my first reaction – in shock – was "I have no future." Suddenly I had no idea of future at all – no sense of direction – no plans. I sat in my doctor's surgery in tears and asked him, "If it was you what would you do?" He said, "I would have surgery and would go to the Gawler Foundation [a complementary cancer support centre in Australia set up by Ian Gawler after he had been given two weeks to live eighteen years ago] . . ." I learned about diets and why, not just what. So, I came back to Perth very well informed, rested and clearer. I had already decided that surgery was absolutely OK, because my obviously misfunctioning immune system did not need to cope with recalcitrant cells in a lump! However, I also . . . did not see the point of nuking this body either . . . I was sixty-one . . . that makes a difference. I think I knew that quality of my life was more important than quantity . . . Here I am (now) hale and hearty with a clean record. I do have a tremendous respect for this disease. I understand what it can do, how it can lie dormant somewhere and – bingo – take off again. So I treat this body much better than I used to. I am much more conscious, though not fanatical, about what goes into it! I am more sensitive to what I need in terms of a stress-free environment. I make sure that I sleep enough. I take antioxidants and vitamin C. There were twenty-one women in (my) group – and without exception they were all, including me, "Doers and Copers". . . . Learn to be selfish, find out what you need to stay relaxed, happy and fulfilled.'

Zoë Lindgren's story

Listening to Zoë tell her story I became very aware of the excitement in her voice as she got to the turning point in her life. She was having a blood transfusion, needed because her red blood cell count had plummeted after chemotherapy, when 'The clouds parted and I realized that I must take charge, must make what I was going through a positive experience and learn something from it all.'

Zoë's story began when she was diagnosed with breast cancer when six months pregnant in 1988 at the age of thirty-one. She already had a nine-month-old son, and eventually her daughter was induced about six weeks early. It had been suggested that she have a termination – which she refused – and she was given a partial mastectomy, with lymph node clearance, while pregnant. Radiotherapy was postponed until after the birth. Zoë's mother died of breast cancer in 1990 and it is difficult to understand the kind of mixed emotions and pressures that accompanied her own experience with the disease at such a vulnerable point in her life.

The next dramatic turn of events came when Zoë was told, in 1991, that she had metastases in her lungs, for which she needed chemotherapy.

From day one Zoë threw herself into the business of getting well, what she describes as a 'healing journey'. As the years progressed she learned more and more about what worked for her and used a number of disciplines alongside her hospital treatment – diet, supplements, acupuncture (which helped to normalize her red blood cell count), meditation, visualization, reflexology and progesterone cream. The day she was informed of her breast cancer she became a vegetarian – 'I think I had always been looking for an excuse to do so.' Zoë attended the Bristol Cancer Help Centre and discovered the power of healing foods including raw foods, soya, and spices such as ginger and garlic. She also started a regime of supplemented nutrients, including high doses of beta-carotene, vitamin C and other antioxidants. The hospital also put her on Tamoxifen, and Zoë has used progesterone cream which offset the resultant menopausal

19

problems and restored her well-being. After her fourth chemotherapy for the lung metastases Zoë went on holiday to New York with her husband, and with no children and the opportunity to think about other things they really enjoyed themselves. On her return she began to work for the same architectural practice as her husband (they are both architects). She felt that the holiday helped to make a shift in her thinking and to normalize her life. Then came the payoff – she was told that no more cancer was showing in her lungs. 'I felt I had conquered the disease.'

Sue Pembrey's story*

'Looking back, my experience of cancer has acted as a great bridge between my old life, working with orthodox medicine for thirty-three years as a nurse in the NHS, and a new one which is embracing wider approaches to health and healing. I retired from full-time nursing at the age of fifty-two (in 1994), having nursed many patients with breast cancer. I discovered my own just two weeks later. Suddenly I was on the other side.

'The whole experience was, at one level, excellent. I felt safe and well cared for; the staff were competent, kind, happy to provide information and supportive when I did not take their advice, for example, not taking Tamoxifen. But inside the good experience and outcome is a more complicated personal story which is about my own responsibility for healing and maintaining good health. The diagnosis of cancer presented a challenge; how was I going to protect my body and delicate healing mechanisms from the assaults of surgery, radiotherapy and possibly chemotherapy? Alternative therapies seemed too extreme; I trusted surgery but felt anxious that the assault on the enemy, which is how Western medicine deals with breast cancer, would over-ride my own healing resources. I did not see the cancer as an enemy but as a messenger.

'What happened next helped me trust more, that the answers would come if I remained open. The day after diagnosis I was struck down with flu. A dear friend who is an orthodox doctor and scientist, and also has some homeopathic training, came to see me. He immediately gave me homeopathic remedies which had amazingly good effects within hours. This integrated physician also gave me remedies that protected my body against harm: such as Arnica to prevent or reduce bruising at the time of surgery, and X-ray and Radium to protect against the ill-effects of radiotherapy. These remedies really worked for me.

Excellent nutrition has also played a vital part in this strengthening of my immune system. Giving up milk encouraged me to eat soya instead. Soya is probably the single most important food that women with breast cancer, or other hormone-dependent cancers, can take. I eat a wide range of natural foods, organic where possible, as pesticides, fungicides and herbicides are implicated in the big rise in breast cancer. I try to maintain a balance between raw and cooked foods and to take as many essential nutrients as possible as food, although some supplements such as vitamin C are necessary. For me, the theory of oestrogen dominance developed by Dr John Lee from twenty years of clinical observation makes the most sense. I take progesterone as there is a family history of heart disease and osteoporosis and I have a low bone mineral density. I feel very well on it – though it has not helped my hot flushes! – but my breasts are much smoother, a point noted by the surgeon.'

*Sue Pembrey now runs workshops for women interested in balancing hormones (see page 245). This extract was previously published as part of a longer article in *Positive Health*, special breast cancer feature, October 1998. For further details, please contact Positive Health Publications Ltd, 51 Queen Square, Bristol BS1 4LH, UK. Tel: 0117 983 8851, email: sandra@positive.u-net.com

Jayne Calgary's story

Jayne thought she was going to die when she was diagnosed nearly twenty years ago, at the age of thirty, with breast cancer. Her reaction was to write tearful goodbye letters to her daughter, aged two, and her son, aged five. Instead, despite two mastectomies and recurrences in 1988 and 1996, she feels incredibly well, holds down a full-time job and has lived to see her children grow up (though sadly her son died two years ago).

By chance Jayne heard about a self-help group for those with breast cancer on the radio – it was newsworthy because it was such a novel idea at the time. This gave her the idea of seeking out a local group and one was just starting – Jayne became a founder member. She also contacted the Bristol Cancer Help Centre and 'felt I was in control for the first time. I had never thought about food as a tool for healing and realized I needed to change my diet radically. It was difficult because the children were already set in their ways, and sometimes I found myself preparing three meals. I was always in the kitchen and sometimes my jaw ached from eating so much raw food. But I have learned how to work with it now and I have no set rules. It is all more familiar. I take high doses of vitamin C alongside lots of other vitamins and supplements. I avoid red meat, eat fish, chicken and pulses, organic if possible.

'The Bristol Centre was a revelation. Relaxation and meditation have played an important part in my health – a time to be still. The thought of healing was initially strange as I had never come across the idea. The Centre offers so much, something for everyone, and it felt so good. The whole experience has changed my life and I am actually glad I had cancer because I've discovered so much and met so many wonderful people.'

The Revd Evelyn Davies's story

When she went into hospital to have a small, 'probably benign', lump removed in 1986, Evelyn Davies – then aged forty-six – had no idea how it would change the focus of her life. Evelyn, previously a teacher and now a trained counsellor, psychologist and vicar, runs the busy Melangell Centre for cancer patients in mid-Wales.

So convinced was she that her hospital visit would entail a weekend in hospital, followed by a return to work on Monday, that she took some urgent work into hospital. As she was coming round from the anaesthetic the sister gently explained to her that she had, in fact, had a mastectomy. In retrospect she believes this was the right decision as it meant that she did not have to be awakened from her anaesthetic for discussion of the procedure and she is happy about what happened, though at the time she was quite unsettled. Chemotherapy was suggested but she decided to reject this treatment.

When Evelyn went to the Bristol Cancer Centre she immediately saw that she could help herself. She addressed her diet, going on a very strict regime initially (after five years this relaxed somewhat but she still applies the principles) and received healing from Canon Pilkington. She began to get more involved with supporting new patients and would talk to them and give talks herself, and even accompany patients on their visits to the hospital.

She is fascinated by the mental realm of dealing with cancer and does not see the need to fight it as if it were a battle – as some people do. Her approach is an altogether gentler one. Evelyn expresses the need to 'get rid of baggage, heal memories, deal with low self-image, learning to say no, not allowing oneself to be a doormat and, above all, restoring balance in all areas of life and learning to build on strong foundations. Restoring balance leads to health.'

The Five Pillars of Health Check-list

The human body is a remarkable self-regulating mechanism. We are not simply made up of separate 'systems' – the digestive system, the nervous system, the immune system, and so on. It is nearer the mark to think of these as components of a complex web of interactions. Human biology is infinitely more complicated than it once seemed when we started categorizing the various parts – almost as if they were the parts of a car engine. We now know that the digestive system has important immune functions – is it part of the immune system? Various organs with other primary functions, including the heart, secrete hormones – does that make the heart a part of the endocrine system? Thyroid hormones affect fertility – does that make the thyroid part of the reproductive system? However, breaking the areas of attention into separate categories can assist in creating a way forward for the individual. As the 'systems' are a part of the web-like structure we call the human being, improving the performance of any one area will impact positively on all other areas of health.

From the holistic perspective there are five areas, or pillars of health, to look at, to give you the best chance of avoiding, or recovering from, breast cancer:

- **Supporting your immune system**
- **Balancing hormones**
  Including blood sugar balance, oestrogen and progesterone balance, thyroid hormone balance and adrenal, or stress, hormone balance
- **Digestive health**
- **Optimizing your detoxification mechanisms**
- **Reducing stress and managing its impact on the body**

The following check-lists will give you an idea of the most important areas for you to examine for clues to improving your health.

By taking this personalized approach to your health you can balance your body's chemistry which in turn optimizes your ability to stay disease-free.

Each of the check-lists corresponds to a chapter discussing the health issues that are at the forefront of each 'system'. Before dealing with any one, or more, of these health issues it will be helpful to read **Your Basic Nutrition Plan** (page 202) which gives the basic 'springboard' which all the other health measures can be built upon.

Building powerful immunity

One of the vital jobs of the immune system is to identify cells that are 'non-self', that is, cells which have mutated into pre-cancerous cells and no longer match the surrounding tissue or cells, cells which have been damaged in some way and need repair, or have to be disposed of. The immune system is well equipped to do this under normal circumstances, but there are times when it does not work effectively, for a variety of reasons.

Do any of the following apply to you?

– Do you take antibiotics more than twice a year?	*1 point*
– Have you done excessive exercise in the recent past? (More than one hour a day of cardiovascular exercise)	*1 point*
– Do you suffer from frequent colds or infections and find them hard to shake off?	*2 points*
– Do you suffer from any allergy-related problems such as hay fever, asthma, migraines, eczema, dermatitis, or reactions to any drugs or chemicals?	*2 points*
– Do you have any food allergies or sensitivities?	*2 points*
– Have you had a major personal loss in the last year or so? (Death, divorce, financial problems, etc.)	*2 points*
– Is there a history of cancer in your family?	*2 points*
– Do you suffer from poor wound healing?	*3 points*
– Have you recently undergone any medical treatment, such as surgery, radiotherapy or chemotherapy (all of which have an immuno-suppressive effect)?	*5 points*

– Do you have a diagnosis of breast cancer, either oestrogen receptor positive or non-oestrogen receptor positive?   *5 points*

If you have a total score of 5 or more, read the chapter **Building Powerful Immunity** (page 239) after you have read **Your Basic Nutrition Plan** (page 202).

Harmonizing hormones

In the last fifteen years breast cancer treatment has concentrated on ways of blocking the effects of the hormone oestrogen on breast tissue, and this approach is beginning to pay dividends, with statistics showing a lowering in mortality.

Whilst this approach seems to be effective up to a point, it may be focused too narrowly. Dealing with breast cancer may require more than simply blocking oestrogen overload – it is the total balance of hormones which we need to seek.

Do any of the following apply to you?

Signs of blood-sugar imbalance which can include:

– A need for frequent meals   *1 point*
– Headaches or migraines which are relieved by eating or drinking something   *2 points*
– Irritability, especially as a result of not having eaten regularly   *2 points*
– An inability to wake up feeling refreshed   *2 points*
– Excessive thirst or sweating   *2 points*
– A lack of energy   *3 points*
– Excessive carbohydrate cravings for foods such as bread, rice, pasta and biscuits   *3 points*
– Drowsiness during the day, especially mid-afternoon or after a substantial meal   *3 points*
– Feeling dizzy especially if after a missed meal or after a sweet snack   *3 points*

– A need for stimulants at regular intervals, such as tea,
   coffee, sweets, sugar, cigarettes, alcohol   *5 points*
– An addiction to sweet foods   *5 points*

If you have a total score of 5 or more, read the section **Blood-sugar balance** (page 246) in the chapter **Harmonizing Hormones** after you have read **Your Basic Nutrition Plan**.

Signs of oestrogen and progesterone imbalance which can include:

– Blood-sugar swings   *1 point*
– Monthly water retention   *2 points*
– Breast swelling and discomfort   *3 points*
– Polycystic ovaries   *3 points*
– A history of pre-menstrual problems   *3 points*
– Unpleasant pre-menopausal symptoms   *3 points*
– Uterine fibroids   *3 points*
– Fibrocystic breasts   *4 points*
– Oestrogen receptor positive breast cancer, or
   endometrial (uterine) or cervical cancers   *5 points*

If you have a total score of 5 or more, read the section **The power of progesterone** (page 250) in the chapter **Harmonizing Hormones** after you have read **Your Basic Nutrition Plan**.

Signs of a sub-optimally functioning thyroid which can include:

– Blood-sugar fluctuations   *1 point*
– Mental confusion   *1 point*
– Thickened skin (especially on face or feet)   *1 point*
– A tendency to being puffy or bloated   *2 points*
– A tendency to put on weight easily   *2 points*
– Feeling more tired than normal   *2 points*
– Always feeling cold when others feel warm   *4 points*

If you have a total score of 5 or more, read the section **The thyroid** (page 257) in the chapter **Harmonizing Hormones** after you have read **Your Basic Nutrition Plan**.

Healthy digestion

You are what you eat? No – you are what you *digest, absorb and assimilate*. This means that you may have an exemplary diet, but if your digestive system is not working at maximum efficiency you run the risk of being sub-optimally nourished. In order to stay free of breast cancer you will want your body's defence and hormone systems to be able to protect you. Providing them with the right nutrients and energy requirements to function properly is critical, and is dependent on a healthy digestive tract. Bowel health, constipation and levels of fibre in the diet have been intimately linked to breast cancer.

Do any of the following apply to you?

– Do you experience anal irritation?	*2 points*
– Do you take antacids or get a burning sensation in your stomach?	*2 points*
– Do you have any food allergies or sensitivities?	*3 points*
– Do you suffer from excessive wind?	*4 points*
– Do you suffer from bloating around the middle that arises during the day or after a meal that is not related to your menstrual cycle?	*5 points*
– Are you constipated, do you get diarrhoea, or do you have irritable bowel syndrome?	*5 points*
– Have you recently had a course of chemotherapy?	*5 points*

If you have a total score of 5 or more, read the chapter **Healthy Digestion** (page 267) after you have read **Your Basic Nutrition Plan**.

Detox your system

We have managed to create an alarming chemical soup in which we live. The air we breathe carries agrichemicals and pollution, the water we drink is laced with chemicals and heavy metals, the food we eat has insecticides and pesticides on it and in it, as well as additives, colours and preservatives. We have to detoxify, and store or eliminate, all these compounds, and this can reduce our physical reserves when we are dealing with other priorities such as fending off breast cancer.

Do any of the following apply to you?

– Do you ever have water-retention problems?	*2 points*
– Do you have 'orange-peel' skin?	*2 points*
– Do you generally eat non-organic produce?	*2 points*
– Do you drink unfiltered tap water?	*2 points*
– Do you live in a city, by a busy road or near a crop-spraying area?	*2 points*
– Do you spend a lot of time in traffic or exercise by busy roads?	*2 points*
– Do you regularly drink coffee, tea or alcohol?	*3 points*
– Do you frequently suffer from mucus in your nose, throat, ears or even in your stools?	*4 points*
– Do you have any food allergies or sensitivities?	*4 points*
– Do you live or work in a smoky atmosphere? Do you smoke or have you smoked in the past?	*4 points*
– Are you having, or have you had, chemotherapy?	*5 points*

If you have a total score of 5 or more, read the chapter **Detox Your System** (page 282) after you have read **Your Basic Nutrition Plan**.

Reducing your stress load

Stress is a word that is hard to define and there is definitely such a thing as positive stress, as well as negative stress. Inevitably, it is the negative connotations of the word that we are talking about in relation to breast cancer.

Stress does not just mean mental stress or, for that matter, taxing life events – such as being diagnosed with breast cancer. It can also mean dietary stress and the stress that chemicals may place on your body.

Do any of the following apply to you?

- Do you set unrealistic goals, are you generally dissatisfied, or do you always do several tasks at the same time? *2 points*
- Do you find it difficult to communicate feelings and tend to 'internalize' problems? *2 points*
- Do you dislike your work or home environment? *3 points*
- Do you tend to over-commit and do too much, or find it hard to say no? *3 points*
- Are you inexplicably fatigued all the time? *4 points*
- Have you recently been diagnosed with, or treated for, a major illness? *5 points*
- Have you suffered a major personal loss in the last two years (death, divorce, financial problems, etc.)? *5 points*
- Are you generally depressed or anxious? *5 points*

If you have a total score of 5 or more, read the chapter **Reducing Your Stress Load** (page 290) after you have read **Your Basic Nutrition Plan**.

These check-lists are signposts to guide you to areas of your health that may need attention. Later in the book each of these topics will be discussed in detail, with ideas for achieving changes in order to minimize your chance of developing breast cancer, or to speed recovery if you have already been diagnosed with the disease. Some sections will be more relevant to you than others. If you get colds frequently and have asthma, maybe your immune system needs more help than that of others. If you have pre-menstrual problems, with sore and tender breasts before your period, perhaps hormone balance is more relevant. In any event, maximizing your health to support these pillars is the key measure needed to load the dice in your favour.

Part 1 **Breast Cancer Explained**

Your Breasts

The female breast, an unending source of fascination and delight to artists, lovers, fashion editors and photographers, has, despite its complex appeal, a fairly straightforward structure which is perfect for its real function – that of suckling infants.

Breasts are composed mainly of fatty tissue which protects the milk-producing glands. There are between twelve and twenty lobes in each breast, which are in turn composed of hundreds of tiny lobules. The milk ducts lead from these and open through the nipple. Ligaments join layers of fibrous tissue to support the breasts and attach them to the muscles underneath. The breast is divided into four quadrants: the inner lower, inner upper, outer lower and outer upper. The outer upper quadrant has a tail, called the axillary tail, which leads up to the armpit.

Breast tissue has a rich blood supply, including branches from the axillary artery which supplies the outer area of the breast leading to the armpit. There are also lymph vessels which drain tissue fluids into the lymph nodes located in the armpits (axilla).

The lymph system

The lymphatic system is a part of the body's defence system, or immune system. It consists of capillaries and vessels, which extend to twice the length of the arteries, veins and capillaries of the blood system, and these serve to drain off the fluid in which cells are bathed. The fluid is passed through lymph glands, or nodes, which are about the size and shape of a dried kidney bean, or smaller. The lymph nodes act as filters, removing bacteria and other substances. Once cleansed, the lymph is drained into the blood for recirculation.

The lymph system is crucial for defence against infections. One school of thought is that lymph nodes become 'infected' with cancer as it spreads. Another is that cancer cells are initially trapped in the nodes as part of the defence system for controlling the spread of the

33

disease, and the nodes are instrumental in destroying those cells. It is because of this that the health of the lymph system is so important.

A lump in the armpit can be a fairly strong indicator of breast cancer and occasionally may be noticed before a lump is found in the breast. However, lumps in the lymph node area can also occur with benign, non-cancerous, breast disease and with infections of the nodes. It could also be that the nodes have swollen in a natural attempt by the body to resist the breast cancer, but this does not necessarily mean that the cancer has spread to the nodes.

Breast cancer cells are believed to migrate, or metastasize, quite early on in the disease process. It seems possible that lymph nodes which do not harbour cancer cells indicate a good level of natural resistance. By the same token, cancer in the nodes may suggest that the woman's natural resistance is at a low ebb.[1]

When surgery is performed on lymph nodes, in about 5 per cent of cases the drainage of lymph fluid is disrupted and results in swelling of the upper arm, or of the breast – this is called lymphoedema. Since the practice of using radiotherapy on the axillary, or underarm, area after surgery to that area has more or less been abandoned, the number of lymphoedema cases has plummeted.

Female hormones

Many women are acutely aware of the effects of hormones on their breast tissue. Many complain of swollen breasts, heaviness, discomfort or even increased 'lumpiness' each month, before menstruation. This is the clearest demonstration of the fact that breast tissue responds to hormone fluctuations, and pre-menstrual problems affect around 65 per cent of women. Three types of cell in the breast are sensitive to hormones: those lining the milk ducts, the glandular cells in breast lobules, and contractile cells responsible for squeezing milk out of the lobules.

The hormones oestrogen and progesterone are responsible for the changes that happen in a woman's body at puberty, during menstruation, pregnancy, breast-feeding and when going through the menopause. The hormone prolactin is responsible for stimulating breast tissue to make milk, and rising levels pre-menstrually may be partially responsible, along with oestrogen and progesterone balance, for breast tenderness at this time. Prolactin levels are high in breast cancer patients and may be an even more potent stimulator of tumour growth than oestrogen.

There is a complicated feed-back mechanism between the hormone control centres (the hypothalamus and the pituitary) as they interact with hormone output from the ovaries. This regulates the quantities of hormones being secreted at any one time.

Oestrogens are secreted by the ovaries, the adrenal glands, fat cells and, in pregnant women, by the placenta. Though oestrogen is usually referred to as one hormone, the term really refers to a group of hormones that have a similar action. There are several types of oestrogen but the three most important are oestrone (E1), oestradiol (E2) and oestriol (E3), all of which have slightly different functions and effects. E1 and E2 are the strong oestrogens associated with an increase in breast cancer risk, while E3 is the milder, benign oestrogen, mainly produced during pregnancy, which is 1,000 times weaker than oestradiol. The relevance of the types of oestrogen and how they affect breast cancer will be discussed later.

Progesterone is produced by the ovaries, and in pregnant women by the placenta. There is only one progesterone hormone produced in the body, although there are many types of artificial progestogens synthesized by the pharmaceutical industry.

Breast symptoms

Common breast symptoms, which can lead a woman to be concerned enough to consult her doctor, include a lump, breast pain, discharge or bleeding from the nipple. All these can be indications of breast cancer, but more often are not.

Eighty per cent of breast lumps are found to be non-cancerous. Usually they are a benign tumour, called a fibroadenoma, or a cyst. The problem with fibroadenomas is that they can feel, to the touch, similar to cancerous lumps. They occur most commonly in younger women, in their late teens and twenties, and typically they move away from the hand during physical examination, earning them the nickname 'breast mice'. Other possible reasons for a benign, harmless lump could be a cyst, caused by blocked ducts, fat necrosis, which is a lump of dead fatty tissue possibly caused by a physical trauma, or lipomas, which are fatty lumps.

Other symptoms that may raise concern can be differences in the size or shape of breasts and nipples. Trauma or blows to the breast can be a cause of worry especially if resulting in bruising or pain. Isolated pain in the breasts is rarely a result of cancer and is most likely to be caused by an abscess – though this is unusual – which needs treatment. Sometimes fibroadenosis, an increase in the fibrous glandular tissue, can also be painful. Occasionally, in older women, angina (heart pain) may be felt as pain in the breast. 'Jogger's nipple', where the breast is rubbing against fabric, causing it to redden, can be a problem for some women. Small swellings around the nipple, called Montgomery's tubercules, are modified sweat glands and can enlarge during pregnancy and breast-feeding. They may become more prominent and tender during sex, and this is a normal reaction.

While all these conditions are usually benign, any changes must be treated seriously, and if you are concerned on any level about breast symptoms, you should go to your doctor for an examination.

Self-examination

There is some controversy on the subject of self-examination. Advocates say that it encourages early diagnosis and therefore an increased chance of early treatment. Those against it say that self-examination does nothing to prevent the disease in the first place and also leads to a lot of unnecessary worry for the great majority who find symptoms which turn out to be benign. I fall into the first camp and believe wholeheartedly that self-awareness in relation to physical symptoms is an integral part of taking responsibility for your own health.

One of the purposes of self-examination is to become aware of what is normal for your body. The object is not to compare yourself to what is normal for other women. Everyone is a different size and shape, with a different nipple type, and the person who is best placed to diagnose changes is the expert – you! Ninety per cent of breast cancers are detected by the women themselves. Mammography in the fifty-plus age group detects very early stage breast cancers, but by far the majority of tumours are still found by the women themselves.

In order to monitor the health of your breasts it is advisable to do a breast check yourself once a month. Ideally, women should start this routine in their late teens or early twenties and continue the habit for life. Breast examination is free, encourages self-awareness, and is the way that most breast lumps are found. This is how to do it:

1. Examine your breasts when you have a quiet moment and the time to do the check properly. It is best to examine your breasts in the week after your period, as hormonal changes prior to your period will probably make the tissue thicker or lumpier, and thus less easy to notice irregularities. Post-menopausal women can make a routine of examining their breasts on the same day every month – the first is easy to remember. If you have had a hysterectomy which has left your ovaries intact, you may be experiencing the stages of your menstrual cycle without accompanying bleeding – in this case choose a regular monthly time when your breasts are not swollen or sensitive.

2. First stand in front of a mirror with your arms by your side, observe the shape of your breasts and determine if there is any change from the last examination. Lean forward and observe any changes. Come upright again and move your arms horizontally to the side and then over your head. All the time you are looking for changes in how your breasts move, in the texture of the skin, for any dimpling or puckering. Look for changes in the nipples as well, such as change of direction or pulling-in.

3. While standing in front of the mirror, physically examine your breasts. This can be done either in quadrants, like the slices of a pie, or in ever-larger circles from the nipples out. Remember to feel under the armpits and also to examine the nipple by pushing downwards with one finger and gently squeezing the nipple to check for any discharge. You should also check above your collar-bone.

4. Repeat the physical examination while lying down on your back. Raise one arm, rest it comfortably under your head and use the opposite hand to check your breast. Many women find it ideal to examine their breasts in the bath or shower as the skin is then

slippery. The whole procedure may take a bit of time at first, but after three or four months you will find it can be done much faster – but not too fast! Thoroughness is important and the examination is a few minutes of time well invested.

5. If you do find a lump or any other symptom, it is important to have it checked by your doctor as early as possible. Early diagnosis is one of the key factors in increasing the chance of survival. However, do not panic – for every five lumps one is cancerous, and the remainder are benign and harmless. Even if a lump is cancerous, six or seven out of ten will be treated without the removal of the breast – the greatest fear for some women.

It is important, for the best chance of early diagnosis, to get away from the idea that you are always looking for a lump. Symptoms that can be a warning of breast cancer are:

- A lump in the breast or any area of thickening
- A lump in the armpit
- Change in the size or shape of the breast
- Inversion (pulling-in) or puckering of the nipple
- A rash around the nipple
- Bleeding or discharge from the nipple (especially one-sided)
- Dimpling or puckering of the breast skin
- Swelling of the arm
- Ulceration of the skin
- Breast pain or persistent tenderness
- Unusually prominent veins on the breast

Even if you have had symptoms where breast cancer has been ruled out previously, say non-malignant breast lumps, you should follow through with any concerns since benign breast disease can co-exist with breast cancer. One does not indicate the other, but neither does one preclude the other.

If you are pregnant, or breast-feeding, your breasts will be undergoing many changes, but monthly examinations are still wise as 3 per cent of all breast cancers are found in women who are either pregnant or breast-feeding. If there are any symptoms that concern you it is best to seek your doctor's advice.

Jasmine Fulcher's story

A frequent misconception is that breast cancer always manifests as a lump; it is not always a lump that you are looking for, but a change from what is normal for you, as Jasmine discovered. In 1992 when she was fifty-five Jasmine was making a wedding dress for her daughter. She put the ache in her arm down to the job in hand and to rheumatism. The pain built up and a few weeks later she was prescribed anti-inflammatory drugs. Nothing worked. Eventually she was sent for a full check-up to include a venogram, mammogram, CAT scan and a bone scan. It was determined that she had breast cancer, despite a mammogram a year earlier that had shown calcifications but had been deemed to be all right. All Jasmine's lymph glands were affected and had attached to a vein, causing a blockage and the pain. At the time Jasmine was furious and vented her anger on all around her. She simply couldn't believe this was happening to her.

Although Jasmine still doesn't like to look at the wound left by the mastectomy, she is glad, as she puts it, 'to have literally got it off my chest'. Despite her fury when she was diagnosed and her reaction of venting her frustration on all around her, Jasmine now has a particularly bright outlook on life and wakes up in the morning saying 'Hello, world.' She has learnt to manage her stress and has decided that many things are simply not worth worrying about. One way of helping herself to feel better about her experience is to do lots of charity work to help others. Jasmine found that meditation helped her enormously and yoga helped her to regain the use of her arm. In the final analysis her husband is less worried about the mastectomy than she is, and he is adamant that he would rather have her with one breast than not have her at all!

Early diagnosis

Finally, remember – apart from prevention in the first place, there is no single tool that is more important in preventing mortality from breast cancer than early diagnosis. If you are suspicious, get yourself checked out, and if you are told that there is nothing to worry about, but you still have doubts, get a second opinion. Do not delay in asking a doctor to check your symptoms out for any reason – there is no reason to be embarrassed, pretend they aren't there or feel that you are wasting your doctor's time. Any competent and caring doctor will not mind examining any irregularities. It is the experience of surgeons that I have talked to that a disquietingly large number of women still come for treatment at an advanced stage, having ignored their symptoms for quite a while. Embarrassment, fear and the hope that it will 'just go away' are reasons that are given. Treatment is much more effective if given during the early stages of breast cancer.

Those Fateful Words

'You have breast cancer.' This is the news that 115 women receive every single working day in the UK. It is not surprising that fear is triggered by these words, and this fear is made worse by the fact that it is, largely, fear of the unknown. So what can you expect to experience if diagnosed with breast cancer? Every person is an individual, and will have an individual experience, but here we will look at the most common issues surrounding this diagnosis, and unravel some of the information about the development of breast cancer.

What is cancer?

Cancer is not just one disease – there are around 180 different types. Even breast cancer is not a single disease. However, most types of breast cancer can be distinguished from other cancers because they are affected by hormones, and this makes the conventional treatment of breast cancer different in some respects, and the nutritional management of breast cancer different in many respects.

Cancer arises when cells begin to multiply out of control, usually developing into a mass which, if left to progress, spreads to other areas of the body. If left unchecked, the expanding cancerous tissue depletes the body of nourishment and may press on body tissues, causing discomfort. Ultimately the cancerous growths may displace healthy tissue to the point where normal body functions can no longer take place.

The word tumour is a worrying one, but a tumour is not always malignant (cancerous). A tumour can simply be an overgrowth of cells that stays localized in one particular area, as in the case of a fibroadenoma. This is called 'benign', and as long as it is not pressing on nerves, ligaments or organs, is nothing to worry about.

There are four stages in the development of cancer and these happen over a long period of time. The average development time for breast cancer is ten years.[1] In some people it may be three years and for others twenty; however, if you take the average, you have a long time to interfere with the process. And interfere you can. Each stage along the way offers opportunities to interrupt the development of cancer. The stages are:

Initiation
The tissue appears normal under a microscope, but important changes have occurred in the cell nucleus, or command centre. Proto-oncogenes, which regulate cell growth and development, are corrupted and switch off the restraints on overdevelopment. Oxidative damage, a major corrupter of DNA (our genetic make-up), can be minimized by nutritional means. The immune system, which searches out and destroys the corrupted cells, can be enhanced, and enzymes which detoxify carcinogens can be boosted.

Promotion
Visible changes to the tissue can be detected under the microscope. This stage is sometimes referred to as a pre-cancerous stage and is reversible. Nutrition can help to strengthen healthy cell membranes, encourage communication between cells at sites called gap junctions (which is necessary for them to recognize their boundaries), enhance the immune system's ability to cope with the pre-cancerous cells, and balance hormones in order to discourage cell proliferation.

Progression
The tumour is still too small to be detected with the naked eye, but has begun to signal to the surrounding blood supply, encouraging it to link the tumour to the blood network, so that it can feed itself and eliminate waste material. This process is called angiogenesis. Some nutritional measures, as well as new drugs that are being developed, can help to interrupt this malignant form of blood vessel growth, and in so doing starve the tumour.

Detectable tumour
This is the stage at which most breast cancers are discovered. To get to this point will have taken several years depending on the 'doubling time', or growth rate, of the cancer. This stage is deemed irreversible,

and the treatment is usually surgical, with radiation, drugs and possibly hormone treatment as well. Nutrition can support the patient's ability to manage conventional treatment and enhance the immune function to help deal with any cancer that the medical treatment may not have totally dealt with. It can change the circumstances that lead to the disease developing in the first place, thereby discouraging recurrence.

Types of breast cancer

In-situ ductal carcinoma	A pre-invasive form of breast cancer which may remain contained or can become invasive. A lump is rarely detectable and usually comes to light with a mammogram. It is estimated that approximately 40 per cent of in-situ carcinomas become invasive.
Invasive ductal carcinoma	The most common type of breast cancer arising in the epithelial (lining) cells of the milk ducts. Invasive duct carcinomas make up 90 per cent of all invasive breast cancers.
In-situ lobular carcinoma	A pre-invasive form of breast cancer which indicates an increased risk of breast cancer. It is usually not treated unless it changes and becomes invasive.
Carcinoma of the breast lobules	The second most common type, also affecting epithelial cells. Lobular carcinomas make up 8 per cent of all breast cancers. The difference between lobular and ductal carcinomas is that with lobular carcinomas there are often several sites affected with either pre-invasive or invasive cancer at the same time.
Paget's disease	An unusual eczema-like scabbing of the nipple and areola (nipple surround) caused by an underlying carcinoma.
Sarcoma and fibrosarcoma	Cancer arising in the connective tissue cells of the breast.

Cystosarcoma	A rare malignant tumour usually found in women with rapidly recurring fibroadenomas (non-malignant fibrous tumours). It does not usually spread to other parts of the body, but tends to invade the adjacent breast.
Melanoma	It is also possible to have a type of skin cancer which happens to be found on the breast.
Inflammatory breast cancer	An uncommon condition found in 1 per cent of all breast cancers. It usually appears as a swollen and reddened breast which looks as if it is infected. There is usually no lump and antibiotics do not resolve the 'infection'. The inflammation is due to the cancer affecting the lymphatics of the skin.

When cancer spreads

When cancer spreads, via the blood or lymph to other areas of the body, this is termed metastasizing, and new tumours are called secondaries. Although the cancer that has spread may be in a new part of the body, it is still referred to as the cancer of origin and treated accordingly. Breast cancer that has spread to, say, the liver is not treated in the same way as primary cancer of the liver.

Some cancer cells develop pseudopodia, or 'feet', to push out into surrounding tissue. They can also secrete an enzyme which dissolves the cement between neighbouring cells, making it easier for them to migrate. Strengthening this cellular cement is an important nutritional tool in the arsenal against breast cancer.

Statistics

While carrying out research, I found that the majority of books dealing with breast cancer started with statistics depicting the mortality rate for the disease. Reading this can be depressing if you have just been diagnosed with cancer, and hanging on to the idea that you are an individual, and not a statistic, is essential. Is a glass half empty, or half full? For every report you read telling you that X per cent die, the fact is that Y per cent live.

Having said this, we are in a crisis at the moment and the incidence of breast cancer is on the increase. The World Health Organization says that worldwide, the breast cancer incidence is set to double by the year 2020.

In less than thirty years incidence has increased by 40 per cent, from around 22,000 cases per year in the UK in 1971 to 30,000 cases at the end of the 1990s. Nowadays one in eleven women can expect to develop breast cancer at some point in their lives in the UK, and one in eight if they live in the USA.

Bad news tends to be more widely reported than good news and the figures of a death rate from breast cancer of 15,000 each year in the UK and 46,000 a year in the USA doesn't make happy reading (in fact during the Vietnam War when 60,000 troops died, 330,000 American women died from breast cancer in the same period). What you rarely see reported is the good news – more than 70 per cent of women who have breast cancer that is operable will be alive and well five years after the diagnosis – and maybe longer: longer-term figures are not available.

It is recognized that advancing years are a major risk factor, with the majority of women diagnosed being post-menopausal. However, around 15 per cent of breast cancers happen in women of child-bearing age and there seems to be an increase in incidence[2] in the twenty to forty age group. In England and Wales the figures[3] for all age groups showed an increase of 28 per cent from 1980 to 1994 (the latest year for which accurate figures are available). And yet younger women, up to the age of thirty-nine, showed a 40 per cent increase, from 1,235 cases in 1980 to 1,713 cases in 1994.

Anna Stopford's story

Anna is now aged thirty-eight, and has a lively sixteen-month-old daughter, Esme: it seems incredible that her first symptoms of breast cancer appeared when she was only twenty-two years old. Anna, a nurse, noticed a white discharge from one nipple and went to her doctor who sent her for a mammogram. The mammogram came back clear and she went away content that she was in the clear. But over the next few years she repeatedly went back to the doctor – she saw a total of five GPs – with a number of classic breast cancer symptoms: orange-peel skin, inverted nipple and a 'fixed' breast. She was repeatedly told that the original mammogram was clear and that she did not need to be referred to a specialist; even a follow-up mammogram was deemed unnecessary. It was also implied that because of her nursing background with all the cancer patients she had tended, Anna was developing slight hypochondria. Finally, she refused to leave the doctor's surgery until she was referred on. Seven years after the first symptom, breast cancer was diagnosed. Anna had a mastectomy, followed by a very successful reconstruction with a silicone implant.

Anna's backlash of anger when she went through the whole experience meant that she began over-eating and, inevitably, put on weight. She has calmed down now and her family's eating habits are pretty good – mostly vegetarian or fish-based meals, lots of fruit and vegetables and organic food dominate the dining table.

When Anna's daughter was born nobody could advise her on the likely problems associated with breast-feeding from one breast, and no literature was available. Finally, she consulted books on breast-feeding twins, had no problems, and continued feeding from her natural breast until her daughter was over one year old. It is astonishing that she was given quite worrying information along the way by well-meaning but misinformed people. It was suggested that there was a chance of passing on cancer in breast milk (you can't) and that another pregnancy would be likely to increase the risk of recurrence of her breast cancer (the opposite is true).

One thing that Anna has learnt through all this is to listen to her own instincts and ignore advice which she believes to be fundamentally wrong. I came into contact with her when she wanted information to resolve a health problem her daughter was experiencing. A paediatrician had said it was definitely not linked to diet – but it was. A nine-month problem was resolved in a few days by a simple adjustment to her daughter's diet. Anna now listens to her inner wisdom.

Breast cancer and pregnancy

When pregnant, the last thing a woman is considering is the possibility of breast cancer. It is usually a happy time of excitement and planning. Women tend not to examine their breasts when pregnant. Apart from anything else, it is not easy to do so, as the breasts are changing in shape and size. Yet it is particularly important to check your breasts at this time.

Sadly, there has been an increase in the number of women with breast cancer during pregnancy.[4] This may be due to the fact that the overall incidence among all women has been increasing, and more women now leave pregnancy until later in life when, statistically, breast cancer is more common. It could also be related to the increase in exposure to environmental pollutants and chemicals which mimic female hormones. Prior use of the contraceptive pill by this age group may be another contributing factor.

It used to be thought that the outlook for pregnant women with breast cancer was worse than for other women, but it is now known that stage for stage, the prognosis is the same. The problem arises when treatment has to be initiated at a later stage than would be the case for non-pregnant women, in order to protect the developing baby.

Treatment options for pregnant women with breast cancer are probably more emotionally fraught than for other women – not that this is ever easy. If the cancer has been discovered in the first trimester, the woman may well be advised to have a termination in order to start treatment, including chemotherapy and radiation which are detrimental to the foetus, as soon as possible. If it is discovered during the second or third trimesters, surgery can safely be performed despite the need for anaesthetics, but radiation will not be used. It may be recommended that chemotherapy be used in the very last weeks of the pregnancy, or that an early delivery is carried out by caesarean section. These are very personal and difficult choices to make.

Male breast cancer

It comes as a surprise to many that men can get breast cancer – a particularly unpleasant surprise both to the men that are diagnosed with it and their families. One in 1,000 men develop the disease at some point in their lives, which accounts for around 200 cases a year in the UK. Male breast cancer is governed by the same hormonal influences as female breast cancers and there are many similarities between male breast cancer and breast cancer in post-menopausal women. Incidence is more likely with advancing years, with most men diagnosed aged sixty-plus, and the condition being extremely rare under the age of thirty. As with female breast cancer, the incidence is lower in Japan and other Far Eastern countries, and more common in the UK and USA. There is a high incidence of male breast cancer in some African countries where the frequency of liver infections is high. Liver problems reduce the ability of the body to process oestrogens correctly.

Men with Klinefelter's syndrome, which affects one in 300 men who have an XXY chromosome pattern instead of the normal male XY chromosomes, have hormonal anomalies, and the incidence rate is similar to that of women. A condition known as gynaecomastia is an excess of breast tissue in men, and is associated with male breast cancer in up to 40 per cent of cases. Chest radiation exposure, testicular injury or inflammation, undescended testes, a history of using drugs which raise prolactin levels, a family history of breast cancer (male and female) and obesity are all added risk factors.[5]

As there is less breast tissue in men, lumps are usually found at an earlier stage than for women. However, the lack of intervening tissue also means that spread to the lymph glands happens at an earlier stage. Men are also less likely to report a lump in the breast area than women, and a delay of eighteen to twenty-four months is common. Bloody nipple discharge is present in about 80 per cent of all male breast cancer cases.

Treatment for men is similar to that for women. This includes surgery, which may also require skin grafts, as there is less 'surplus' skin to work with, and sometimes Tamoxifen. There is some evidence that men do not tolerate Tamoxifen as well as women, and in one study one in five men stopped treatment because of unpleasant side-effects, compared to one in twenty women.[6]

Dick Hill's story

When Dick, aged forty-five, found a lump on his chest, he was not especially concerned. It was not examined until nine months later when he went for a health check on his company's private health scheme. The report said it was of no consequence and was probably fibrous tissue. Several months later Dick mentioned the lump in passing to his doctor, who decided that it needed to be biopsied immediately. Events escalated, and it was decided to remove the lump. A letter arrived giving a date for ten days' stay in hospital. Up to, and including, this moment nobody had mentioned the words breast cancer to Dick, and he had absolutely no idea that men could be afflicted with this disease. It was the ten-day hospital stay that finally alerted him to the fact that this was more than just a routine procedure.

He had a mastectomy, and what then followed was a trek from oncologist to oncologist to find someone who knew anything about the problems of male breast cancer – time after time the doctors had never dealt with it. Nobody seemed to have a clear idea of how best to treat the problem, but finally Dick found a physician who had researched male breast cancer extensively and it was agreed that he should have chemotherapy and he later had radiotherapy and was put on Tamoxifen.

His wife, Linda, became fascinated by nutrition and cajoled Dick into investigating the possibilities. After a visit to the nutritionist and a two-week period of avoiding dairy products, Dick's chronic, lifetime, asthma totally disappeared, never to return. The assumption has to be that this step, as well as being a preventive measure against breast cancer, also supported his immune system as a whole. Dick also decided it made sense to take an array of supplements during his chemotherapy regime to minimize side-effects, though he has now cut back to around seven capsules a day. He has no doubt that these supplements carried him through the experience and nine years on, he still swears by them.

Seeking Medical Help

Visiting your doctor

The majority of women who notice symptoms will initially consult their GP. An assessment should take place involving questions about the symptoms being experienced, general health and family history. Your doctor should also examine your breasts and underarm areas and will then decide whether it is necessary to refer you on to a specialist. This is a delicate subject to touch on because doctors are human and do make mistakes from time to time. Also there is great pressure on resources – if every woman who had a lump (remember, 80 per cent are non-malignant) had to be referred to a specialist, the system could probably not cope. Nevertheless, if you are unhappy that you are not being referred on, it is important to press the point or to seek a second opinion because mistakes are sometimes made. Some women are reluctant to 'make a fuss', or may even be embarrassed to visit their doctor in the first place, but it is still important to overcome these worries and initiate whatever steps you think may be necessary.

Aida Morris's story

In 1991, at the age of thirty-eight and with a five-year-old daughter, Aida was diagnosed with breast cancer. 'When my GP examined my breasts he told me to go home and forget about it – that it was just a hardening of the tissue – but to come back three weeks later. At the next appointment he sent me away once again, but as I was leaving his office I had a surge of courage and insisted on a mammogram. When I rang for the results (I had been told not to bother with an appointment as it was undoubtedly benign) he had a very different humbled and hushed tone. I had surgery within days and, once again, was at home on my own when the malignancy was confirmed over the telephone – which left me pretty devastated. Just as I was about to start radiotherapy

I heard news of a friend, also thirty-eight, who had just died from breast cancer. She had also been told, a year previously, that there was nothing to worry about – but obviously there was. I was really knocked back by this news and shocked by the parallels. At some point later when I was asking some questions, having done a little research, the doctor, who had been perfectly nice in the past, actually asked me, 'Don't you think we know what we are doing?' I felt like a naughty little girl who had stepped over some invisible boundary. I feel exasperated that at every turn I was not taken seriously. I feel much stronger now and am convinced that taking some control over my fate was the most important thing I could have done.'

Seeing the specialist

Your first appointment will be with either a consultant surgeon or a senior member of his or her team.

A case history and examination much as described above will take place, though probably in greater depth. The main objective of the physical examination is to determine if there is an obvious and separate lump or if there is general lumpiness in the breast tissue. Each quadrant of the breast is checked in turn, as are the glands in the armpit and above the collar-bone. The specialist will probably also listen to your chest and feel your abdomen. A visual check is made to see if there is a difference in size or shape of the breasts, if there is any skin dimpling, or if the nipples are retracted.

If no obvious lump is found and you are under forty, the specialist may well take a wait-and-see approach, suggesting that you return in six to eight weeks to re-check the breasts. If no lump is then found you will probably be told there is nothing to concern you.

If you are over forty, a mammogram may be suggested to check for any cancer that may not be detectable by physical examination.

There are several methods of further examination if the specialist is suspicious that breast cancer may exist.

Triple assessment

This is the current term to describe an initial examination of a woman with suspicious symptoms. The three assessments are: examination, mammogram and/or ultrasound investigation, and core biopsy, which allows for grading and hormone status of any tissue if it is cancerous.

Discharge

If a discharge from the nipple is one of the complaints, some will be expressed in order to examine it under a microscope.

Fine-needle aspiration

This is when an ordinary hypodermic needle is inserted into a lump – the procedure may be a little uncomfortable, but it is not painful. If the lump is solid, a few cells can be withdrawn for examination under the microscope. If the lump turns out to be a cyst, the cyst can be drained and usually will not recur. The cyst fluid should be checked for blood (which occurs in about one out of 2,000 samples); if this is found, further investigation will be needed. Fine-needle aspiration has more or less been given up in favour of core biopsies (see below).

Core biopsy

Also called cutting-needle biopsy or wide-bore biopsy. This is performed with a local anaesthetic to numb the area and is often done with the help of ultrasound to get to within 1 mm of the area in question. A special tool, like a punch, will retract a sample of tissue from the lump, which will then be sent to the histology laboratory to be investigated. Both fine-needle aspiration and core biopsy can be useful to detect cancer, but they are not necessarily conclusive. The tissue taken may be non-cancerous while cancer is lying in immediately adjacent tissue. If there is still uncertainty, the specialist may suggest a mammogram, an ultrasound or an open biopsy under a general anaesthetic.

Mammogram

This is a specialized breast X-ray where the breast is sandwiched between two X-ray plates. I joked once, when having a mammogram myself, that if men had to have them, they would never have been designed the way they are. The radiographer told me that unfortunately men with testicular cancer do have to go through exactly the same routine, only it isn't their breasts – keep that in mind as you go through the minor indignity of a mammography check. It is a slightly uncomfortable (not painful) procedure, less so for post-menopausal women whose breast tissue is less active than in younger women. Usually four X-rays are taken, two of each breast – one compressing the breasts horizontally and one vertically.

Mammograms are more useful for women beyond the menopause when the breasts lose volume and ducts shrink and eventually atrophy. There is less to confuse the eye when interpreting the results and so it is more successful at picking up small cancers. Mammograms will only show the breast itself (i.e. not the axilla tail or underarm area).

If you are unhappy with a mammogram result, have the situation reviewed by a breast surgeon, as about 10–15 per cent of the time a malignant lump will not show up on a mammogram. A persistent lump, which does not go away or which changes in nature, should always be investigated further.

To improve the chances of the mammography being accurate, make sure that you point out to the radiographer the location of any lump, and if you are uncertain that the positioning on the film plate prior to taking the X-ray is appropriate, say so. Do not be embarrassed about discussing these questions with the technician.

Mammography is also used for routine screening of post-menopausal women, as well as for investigating suspicion of breast cancer. Calcification of tissue can be seen in very early development of breast cancer and is one of the signs that are looked for with mammography. However, calcium flecks, known as calcifications, can also result from stagnant milk secretions within breast cysts and are totally harmless. Micro-calcifications are more suspicious if they are clustered in one section of the breast than if they are scattered throughout the tissue, and around 20 per cent of micro-calcifications turn out to be cancerous.

Ultrasound imaging

This is another investigative option which is available in most clinics. Sound waves build up a picture of the breast and the procedure is good for showing up cysts. This can be useful for younger women who have dense breast tissue making mammography less effective, but because it does not reveal micro-calcifications it is not useful for routine screening of older women. (Ultrasound is so safe that it is used routinely during pregnancy to view the developing child.) The breast is covered in jelly and an instrument is slid across the surface – the result is then viewed on a screen.

Magnetic resonance imaging (MRI)

A method to produce a three-dimensional picture of a tumour in the body using a safe form of radiation and a large magnet. It is, at this stage, an experimental tool for acquiring information about the breast but is frequently used for other parts of the body.

Timing

In the most efficient clinics results can be given the same day, or within just a few days. In any event guidelines[1] say that a woman should have initial screening results within seven to ten days. It is possible that the results will be inconclusive, in which case the consultant may suggest additional testing such as biopsy under general anaesthetic.

If the test results show breast cancer, the next appointment will be with the consultant surgeon or with the oncologist, to decide on a treatment plan. You should also have a specialized breast nurse available to you, though you may have to ask to see one as this may not be offered automatically. As there are only about 350 specialist breast consultants in the UK and each one sees around 600 new patients a year (compared with seventy-five a year in the USA), there is pressure on resources and the time spent with the surgeon discussing your situation can be as little as fifteen minutes. However, the breast-care nurse-counsellor who works alongside the consultant is authorized to answer any medical questions that you may have forgotten to ask or any other questions that arise, to explain treatment options more fully and to advise on practical matters. It is probably a good idea to take a relative or friend with you for the next appointment, and any following. You may want to go in with a list of questions, or take notes and raise questions later. In any event, moral support is often needed at this point, and a second person to recall what was said, or who can help to think of questions at the time, is useful – I found that my appointment was a blur and I could not remember much of what was said – I had to rely on my parents, who accompanied me, for accurate recall.

Staging

Cancer cells invade and spread at vastly differing rates and it is this speed which determines how malignant, and therefore how danger- ous, a tumour might be. To work out how aggressive a breast cancer is, grading and staging tests are done. These tests also help in deciding on a treatment plan and will help determine if conservative treatment can be used or if a more radical treatment plan needs to be considered.

The classification system for cancer is complicated and there are differences from country to country. The following is based on an international classification system and will help you to discuss your treatment and risk status with your doctors.

The classification is expressed as a stage, according to a system called the TNM system – T for Tumour, N for Nodes, M for Metastasis.

Stage 0	Tumour in-situ (i.e. contained), no lymph nodes involved and no metastasis
Stage I	Tumour under 2 cm/¾ in, no lymph nodes involved and no metastasis
Stage II (a)	Tumour in-situ or under 2 cm/¾ in, lymph nodes involved but moveable and not fixed in place by spread, or tumour 2–5 cm/¾–2 in without lymph node involvement, no metastasis
Stage II (b)	Tumour 2–5 cm/¾–2 in, lymph nodes involved but

	moveable and not fixed in place by spread, or larger tumour without lymph node involvement, no metastasis
Stage III (a)	Tumour in-situ or under 5 cm/2 in, lymph nodes involved and attached to each other or neighbouring blood vessels, or tumour under 5 cm/2 in with lymph nodes involved and moveable or fixed, no metastasis
Stage III (b)	Tumour of any size (with any lymph node status and no metastasis) accompanied by any of the following characteristics: – Fixed to the pectoral muscle or the chest wall – Involvement with the lymphatics of the skin of the breast – Infiltration of the skin by malignant cells – Skin ulceration (excludes tumours where nipple is retracted or skin pulled due to position of tumour, rather than skin invaded) – Spread to nodes over the collar-bone
Stage IV	Tumour of any status, lymph nodes of any status, has metastasized

It is obvious to anyone that the later the staging, the more invasive the cancer; however, it is still dangerous to make predictions of the outcome. The downside of reading information such as that above is that a woman might decide to start writing her will. Keep an open mind, be determined to fight, and you may well win through. I had a Stage III breast cancer with eight out of fifteen nodes affected, but ten years on I am still here to tell the tale.

Hormone receptor status

The pathologist will check on the receptiveness of the breast lump and tissue to the hormones oestrogen and progesterone. The tissue will either be ER positive or ER negative (oestrogen receptor positive or negative. In the UK we use the American abbreviation ER, for estrogen receptor, instead of OR which could be confused with operating room). About 75 per cent of breast cancers are ER positive. The tissue is also classified for progesterone receptiveness, either positive or negative. It usually takes a couple of weeks to get this information. Two tumours existing at the same time, from the same breast, can have a different status. The oestrogen and progesterone status will be used to determine the likely success of response to the hormone therapy Tamoxifen.

You will probably be told the ER status, although progesterone receptor status is rarely given to patients unless they ask. The chief interest for the oncologist in determining if breast cancer is progesterone receptor positive is to help determine the success of Tamoxifen; however, it is always possible that, in the future, this information may be used to examine whether breast cancer may respond to the use of natural progesterone products (see the chapter **Harmonizing Hormones**, page 245).

The Impact of Oestrogen on Breast Cancer

Oestrogens are very important in understanding the development of breast cancer. All cells have hormone receptor sites on their surface. The type of cell will determine the type of receptor site. So a hormone will circulate in the blood, and visit all cells, but only those with receptor sites for that particular hormone will respond to it. Breast tissue has a strong affinity for oestrogen and progesterone hormones.

Oestrogens can be grouped into two categories in terms of their impact on breast cancer – bad oestrogens and good oestrogens (not accurate medical terminology, I agree, but it gets the picture across). Oestrogens are certainly not all bad, even though when talking about breast cancer they tend to be viewed that way. The real problem relates to their balance and the dominance of some types of oestrogen over others. On the plus side, oestrogens are responsible for sexual maturation, protecting against heart disease, maintaining bone density and keeping tissues plump and lubricated. On the downside, if the wrong oestrogens are produced to excess and not eliminated properly, they can become a major contributing factor to most breast cancer and other hormone-related diseases such as uterine and ovarian cancers.

The main natural oestrogens that we manufacture within our bodies are oestrone (E1), oestradiol (E2) and oestriol (E3). Oestradiol is a strong oestrogen which has generally been found to be raised in women with breast cancer. As a rule Asian women, with their low incidence of breast cancer, have lower E2 levels.

Oestrogens are carried around the bloodstream on carrier proteins, called sex-hormone carrier globulin, almost like little boats securely carrying their cargo. Some oestrogens, however, are free oestrogens, not bound to carrier proteins, and are therefore readily available to bind to the receptor sites on cells. Insulin, the hormone produced mainly in response to carbohydrates in the diet, and produced to excess in response to refined carbohydrates or sugar, is a key regulator of oestrogen carriers. The more insulin produced, the fewer oestrogen carriers are manufactured, and the more damaging free oestrogens are left circulating.

In addition to oestrogens being produced by the ovaries and the adrenal glands, they are also produced by fat cells, meaning that women with excess body fat are likely to be producing more oestrogen than their lean sisters. In particular this effect is pronounced with weight gained in adult life, and may help to account for a percentage of post-menopausal women diagnosed with breast cancer. Women who gain weight on their upper body, abdomen and breasts are at even higher risk, possibly because the fat is in the area where the oestrogen production can do the most mischief. Fat cells secrete an enzyme called aromatase which converts some of the circulating male hormones, androgens, into female oestrogens. This extra female hormone load may help to tip the balance into breast cancer. (All women have a small amount of male hormones, and all men have a small amount of female hormones.)

Oestrogens are metabolized, or altered, within the liver where a process called hydroxylation converts E1 and E2, the 'bad' oestrogens, into E3, the 'good' oestrogen. The thyroid hormone, thyroxine, helps positively to influence this process. E1 and E2 are capable of being converted into carcinogenic catechol oestrogens, whilst E3 goes down a different metabolic pathway and cannot be converted into these harmful oestrogens.[1] Catechol oestrogens can also be promoted by carcinogens, such as Dioxin, while beneficial plant oestrogens are incapable of going down this route – the relevance of this will become apparent later.

Once they have been metabolized in the liver, oestrogens are taken to the bowel for elimination. If there is insufficient fibre in the stools and digestion is sluggish, they hang around for longer than is desirable and can be reabsorbed into the body, increasing the woman's oestrogen load. On the other hand, if elimination time is speeded up, oestrogens have less time to be reabsorbed and are passed out of the body much more effectively.

Another category of oestrogens which is causing huge concern in the area of breast cancer management are artificial oestrogens and chemicals which mimic the effects of oestrogens. These are called xenoestrogens (*xeno* meaning outside, thus oestrogens which are not naturally made in our bodies). Sources of these strong and 'bad' oestrogens include pesticides, insecticides, herbicides and pliable plastics as used in food wrapping and containers. Because breasts are largely composed of fat, they are particularly good storage sites for these fat-soluble chemical oestrogens, which are then ideally placed to do more damage to the breast.

Oestrogens cause the cells in the breasts to multiply. The more oestrogens that are around, the more often, and the more speedily, the cells replicate themselves. If the speed and frequency of multiplication are too high, there is more room for error. Cells can be formed with incorrect DNA coding, or they may not fully divide so that cells will have two nuclei. The more damaged cells that are produced, the more difficult it is for the body's 'search and destroy' mechanisms, or immune system, to deal with them. If the mutated cells begin to divide under the influence of too much oestrogen, breast cancer can develop.

Could progesterone be part of the answer?

Progesterone is the hormone which complements, and balances, oestrogen. The hormone is secreted in the second half of a woman's cycle and its main purpose is to PRO-long GEST-ation – hence its name. But it has other interesting effects including tempering the effects of oestrogen and slowing down cell proliferation. As the majority of breast cancers are, at least in part, related to excessive exposure to oestrogens, whether they are oestrogens we produce in our bodies, oestrogens from chemicals in our environment, or pharmaceutical oestrogens, it could be that progesterone will have a major role to play in reducing the impact of these oestrogens. Progesterone can have the effect of balancing excess oestrogen and countering some of its negative effects. This is an interesting story and the whole topic is dealt with in more detail under **The power of progesterone** (page 250) in the chapter **Harmonizing Hormones**.

Minimizing Risks

Why me?

One of the dangers of writing a book looking at the nutritional and environmental contributions to breast cancer is that some people may conclude that they are to blame for the breast cancer – in much the same way that smokers may be considered to blame for their diagnoses of lung cancer. But there is no way that we can know this on an individual basis and it is likely that each case is a reflection of various historical factors. The emphasis has to be, if not prevention because cancer is already diagnosed, prevention of recurrence – a much more positive framework in which to work.

Reprogramme your genes!

'It's in my genes' seems to have taken over from 'It's in the stars' as a way of explaining our fate.

But is the likelihood of developing cancer mainly due to the genes we inherit, or to the way that we choose to live our lives? It is now believed that genetic programming does not necessarily imply genetic determination. Dr Jeffrey Bland, a leading clinical nutritionist, said in his highly respected audio magazine *Functional Medicine Update*, 'We are given a genetic map, but within that map there are many different routes.' Which route we take can depend on the lifestyle and dietary choices we make – we have more control than we think over how our genes manifest themselves.

While the area of genetics is important and, compared to other fields, is developing rapidly, there are 100,000 genes in the human cell, and a human genome, or set of genes, contains 3 billion component 'letters' – the permutations are huge and it will probably be quite some time before we can have any usable therapy from this. It is tempting to believe that this is going to be the answer to the cancer problem, but we have been disappointed in the past with 'great white hopes'.

Immunotherapy was seen as the magic bullet that would act as a key solution in the 1980s – but nothing much came out of it. And the practical application and benefits of gene therapy, if there are going to be any, remain theoretical.

Genetic predisposition to breast cancer is seen as a key area of research for scientists in the fight against the disease. Imagine a world where the geneticist could manipulate a person's genes to reduce their susceptibility to a particular disease. It is indeed an exciting prospect, but one which gives rise to anxiety as well as hope. This new area of inquiry has led to intense debate on medical ethics, and wars are raging in the popular press between those who see this as the solution to much human misery, and those who are nervous of misuse, imagining the potential to abort foetuses which carry rogue genes.

In the case of a woman with a near relative (sister, mother, grandmother or aunt) who has had breast cancer before the age of fifty the statistical risk of developing breast cancer is doubled.

In the meantime women who find that they do have a genetic susceptibility, and are carriers of the BRCA1 or BRCA2 gene, are subject to great anxiety. A number of these women may be persuaded, or persuade themselves, that preventive treatment is a good idea despite the fact that they are currently disease free.[1] This treatment could be the hormone-blocker Tamoxifen, or even a double mastectomy.

Margaret Carey's story

In 1988, when Margaret was fifty-one, she found a lump in her breast. As her mother had been diagnosed with breast cancer this raised clanging alarm bells and she went for investigation. Her treatment was swift and effective – she was given a mastectomy, had radiotherapy, and was one of the first women to be put on Tamoxifen. At the time, Margaret became quite low emotionally and was convinced that she had, at best, three years to live.

'In retrospect I realize that I need not have felt this as my mother, who was diagnosed at the age of sixty-four, went on to live another eleven years and eventually died of heart failure, not breast cancer.

'My daughter will now be going for genetic testing, but we know that if she carries the wrong gene she can do a lot to prevent it with her diet. It would probably be a bad decision to do anything more radical as both I and my mother have survived our own diagnosis by a significant number of years. I eat a lot more vegetarian-based meals using all the pulses, and keep to a low-fat diet. I make all my own meals so that I know what goes in them, take antioxidant supplements and do yoga. It is never too late for a new career and I now teach yoga – it's a shame I had to have cancer to start thinking about life and living for the moment.'

In all this debate one key issue seems to have been forgotten. Our genetic make-up has probably not changed significantly over the last couple of centuries yet there has been a massive increase in the incidence of breast cancer – more than can be accounted for by the increase that might be expected from our longer average lifespan. Scientists can't give us all the answers yet, but while some people do have a higher genetic risk, it is likely to be lifestyle which dictates whether they actually develop the disease. It isn't simply a question of the genes that predispose a person to breast cancer being present, but whether these genes are triggered into action so that they can then disrupt normal cell division. Hormones, diet and exposure to various chemicals are the triggers – and some of these can be the protective factors. So preventive treatment *is* appropriate, but rather than taking drugs or having surgery, the less heroic measures of altering diet, lifestyle and environmental factors may well prove to be as useful, though less newsworthy. Donald C. Malins, director of molecular epidemiology at the Pacific Northwest Research Foundation, in Seattle, USA, blames most breast cancer on free-radical damage to breast cancer DNA, and says that such DNA damage is likely to be what turns BRCA1 and BRCA2 bad as well. 'Diets rich in antioxidants that neutralize free radicals may well be helpful at early stages of DNA damage,' and later on more powerful and concentrated antioxidants may be necessary to repair the damage.[2]

Women's families with the BRCA1 or BRCA2 gene will probably have had them for many generations. Yet breast cancer incidence has risen sharply in the last half of this century. Another gene, the p53 gene – which is normally responsible for pre-programmed, natural cell death – is estimated to be mutated in 20–40 per cent of breast cancers, thereby allowing cells to grow out of control. The point is that it is the *expression* of these genes that has changed, which in turn affects cell repair, renewal and growth. In other words, exposure to other influences, such as hormones, diet, smoking and radiation, are likely triggers of breast cancer genes[3] – and women with a genetic tendency are more susceptible to these triggers than other women. Remove the triggers, however, and the genetic tendency does not have as much opportunity to express itself – the woman remains healthy.

An excellent example is evidence shown by recent research that long-term smokers, with a twenty-a-day habit, are four times as likely to develop breast cancer if they have a particular mutation of the NAT2 gene. This mutation predisposes women to be slow to break down carcinogens. Around 50 per cent of white women have this gene mutation, 35 per cent of black women, 20 per cent of Chinese women, and 10 per cent of Asian and Japanese women. Additionally we are seeing a massive upswing in the number of teenage girls who smoke, and it is the breast tissue of younger women that is most sensitive to carcinogens.

There is a massive amount that any woman can do, right now, to modulate her own individual genetic expression through diet, exercise and environment. Antioxidants, B vitamins, foods such as soya and the brassica family of vegetables, which includes broccoli and Brussels sprouts, have all been shown to help to positively influence gene expression – the way that genes behave. Diet can help to modulate a woman's susceptibility to her 'genetic fate'.

While we can do nothing about choosing our genetic background, we can do everything about our lifestyle choices – and these are of crucial importance in determining our future.

Other factors which influence breast cancer risk

There are other factors, apart from genetic risk and diet, to take into account when considering the risk of breast cancer. Some aspects you can do something about, like smoking or exercise, others you just have to put down to experience. Frankly, at the age of thirty, forty, fifty or more, it is pretty pointless to be told that early onset of periods is something that increases your risk of breast cancer. Younger women – teenagers and young adults – seem to be particularly susceptible to environmental cancer-causing influences. Exposure to, for instance, smoking, alcohol and radiation, seem to have the greatest impact on this age group – and unfortunately this is the age group that is likely to be most blasé about the risks. The *mañana* viewpoint is not helped by the fact that breast cancer usually progresses slowly from its initiation and only appears in a detectable form many years later, meaning that cause and effect are too remote from each other to make a significant impact on this age group.

Many of the risk factors below rank as the straw that breaks – or may break – the camel's back and they are small contributors when compared to diet, environment and lifestyle. To paraphrase St Francis's Prayer: it is helpful to change what you are able, not worry about what you can't change – and have the wisdom to know the difference between the two.

Early starters

The early onset of menstruation in a girl's life increases her risk of breast cancer. At puberty a girl's secondary sexual characteristics begin to develop, including breast development. A girl reaches a 'set weight', usually around 40 kg/88 lb, before puberty begins. Fat and calories in the diet, and general nutritional status, are factors contributing to when this point is reached. Girls are now reaching puberty much earlier than previous generations. In the UK at the turn of the twentieth century, on average girls entered puberty at around fourteen and a half years of age, and only 100 years later the average age is eleven. Japanese women have shown similar trends as they adopt the Western habit of increasing fat in the diet. In the 1870s girls in Japan had an average puberty age of sixteen and a half, it has now dropped to twelve, and this could be related to the fact that, since the Second World War , their traditional rice and vegetable diet has been replaced to some extent by a diet much higher in animal fats[4] – although they are still way behind us in the West in animal fat consumption!

Exercise is a protective factor against breast cancer (see below) and it is also interesting to note that young girls who do a lot of sport before puberty tend to start their periods (menarche) at a later age.

Good breeders

When compared to the variations of hormone levels during menstruation, with oestrogen and progesterone peaking and troughing every four weeks or so, pregnancy and breast-feeding can actually be a mercifully peaceful interlude for the female breast. Western women's lifestyle, with early onset of menstruation and relatively few pregnancies, contrasts starkly with the way of life in developing countries where there is generally a much later onset of menstruation and more pregnancies. Both these factors have a profound effect on the incidence of breast cancer. With each pregnancy a woman is exposed to progesterone and oestriol (E3), both of which have a protective effect against breast cancer.

The differences can be quite striking: a girl in the West who starts menstruating at the age of eleven, and has, on average, two full-term pregnancies, will have about 400 menstrual cycles during her reproductive life. On the other hand, a South American woman whose puberty is delayed to around the age of sixteen, and has repeated pregnancies throughout her life, may have fewer than 100 menstrual cycles, due to the pregnancies followed by prolonged breast-feeding, which inhibits the return of menstruation. These differences account, at least in part, for the higher incidence of breast cancer in the West, and this is one of the few 'definites' about breast cancer. Women who have no children at all, for instance nuns, are considered high-risk as they consistently have higher oestrogen levels than women who have borne children.

Young mums

Having a family, with first pregnancies before the age of twenty, decreases the risk of breast cancer – again there is earlier exposure to progesterone and oestriol (E3). In the West the average age at which women have their first child has been steadily increasing since the Second World War and it is not unusual these days for women to put off starting a family until their thirties, or even their forties. One in five women in the UK remains childless.

Breast is best

Breast-feeding for a minimum of three months is protective against breast cancer – so not only does your baby benefit, you do as well. The good news is that breast-feeding is on the increase – about two-thirds of women now breast-feed. The bad news is that only 20 per cent of women continue to breast-feed beyond three months. It is ideal, from both the baby's and the mother's point of view, to carry on breast-feeding for as long as possible, preferably for at least a year. Even greater protection is conferred by breast-feeding for this long. Among Hong Kong boat women, who traditionally almost always suckle their infants on the left breast, any breast cancer tends to occur in their right breast.

Race debate

It is always possible that race is a factor in determining a woman's susceptibility to breast cancer, although it seems that dietary and environmental issues are more likely to be the explanation where there are racial divides in the statistics. For instance, there is a higher incidence of breast cancer in African-American women compared to European-American women. The African-American women, generally speaking, fall into a lower-income group, with eating, smoking, and exercise habits which are more likely to be risk factors for breast cancer. If you then look at African women who are on a well-nourished diet, the incidence of breast cancer is relatively low. Japanese women have a low incidence, and Eskimo women a barely existent incidence of breast cancer, until they move to the West and adopt a Western diet, when their levels equalize with those of women in their host country. Even in Japan, where adopting Western dietary habits has been on the increase amongst the well-to-do since the 1950s, there is an eight-fold higher incidence of breast cancer among affluent women when compared to poorer women who rarely eat the meat and dairy products that wealthier women have adopted. Indeed, the window of opportunity to study the dietary differences between industrialized Japanese and Western populations may well be closing fast, and we will probably need to turn to rural Eastern cultures for the information that is needed.[5]

Nevertheless, there is one common genetic difference which is relevant and that is the NAT2 gene mutation we discussed previously, which has different incidence rates among various racial groups.

Invisible foes

Breast tissue is sensitive to radiation damage, and the experience following the atomic bombs at Hiroshima and Nagasaki have highlighted this – a high proportion of female survivors later developed breast cancer. Questions are now being raised regarding EMFs (Electro-Magnetic Fields) created by computers, faxes, pylons and mobile phones and their impact on breast cancer. There is enough concern for the World Health Organization to have set up a five-year study examining all the health issues relating to EMFs.

Part 2 **The Nutrition Connection**

Basic Nutrition

The news lines about cancer prevention are buzzing with talk of broccoli and Brussels sprouts, tofu and tempeh, flax and fennel, apricots and artichokes. There are dozens of newly identified phyto (plant)-chemicals in familiar fruit and vegetables, which are proving to have varied and quite remarkable properties, enabling them to disrupt the progress of cancer. As we learn more about the make-up and chemistry of nature's bounty there is great hope that we will be moving into a new era of cancer prevention and treatment. But before we get too excited about the long list of high-tech names of food components, what about the basics?

Here we will look at the information that is available to judge the effect of specific factors in our diet in preventing breast cancer or in helping to arrest its progress. The basic 'ingredients' of our foods are carbohydrates, fibre, fats, proteins, water, vitamins and minerals. There are also a number of other constituents such as antioxidants and phytoestrogens which are the subject of intense interest in the fight against breast cancer.

But let's start at the beginning.

Keep It Complex

I like the KISS principle – Keep It Simple Sweetheart. But when it comes to carbohydrates the opposite is true. Carbohydrates are the most readily available source of energy in our food. They always come from plant sources and are, in effect, energy from the sun trapped by the plant in a form we can then use. The idea of eating trapped sunshine is great! Carbohydrates can be either complex or refined.

Sources of complex carbohydrates are:

- Whole grains, such as brown rice, wholemeal flour products (bread, brown pasta), porridge oats, whole rye, millet, corn and buckwheat
- Beans, pulses, lentils
- Potato skins
- Vegetables

In short, any starchy food which has not been processed in any way and is close to the form in which it came out of the ground.

Sources of refined carbohydrates are:

- White flour products such as white bread, white pasta, most pies, pizza bases, cakes and biscuits (unless made from wholemeal flour)
- White rice
- Sugar, honey, treacle

In short, any starchy food that is processed and is not in its original form.

Sugar has become a significant feature in the Western diet. In the UK around 45 kg/100 lb are consumed annually by every man, woman and child, and the situation is even worse in the USA where the figure is 67.5 kg/150 lb per person.

A large part of the sugar in our diet comes from convenience foods. It is added to breakfast cereals, sauces and canned foods.

You can check this by looking at ingredients lists – anything ending in an -ose or an -ol, or which is described as syrup or honey, is sugar.

There are key differences between the two types of carbohydrate, complex and refined, from a health point of view. Complex carbohydrates provide the nutrients which are necessary to digest and process them, and which contribute to general health. In refined carbohydrates nutrients such as calcium, magnesium, chromium and selenium are stripped out, by 70–90 per cent. This happens when whole grains are refined to produce white grain products such as white bread, white rice, pasta, pies and biscuits. In the UK cereals and white bread are, by law, fortified with nutrients to put back some of what was taken out. B vitamins and iron are added to breakfast cereals, and calcium to white flour. However, this in no way matches the full complement of nutrients that the whole grain originally contained, let alone its fibre content.

Another key difference relates to the speed with which energy is released from carbohydrates into the bloodstream. Complex carbohydrates provide a slow release of energy over a sustained period of time. This gives cells a steady source of energy without significant peaks and troughs. Sugar and refined, or simple, carbohydrates, on the other hand, are like rocket fuel. They give a 'quick hit' of energy which peters out just as quickly, leaving a void that has to be filled. This means that another quick hit is needed to stop the person going into an energy trough or blood sugar low. The effect of refined carbohydrates is to trigger insulin more often and with greater impact than complex carbohydrates. Additionally, if sugary foods are eaten too often, over many years, this can lead to a condition known as 'insulin resistance' in susceptible individuals, where cells do not respond to insulin as sensitively as they ought to. This leaves a lot of free insulin floating around in the body with nowhere to go. One of the effects of insulin is to act as a growth enhancer and encourage cells to multiply.[1] The combination of this excess free insulin, plus oestrogen, has the effect of instructing the cells to divide at a faster rate than is normal.

From the point of view of breast cancer there are many reasons to favour complex, or whole, carbohydrates over refined sources:

- Sugar is associated with breast cancer in several studies.[2]
- High blood-sugar levels encourage oxidation of, and therefore damage to, body tissues. See the chapter **Antioxidant Armoury** (page 99) for information about the effects of oxidation and free radicals.
- To prevent breast cancer, or when aiming for recovery, the individual needs all the naturally occurring sources of vitamins and minerals that she can get. While supplements can be a useful adjunct, the nutrients derived from food are more valuable. Food sources of nutrients come in forms which are most readily used by the body and with an assortment of co-factors (helping hands) that we are only just beginning to appreciate fully. Refined carbohydrates are largely stripped of these nutrients.
- Malignant tumours are mainly 'sugar-feeders' – an excellent reason to keep sugar out of the diet as much as possible. Cancer cells are principally fuelled by blood sugar, rather than by fats or proteins, and tumours have abnormal energy requirements which resemble a primitive yeast organism in fermenting sugar. Keeping blood-sugar levels regulated at a lower level helps selectively to starve cancer tumours.
- High blood-sugar levels cripple the mechanisms for regulating oestrogens by interfering with prostaglandin metabolism. Prostaglandins are hormone-like substances which are critical for controlling inflammation. The body makes its own oestrogen binders, which lower circulating oestrogens, as a by-product of healthy prostaglandin production.[3]
- Constant exposure to elevated blood-sugar levels, engendered by a high-sugar and high-refined carbohydrate diet, depresses the immune system.
- A major study in Italy, where the majority of carbohydrates are consumed as refined products, such as white bread and pasta, showed that a high starch intake was associated with a risk of breast cancer.[4]
- High-sugar, low-protein intravenous hospital feeding accelerates cancer growth, whilst the opposite, low-sugar, high-protein formulas (which are tailored to cancer), seem selectively to starve the tumour.[5]

- Sugar and refined carbohydrates are more readily turned into body fat than complex carbohydrates. This means that if a person is inclined to put on weight, the chances of sustaining a high body weight are greater if sugar or refined carbohydrates feature significantly in the diet. Excess weight is a factor to consider with breast cancer.
- Sugar triggers insulin and high insulin levels have been linked to a greater risk of breast cancer, independently of body weight or fat distribution, which would normally be considered the more important factor.
- International studies have shown a direct correlation between breast cancer mortality rates and national statistics for sugar (sucrose and glucose) consumption.[6]

The way forward

There is no doubt that it benefits breast cancer patients to consume the major portion of their carbohydrates in a complex, unrefined, form. This argument has been used to promote vegetarianism as a key way to reduce risk of breast cancer – and certainly it would appear that vegetarians on a healthy vegetarian diet enjoy hormone profiles which indicate a lowered overall risk. However, many women find that they are unable to adopt a strict vegetarian diet, and should not feel that they are deficient in willpower for this reason.

What may be most important about a good-quality vegetarian diet is the increased intake of grains, pulses, vegetables and fruits, and not necessarily the complete avoidance of meat. To reap the rewards you may not have to give up meat, just treat it as a condiment and enjoy more vegetarian-based meals a few times a week – after all, you do not need to be Jewish to enjoy chicken soup, and you do not need to be a vegetarian to enjoy some vegetarian meals. A diet based on vegetables, whole grains and pulses is one that helps to regulate blood-sugar and insulin levels, improve bowel health, minimize oxidation damage and selectively starve tumours. Not a bad menu!

The Fibre 'Movement'

Fibre is the other component of carbohydrate foods and all the authorities agree that the quantity of fibre in the diet is intimately related to breast cancer incidence. Fibre is found naturally in all plant foods – fruits, vegetables, roots, pulses, grains, nuts and seeds. There is no fibre in meat, fish or dairy products.

In less developed countries, where there is a low incidence of breast cancer, carbohydrates which contain fibre make up 50–80 per cent of calorie intake. In developed countries the figure has dropped to around 35–45 per cent carbohydrate intake, with a significant part of those carbohydrates coming not from fibre-rich starches, but from sugars and refined carbohydrates.

It was once thought that as fibre passes through the body largely undigested, it was a superfluous component of the diet. The rise in digestion-related problems, including colon cancer, that were not observed in countries which maintained a high degree of fibre in their diet served to convince the nutritionists and the medical establishment of the day that fibre was indeed needed as a regulatory substance for digestive health. It is now accepted that fibre has a beneficial effect on overall health and can help to reduce the risk of diabetes, cardiovascular (heart) problems, and hormone-related cancers such as breast and prostate cancers in addition to colon, rectal and pancreatic cancers. The reason why hormone-dependent cancers are reduced with high-fibre diets is that oestrogens are eliminated more efficiently from the bowels, and fibre levels of 25 g daily, or more, eliminate sufficient oestrogens to lower risk dramatically.

Fibres are insoluble non-cellulose polysaccharides, cellulose and lignans (together these are called insoluble fibre), and soluble non-cellulose polysaccharides (soluble fibre). Both main types of fibre – soluble and insoluble – are necessary for good health. Soluble fibre dissolves in water when heated up – porridge goes sticky and fruit goes gooey. Insoluble fibre, such as wheat bran, does not dissolve in water.

What are the facts about fibre and breast cancer?

- Fibrous foods are usually also low-fat foods, for example grains, vegetables and pulses, and a diet that is high in fibre will tend also to be low in fat, in particular saturated fats. Fat intake has been correlated to breast cancer risk, and this is possibly because of the high calorie content of fats, their effect on weight, and the chemicals that fats accumulate (see **A sea of chemicals** in the chapter **Organic Food** (page 106).

- Fibre helps to eliminate excess oestrogens. It prevents reabsorption of oestrogens in the intestines, and the oestrogens are then excreted in bile.[1] Fibre speeds up the transit time of stools, making it difficult for the oestrogens to be reabsorbed. Levels of up to 36 per cent less oestrone (E1) have been reported in women on high-fibre diets.[2] (Oestrone is a strong oestrogen which is linked to increased risk of breast cancer.)

- Higher stool weights in women (which indicates fibre in the diet) means lower levels of circulating oestrogens, and constipated women are more likely to have pre-cancerous cellular changes in breast tissue than are non-constipated women.

- It is also possible that fibre acts indirectly on breast cancer risk by reducing obesity or improving insulin sensitivity.[3] It is probable that high insulin levels are involved in the development of breast cancer as insulin is an important growth factor for breast cancer cells.[4]

- A diet high in fibre-rich foods ensures that you are getting other valuable 'bioactive' components of foods, such as carotenoids, iso-flavones and lignans, which almost certainly play a role in reducing breast cancer risk.

The way forward

Fibre is acknowledged as a factor which decreases the risk of breast cancer.[5] It is best to get fibre as an integral part of the food, rather than as an add-on, and a diet high in fruits, vegetables, roots, pulses, beans, nuts and seeds is protective. Twenty-five grams a day is the amount of fibre to aim for – you will find a chart of the fibre contents of foods in **Your Basic Nutrition Plan** on page 215. Added wheat bran can irritate the digestive tracts of many people and is best avoided in excess. There are other forms of added fibre which are not irritating to the gut wall for people who have particular digestive problems; see **Healthy Digestion** (page 267).

While both soluble and insoluble fibre are necessary, we have a tendency to over-use insoluble wheat-bran fibre in the West. Many of our cereals are advertised with 'added bran' and we may even be encouraged to add spoonfuls of bran to our cereal in an attempt to increase the fibre in our diet. The problem with this approach is that added insoluble bran of this type, in excess, tends to be an irritant and 'loosens the bowels' precisely because it irritates them. This type of fibre does not work as mixed fibres in whole foods do, by increasing the bulk of stools. To sum up this problem, we make ourselves constipated by eating low-fibre refined carbohydrates, and then try to remedy the damage by introducing an excess of one type of fibre over another. This is marketing genius on the part of the food manufacturers who sell us the fibre which was integral to the food in the first place, but removed in the refining process.

Kitchen-sink Salad

So called because if you put in *all* the ingredients you would need a kitchen sink to mix it up in. The average salad can be a sad affair, consisting of a few lettuce leaves, slices of tomato and cucumber. The kitchen-sink salad, on the other hand, can be a 'fibre giant' and contribute 10–15 g of fibre to your daily total if you make sure that you always include pulses, whole grains, or even dried fruit.

The kitchen-sink salad makes an excellent main meal, and can be put into a container and taken to work easily. The more 'filling' ingredients (rice, pasta, boiled potatoes, legumes) can be prepared in advance and put into the fridge ready to arrange on a plate or mix in a bowl when required. A good kitchen-sink salad will have at least ten ingredients representing a balance of pulses, vegetables, salad ingredients, grains, seeds or nuts. If you put in enough grains and legumes then it becomes a main-meal salad which will fill you up even at your hungriest.

A perfect example of a good kitchen-sink salad with a more formalized recipe is the salad Niçoise. On a bed of crispy lettuce (I like cos or little gem) which has been pre-tossed in a little dressing, pile up individual mounds of: sliced or baby tomatoes, green or white flageolet beans, tuna, grated carrot, whole steamed baby potatoes, steamed French beans, and intersperse with quartered eggs, black and green olives and anchovies. No more dressing is needed. This is a visual and taste sensation.

Your kitchen-sink salad could include:

- Brown rice on its own as a base for the salad, or mixed with raisins or chopped nuts. Try quinoa or barley for a change (both cook like rice)
- Any type of legume: beans, peas, lentils, chick-peas
- Pre-cook pasta shapes – shells, twists or bows. Use wholewheat pasta, or to ring the nutritional changes, or if you are gluten-intolerant, experiment with other types of pasta available from health food shops – buckwheat pasta (not wheat despite the name), rice pasta or corn pasta
- Grilled vegetables: aubergines, fennel, peppers, onions, spring onions, courgettes
- Grated beetroot or carrot (no need to cook the beetroot, just wash, peel and grate – yummy – wear rubber gloves or you will end up with purple hands)
- Coleslaw (shredded cabbage, carrot and onion with half-vinaigrette and half-yoghurt dressing – takes seconds in a food processor)
- Florets of raw or lightly steamed broccoli or cauliflower are ideal additions whenever possible
- Fresh pumpkin or sunflower seeds for their valuable essential fats. Don't forget to take every opportunity to add in a tablespoon or two of flax seeds as well. Freshly chopped nuts or pine nuts should be used in moderation
- Fresh or canned fish, packed in spring water, brine or tomato juice. A couple of ounces of skinless chicken breast, shredded or cubed. Hard-boiled eggs

- Marinated tofu, cut into cubes (available from health food shops)
- Seedless or halved and seeded grapes, orange segments, chopped dried figs or dates, apple chunks
- Olives, cucumber, tomatoes, avocado, celery, potatoes, green beans (as in the salad Niçoise)
- Bean sprouts, alfalfa or other sprouted seeds, grains or beans
- Goat's, feta or cottage cheese
- Seaweed flakes, or toasted seaweed strips, crumbled and sprinkled on
- Mushrooms, raw and sliced, or marinated in tomato, garlic and vinaigrette dressing, or oriental mushrooms steamed and tossed in lemon juice
- Many different types of green leaves: arugula, lamb's lettuce, red lettuce, watercress, cress, curly lettuce, baby dandelion leaves, Chinese lettuce

Ideas for dressings

- Flax oil, mixed with olive oil, lemon juice or vinegar, garlic, pepper and herbs (such as tarragon, coriander leaves, parsley, thyme, lemon thyme)
- Flax oil, mixed with olive oil and flavoured with honey and mustard – strong-tasting so a little goes a long way
- Anchovy dressing: in a food processor blend a can of anchovies with several garlic cloves, mixed dried herbs, olive oil and lemon juice. This keeps in the fridge for a few days and is so strong-tasting that only a little is needed. It is ideal to jazz up greenery such as curly kale, collard, green beans and perpetual spinach, and dignifies them enough to serve them on their own as a first course
- Salsa – available from supermarkets and containing, variously, tomato, green pepper, onion and vinegar – or make your own
- Live yoghurt with onion or chives, or grated cucumber and turmeric and cumin
- A squeeze of lemon is enough with some ingredients (for example beans or grated carrot or beetroot)

Fats – Friends or Foes?

There are different types of fat which can either contribute to an increased risk of breast cancer or, surprisingly to many, help to protect against breast cancer. Some fats have even been shown to discourage tumour growth. In our bodies there are two types of fat: storage and structural.

Storage fats are visible with the naked eye and are the sort that pad out our waists and hips. They act as storage for energy – surplus calories that we keep for future energy needs, and they are saturated fats.

Structural fats are invisible to the naked eye, and only show up under the microscope as part of the structure of our cells and nerve tissues. They are also used for hormone production. The type and health of these fats are intimately linked to the health of cell membranes. Cell membranes are not just an envelope surrounding the contents of cells, but are actively involved in breaking down and transporting raw materials into the cells and eliminating waste products. The ability of cells to divide healthily is significantly dependent on the health of the fats that make up a large part of the cell membranes. These fats are unsaturated fats.

These two categories of fat, saturated and unsaturated, are also the main divisions of our dietary fats.

Saturated fats

These come principally from animal sources: meat, cheese, milk, cream, eggs, butter, lard. They are all solid at room temperature (milk, cream and egg fats are in suspension) and are very 'stable' fats, which makes them useful for cooking. We do not actually need saturated fats in the diet as we are able to make them from carbohydrates, especially refined carbohydrates and sugar, which convert very readily into energy stores, i.e. our spare tyres. Saturated fats are the fats that pad our hips and protect our organs internally – and some people are better at making them than others! Coconut and palm-kernel oils are vegetable sources of saturated fats, although they do not behave in quite the same way as animal fats and do have health benefits.

Consumption of animal fats has changed quite a lot in the last 100 years. Animals are bred for high weight because they fetch the best prices. The best way to increase an animal's weight is to increase the amount of fat it carries, and animals have been getting progressively 'fattier' over the years – for example we have increased the percentage of fat in chickens from 2.4 per cent at the turn of the century to 8 per cent in the early 1970s, rising to a staggering 22 per cent fat in the early 1980s. In the earlier part of the twentieth century surplus white fat from animals would be used to make candles, and homes were lit by them in many rural areas until electricity or oil became available. Animal fats which did find their way on to the plate would have been of more use to our grandparents because, on average, they were more active than we are today with our sedentary lifestyles, cars and energy-saving gadgets. Nowadays we do not use candles as a matter of course, and those that are manufactured are mostly made from paraffin wax. Surplus white animal fat now goes into the manufacture of sausages, pies, cooking fats, pastries, ice-cream, biscuits, cakes, crisps, and all manner of convenience foods. We are now eating the candles![1]

Unsaturated fats

Our main sources of unsaturated fats are vegetables, nuts and seeds, and their oils. The other major source of unsaturated fats is fish, especially oily fish such as tuna, sardines, salmon and mackerel. At room temperature these fats are liquid and they are susceptible to rancidity if not refrigerated. This is why fish 'goes off' – really fresh fish smells wonderful, but if the fish oils go rancid the fish smells awful quite quickly.

Unsaturated fats are used for a number of different functions in the body, all of which are essential for good health: hormone production and balance, cell membrane structure and nerve tissue. Cell membrane structure and hormone balance are critical from the point of view of breast cancer. The health of the cell membrane can make a difference in whether it divides correctly to make two healthy cells, or divides incorrectly, possibly to start the process of cancer. Hormone balance is vital for optimal protection against breast cancer and fats have a major role to play in this.

There are three main categories of unsaturated fat: omega-9, omega-6 and omega-3. Omega-9, most readily available from olive oil, is also called mono-unsaturated, or oleic acid, and the dark green cold-pressed olive oil also provides potent antioxidants.

Unsaturated fats are also the source of the two essential fats, linoleic acid and gamma-linoleic acid, which we have to obtain from our diet (we cannot manufacture them in our bodies as we can with other types of fat). These omega-6 and omega-3 fats come from a wide variety of foods and have an important role in keeping down inflammation by regulating substances called prostaglandins, which can have either an inflammatory or an anti-inflammatory effect. Deficiency of these two fats has serious health implications, as would a vitamin deficiency.

Here are the main sources of the three types of unsaturated fat (some foods provide significant amounts of more than one type)[2]:

Omega-9	Omega-6	Omega-3
Almond (78 per cent)	Evening primrose oil (81 per cent)	Oily fish (EPA and DHA fats)
Olive oil (76 per cent)		Flax oil (58 per cent)
Macadamia nuts (71 per cent)	Safflower oil (75 per cent)	Hemp seeds (25 per cent)
Cashew nuts (70 per cent)	Grape seed oil (71 per cent)†	Pumpkin seeds (15 per cent)
Pistachio nuts (65 per cent)	Sunflower oil (65 per cent)†	Soya bean oil (9 per cent)†
Pecan nuts (63 per cent)	Corn oil (59 per cent)†	
Beech nuts (54 per cent)	Hemp seeds (55 per cent)	
Brazil nuts (48 per cent)	Wheat germ oil (54 per cent)	
Rice bran (48 per cent)	Walnut oil (51 per cent)†	
Peanut oil* (47 per cent)	Soya bean oil (50 per cent)†	
Pumpkin seeds (42 per cent)	Sesame oil and seeds (45 per cent)	
Walnuts (28 per cent)†		
Soya beans (26 per cent)†	Pumpkin seeds (42 per cent)	
Sunflower seeds (23 per cent)†	Rice bran (35 per cent)	
	Beech nuts (32 per cent)	
	Peanut oil* (29 per cent)	
	Brazil nuts (24 per cent)	

* toxic fungus, aflatoxins
† not recommended for use as oil, unless specified cold-pressed and available in dark glass bottles (to protect against light damage), since the extraction process usually damages the oil. Alternatively, eat very fresh nuts or seeds.

From the point of view of breast cancer, and to simplify the matter, omega-9 fats and omega-3 fats have been found to be protective – as evidenced by the Mediterranean and Japanese diets – while an excess of omega-6 fats is suspected of contributing to breast cancer (suggesting that omega-6 should be kept to a low level in the diet when compared to the other two groups).

Trans-fats

One of the reasons why omega-6 fats may be a problem for breast cancer is that as they are so unstable, and are often the subject of chemical extraction processes that damage the oils, they may become the source of rogue 'free radicals' – damaging compounds which corrupt healthy cells (see the chapter **Antioxidant Armoury** (page 99)). In this way they may initiate cancer in the first place, and also burden the body's immune system. Another reason may be an excess of omega-6 fats when compared to omega-3 fats, probably due to our reliance on margarines and vegetable cooking oils.

Under particular suspicion are the so-called unsaturated fats – hydrogenated or partially hydrogenated margarines. These have undergone a process to turn a liquid oil (such as sunflower oil) into a fat which is solid at room temperature. This is why I call them 'so-called' as they have become 'honorary' saturated fats by processing. They are even more problematic than natural saturated fats since they contain 'trans-fats' which are highly damaging. Margarines are cheap and stable and are therefore beloved of food manufacturers. Manufactured products such as biscuits, potato crisps, pies, cakes and pastries will have hydrogenated fats as an ingredient because they allow for a long shelf-life. While manufacturers claim that a small percentage of their overall ingredients have been turned into trans-fats (2–17 per cent), what they don't tell you is that it has been shown that these fats accumulate in women's breasts, and particularly so in women with breast cancer. Here they can damage cell membranes and interfere with correct hormone and prostaglandin function.

Trans-fats are also created when oils are extracted by chemical processes, a process which is used as an alternative to pressing which would provide a low yield, or where the appearance or flavour of the oil needs to be altered. For example, grape seed oil or avocado oil is naturally dark and unpleasant-tasting in the raw, so chemical solvents are used to extract the oils. As corn has a low fat content, extremely high temperatures and toxic solvents are used to extract the oil efficiently, and the same is often true of soya oil. These processes make the oils high in trans-fats and chemical residues.

What can I spread on my bread?

This is the lament I frequently hear when people want to reduce animal and hydrogenated fats, and butter and margarine are first off the list. If you still want something to 'moisten' your bread, here are some ideas for spreads, all of which can be bought at health food shops or supermarket delicatessen counters, or made in seconds to keep in the fridge.

100 per cent fruit jam, available from health food shops
Prune purée
Tahini or sunflower seed spread
Mackerel pâté
Hummus
Guacamole
Salsa – green or red
Mashed garlic steeped in olive oil (on toasted bread)
Anchovy or olive tapenade
Sun-dried tomato tapenade

Prune purée

Great for spreading on bread or crackers as a fat-free spread. Prunes came out tops, in research at Tufts University, USA, at raising blood levels of antioxidants when compared to other fruits and vegetables. Plums scored one-sixth as high as their dried counterparts.

Put 225 g/8 oz pitted prunes into a blender with 6 tablespoons of water and whizz to a purée. Keeps in the fridge for two months in a covered container and freezes well.

Tapenade

Tapenade can be made in seconds in a food processor. Blend some or all of the following to a purée. It keeps in the fridge for a week in a covered container and freezes well.

Anchovies, black olives, sun-dried tomatoes, a little olive oil to moisten. These are the basic ingredients and you can emphasize one, or add them in equal parts. To this mixture add, according to taste: minced garlic, dried mixed herbs, fresh basil, capers.

Quantity of fat in the diet

The overall quantity of fat in the diet is important from the point of view of breast cancer. It is probable that fat in the diet increases breast cancer risk by contributing more calories overall.[3] Reducing calories can most easily be accomplished by lowering overall fat intake. Fewer calories in the diet means that there is less oxidation damage from metabolism, and this may be one mechanism where reducing calories by restricting fat intake works to the advantage of those wanting to minimize breast cancer risk. In the West, around 40–45 per cent of our calories comes from fat, despite Government recommendations that fat intake should not exceed 30 per cent of total calories. Countries with the lowest incidence of breast cancer consume around 20–25 per cent of calories from fat. The higher level of fat in the diet, especially when combined with a high intake of refined carbohydrates and sugar, contributes to excess body weight which is a risk factor for breast cancer, especially in post-menopausal women. Of course, percentage of dietary fat is not the whole picture and it must be remembered that quality of fat is important. To quote one paper: 'Some oils, including those rich in mono-unsaturates (olive oil), medium chain fatty acids (coconut), or omega-3 fatty acids (fish and flax oils) appear to lack tumour-promoting effects *despite their presence in the diet at high levels.*'[4]

Fats and oestrogens

Another reason why a high-fat diet, and particularly a high-animal fat diet, may be a problem for women with breast cancer is because it is fat in which animals store, and we store, chemical residues – herbicides, pesticides, fertilizers, growth enhancers, hormones and antibiotics, to name a few. Like water, fat is a universal solvent – when a cow grazes, it consumes whatever has been sprayed on the grass which is then stored in its body fat, including its milk. When we eat a steak, drink milk or eat butter or cheese, we consume the same chemicals. We do not eliminate them efficiently either, but store them in our own fat cells. The fats may also become more concentrated as you go higher up the food chain. Breast tissue is largely fatty tissue and is a storage area for these chemicals in the body. Many of these chemicals have an oestrogenic effect to which breast tissue is particularly sensitive. The reason why these chemicals are stored in fat is that they are fat-soluble chemicals. For example, in the case of pesticides, if they were water-soluble they would run off in the rain and not do the job for which they are intended – you will notice that the waxy residue on apples is greasy, because it is a fatty compound.

The other important thing to remember in the relationship between fat and breast cancer is that our fat cells encourage the production of oestrogens. Fat cells secrete an enzyme called aromatase which converts some of the circulating male androgen hormones, produced by all women, into female oestrogens. The heavier a woman, the more oestrogen she is making. Excess weight is therefore a contributing factor to breast cancer in post-menopausal women.

What is the evidence for and against different types of fats in the fight against breast cancer?

- Japanese women, who eat a traditional diet, have a quarter of the breast cancer incidence of British and American women. This is an interesting comparison because the Japanese have a similar level of industrialization to that in the West. The majority of their fat intake is from oily fish while in the West the majority of our fat intake is from saturated animal fats and from vegetable and seed oils. Any likelihood of there being a genetic influence is eliminated because, when Japanese women emigrate to the West and adopt a Western diet, their breast cancer levels match those of the host country,[5] and the reverse applies – when women migrate to the East and adopt a local diet their breast cancer incidence drops. It is true that the differences between the two diets encompass other aspects – fibre levels, vegetable intake and carbohydrate sources – but type and level of fat are inextricably linked to the overall eating differences.

- The much-publicized 1992 Nurses' Health Study[6] found no link between fats and breast cancer risk and, although the results have been questioned, many have accepted the study's findings unconditionally. This has caused controversy over one of the 'holy cows' of breast cancer causation. It may be nice to believe that fat-loaded convenience foods such as crisps, mayonnaise, hamburgers and ice-cream do no harm, but when you look at cross-national differences you may get a truer picture of the effect of fat on breast cancer. One of the flaws in the study may have been that the authors were comparing high-fat diets with moderate-fat diets (as opposed to low-fat diets). When you compare a moderate-fat intake of around 30–35 per cent of calories to a high fat intake of 40–45 per cent, you may not get much useful information. However, comparison with a very low-fat diet of 20 per cent fat, which is hard to find in the West, may reveal more meaningful data. Incidentally, 20–25 per cent fat intake is the range in countries with very low breast cancer rates, while 35–45 per cent is the range in countries with a high incidence.

- The 1998 report from the World Cancer Research Fund together with the American Institute for Cancer Research concluded, after exhaustively reviewing the available data, that diets high in total or in saturated fats may increase the risk of breast cancer.[7]

- A very low-fat diet of 15 per cent of calories from fat pursued over two years has been shown to lower oestradiol (E2) levels (the most troublesome oestrogen with breast cancer) in women by 20 per cent. (However progesterone levels were also lowered and this may be too low a level of fat to aim for to maintain a healthy diet.[8])

- Research has suggested that women with breast cancer who had lower saturated fat diets, suffered less DNA damage to their breast tissue cells.[9]

■ Animal studies (mice and rats) show that omega-3 fish oil fats significantly reduce tumour incidence, number, growth and metastases, and reduce tumour prostaglandin production.[10]

■ Women who eat fish, and therefore fish oils, have a lower breast cancer risk than those who do not.[11]

■ Fish oil interrupts the manufacture of a type of 'local hormone' called prostaglandin E2 (PGE2). On average breast cancer patients have excess levels of PGE2. Excess PGE2 suppresses the immune system and makes the fight against breast cancer more difficult,[12] so bringing levels of PGE2 down is beneficial.

■ Low levels in breast tissue of the vegetable sources of omega-3 fats, called alpha-linoleic acid, principally found in cold-pressed flax oil, was found to be the best predictor, along with tumour size, of the risk of breast cancer spreading into the lymph nodes, vascular invasion and metastasis.[13]

■ Olive oil and its major constituent, oleic acid, have not been found to promote cancer in animal studies as do other fats[14] and olive oil is associated with a decrease in death rates from breast cancer.[15] Countries with high olive oil intake have lower breast cancer rates than those which do not consume much olive oil.[16] One study suggested that oleic acid may increase the risk of breast cancer; however, in this study the oleic acid was not sourced from olive oil as it was in the other studies.[17] It is presumed that it is the high level, and the specific type, of antioxidants contained in olive oil that are so beneficial.

■ While a deficiency of the essential omega-6 fat (linoleic acid) is detrimental to health and will depress antibody response and cause lymph tissue to atrophy (waste away), an excess of the omega-6 polyunsaturated fats, such as is found in corn and soya oils, can be detrimental by lowering T-cell immune response. Obviously, getting the correct balance of these omega-6 fats is important, though an excess is most likely on a Western diet, because of the quantities of vegetable oils and margarines in the diet.

■ A low-fat diet has been shown to be accompanied by a decrease in circulating levels of several types of oestrogen (total oestradiol, weakly bound oestradiol, oestrone and oestrone sulphate), lower levels of which decrease breast cancer risk.

■ Data show that breast cancer patients report significantly shorter menstrual cycles than women without breast cancer. A study looking at restricting calories from fat concluded that there was a significant increase in length of the menstrual cycle,[18] which may be beneficial to pre-menopausal breast cancer patients.

■ One study showed that when women adopted a low-fat diet for a period of two years, with 21 per cent of calories from fat, the density of their breasts lowered by an average of 6.1 per cent. Those on a 32 per cent fat diet had a drop of 2.1 per cent in breast density. Breast density is considered a possible risk factor for developing breast cancer.[19]

The way forward

It is probably wise to keep overall fat levels in the diet to 30 per cent or below – more about how to do this can be found in **Your Basic Nutrition and Supplement Plan** (page 197), but what this means is that for an average woman on 2,000 calories a day, 30 per cent fat is equivalent to 600 calories coming from fat, or 65 g/2½ oz of fat. It is desirable to keep saturated fats from animal sources to a minimum and any that you do eat should ideally be organic to minimize exposure to oestrogen-mimicking chemicals which concentrate in animal fats. Increasing fish in the diet is highly beneficial. The best source of oil for most cooking or salad uses is cold-pressed extra-virgin olive oil. For salads and other cold uses (i.e. when not heated) flax oil, which is high in omega-3 fats, is ideal. Avoiding hydrogenated fats from packaged foods and margarines is of paramount importance. Omega-6 oils should be ultra-fresh and kept to a very moderate level, and the best sources are fresh, unroasted nuts and seeds.

Easy Fish Dish (1)

1 portion of fish (salmon, tuna, cod, halibut, haddock, or other fish) per person, cleaned, descaled and filleted
olive oil
white wine
garlic cloves, chopped
freshly ground black pepper
fresh or dried herbs (parsley, chives, basil, fennel, tarragon)

Pre-heat the oven to 180°C/350°F/gas mark 4.

Drizzle some olive oil into a ceramic or stainless-steel baking dish and put in the fish skin down. Splash some white wine on top (allow half a glass for two people, and adjust accordingly) and sprinkle with the garlic, pepper and herbs. Bake in the oven for 10–20 minutes, depending on the thickness of the fish. Spoon the cooking juices over the fish half-way through cooking to avoid drying out. Serve with salad or vegetables and lentils.

Note: If you are using salmon or tuna, cook some extra which will be delicious served cold the next day for an instant healthy meal.

Easy Fish Dish (2)

Serves 1
1 portion of fish
½ × 400 g/14 oz can chopped tomatoes
½ red pepper, deseeded and cut into strips
½ onion, chopped
1 garlic clove, chopped
mixed Italian herbs, dried or fresh
freshly ground black pepper
½ glass white wine
drizzle of olive oil

Pre-heat the oven to 180°C/350°F/gas mark 4.

Put the vegetables, garlic, herbs, pepper, wine and oil into a ceramic or stainless-steel baking dish and bake in the oven for 15 minutes. Place the fish on top, spoon over the vegetables and liquid, and bake for a further 10 minutes, depending on the thickness of the fish. Serve with vegetables or salad and crusty wholemeal bread to mop up the juices.

Pick Your Proteins

We use protein for building body tissues – muscles, skin, organs, for the immune system, and for internal messengers and regulators – enzymes, hormones and brain chemicals. In order for us to manufacture the proteins we need, we must have an adequate supply of protein building blocks, called amino acids, in our diet. When we consume protein from either animal or vegetable sources, we must first break these down into amino acids, and then build them up again into the types of protein that are needed at that moment by the body.

Our meals are often centred on meat and the average person gets twice the Government recommended amount of total protein per day. The excess protein is stored as fat as it cannot be used immediately for tissue growth and repair, and processing it involves a detoxification cycle, called the urea cycle, which is a taxing and difficult process for the cells to deal with. It uses energy that could serve us better, repairing tissues and fending off invaders.

And there is another problem with excess protein – it forms an acid residue. We are principally alkaline entities. We have only three areas in our body that are meant to be acidic: our stomach; the surface of our skin; and inside our large intestine (colon), which is mildly acidic in order to support the right balance of helpful bacteria. But all our cells have to be alkaline, and they cannot tolerate acidity at all. The residue that is left at the end of using proteins is acidic, which then needs to be made alkaline as a matter of priority to avoid damaging cells. Excess protein overloads this mechanism and ties up cellular activity, using up valuable energy and nutrients which could be used to better advantage for other functions.

Many anti-cancer diets recommend a vegetarian, or vegan or macrobiotic, eating programme in the fight against cancer, precisely because more vegetables in the diet support the alkaline environment of the cells. Vegetarian diets will exclude meat but include eggs and dairy products, whilst vegan diets will exclude all foods of animal origin. Macrobiotics is more of a 'philosophy' of eating which is based on

Eastern yin and yang principles – however, it is often vegetarian or vegan in practice and is centred on large amounts of brown rice and vegetables.

Animal sources of protein are meat, fish, cheese, milk and eggs. Vegetarian protein-rich sources are beans, nuts, soya products and grains. One of the key *raisons-d'être* for recommending little or no animal protein in these special anti-cancer diets is that it is far easier to overdo protein intake on a meat-eating diet than on a vegetable-based one. The detoxification process, and the alkalization process of excess proteins increases the body's overall work-load resulting in the healing process being compromised.

There does not seem to be any evidence suggesting that protein from a mixture of vegetable and animal sources[1] compromises health from the point of view of breast cancer, but there does appear to be some evidence against excess animal protein in the diet.[2] A link has been made between high animal protein consumption in young girls at the time of sexual maturation and increased breast cancer risk later in life.[3]

When we talk about animal protein we are also, inevitably, talking about the fat content of meat and dairy produce, since all animal proteins come with fat as an integral component. Quantity and type of fat is important in the fight against breast cancer and it is hard to divorce this issue from the subject of animal protein. On balance the evidence is against a high quantity of saturated animal fat in the diet, which may be one of the key reasons why animal protein in the diet is best reduced. Conversely there is a quantity of evidence which shows that omega-3 fish oils are protective against breast cancer and can be instrumental in helping to shrink tumour growth. See **Fats – Friends or Foes?** (page 81) for detailed information about meat, dairy and fish fats.

However, in the developing world, where breast cancer is statistically much lower than in the West, most protein consumed is of vegetable origin. In the developed world, where breast cancer statistics are soaring, most protein consumed is of animal origin. Yet there are exceptions that disprove every rule: Eskimos on a traditional diet, who have a high protein intake from oily fish and a very low vegetable intake, have nil incidence of breast cancer, perhaps because of the protective effects of the fish oils; the Masai tribe, for whom cow's blood and milk are the staple diet, also have a low breast cancer incidence (possibly due to the fact that these foods are uncooked and unpasteurized and are therefore easier to assimilate due to the enzymes they contain).

During an active fight against cancer, it is necessary to have sufficient protein to use as building blocks for the immune system, so it is important to get the balance right. What does research tell us about protein, in particular animal protein, in the diet in relation to breast cancer?

- Advocates of a largely vegetable- and fruit-based, predominantly raw diet, such as the Bristol Cancer Centre's, are careful to point out that eating in this way is likely to cause a rapid weight loss and that it is therefore important to include sufficient proteins, as well as carbohydrates and fats.[4]
- All healing and repair activities in the body require a balance of nutrients. Protein is required in greater quantities (but not to excess) when there are increased healing and repair tasks, than the amounts needed just for maintenance.
- Excessive restriction of dietary protein does not affect the growth rate of a tumour, but does restrict the well-being of the individual.[5]
- Some studies suggest that a vegetarian diet is not protective against breast cancer. This is thought to be due to vegetarians being more likely to have significantly higher intakes of vegetable oils and hydrogenated fats than non-vegetarians. Many are also likely to rely on dairy sources of protein such as milk and cheese, which can be very high in saturated fat. High vegetable oil, hydrogenated fats and saturated fats may contribute to increased risk of breast cancer (see **Fats – Friends or Foes?**).
- Links between animal protein intake and breast cancer have been widely suggested[6] and in particular, a lowering of risk for pre-menopausal women who avoid animal protein has been reported.[7]
- Animal protein is devoid of fibre. Fibre has been shown in many studies to be protective against breast cancer, as we have already seen.
- In vegetarian women, oestrogen hormone profiles can be different to those of their meat-eating sisters. Studies have shown vegetarian women to have lower levels of plasma oestrone and 17β-oestradiol,

lower levels of urinary oestrogens, higher faecal oestrogen levels and lowered metabolism to 16-hydroxylated oestrogen compounds – all these are associated with decreased risk of breast cancer.[8]

Chilli without Carne

Spanish onions, roughly chopped
green and red peppers, roughly chopped
tomatoes, roughly chopped, or canned tomatoes
garlic, minced or sliced
olive oil
tomato paste
cayenne pepper, paprika, cumin, oregano, pepper, or other spices
vegetable stock or water
Soya mince (TVP, textured vegetable protein)
kidney beans, cooked from dried or canned, drained and rinsed
fresh chilli pepper, deseeded and finely chopped, or dried

Cook the fresh vegetables and garlic in olive oil until softened, then add the spices, tomato paste, stock or water and heat up. Add the soya mince and kidney beans. Simmer for at least 30 minutes, longer if possible. Add more stock or water if the mixture shows signs of drying out.

Serve with baked potato, tortillas or brown rice. Add toppings: sliced mild onions or spring onions, sliced tomato, sliced avocado, plain yoghurt.

■ Overcooked meat is four times more likely than rarer meat to contribute to breast cancer among meat-eating women. This is probably linked to the formation of HCAs (heterocyclic amines), a chemical that results when amino acids react with creatine, a chemical found naturally in muscle. This reaction takes place at the high temperatures caused by frying, grilling and barbecuing. Boiling, stewing and poaching at lower temperatures create negligible quantities of HCAs. Conversely, eating undercooked meats does have risks, with *E. coli* and salmonella outbreaks becoming more common. Cooking meat by the least harmful methods until thoroughly cooked through is probably the best option.[9]

- Excess protein from dairy sources (milk and cheese predominantly) causes, in susceptible people, an excess production of mucus. This can lead in turn to an increased tendency to infections, especially respiratory infections, bowel disorders and allergies. These can over-load the immune system and reduce its overall effectiveness.

- Another issue that has yet to rear its unattractive head in Europe, but is a problem in the USA, is the use of growth hormones in animals. So far the European Union has resisted the pressure placed upon it by the USA to accept meat and milk products which use these growth enhancers. However, the debate continues, and it is always possible that economic pressures will prevail. Resistance to changing this policy has looked weak recently. It is suspected that in the USA breast cancer is accelerated by levels of IGF-1 (Insulin Like Growth Factor) from milk. Humans produce IGF-1 and it is known that breast cancer is stimulated by human production of this powerful hormone.[10] And the bovine version is very similar to the human version. These facts should not be taken lightly as the incidence of breast cancer in the USA is quite a bit higher (one in eight women) than in the UK (one in eleven), and it is entirely feasible that IGF-1 in dairy products can, at least partially, account for the difference in incidence. If imports of hormone-treated meat ever reach Europe they should be avoided at all costs.

The way forward

A diet that maintains sufficient protein levels to nurture the individual is essential. However, it is preferable to reduce the amount of animal protein from the levels typical of a Western diet and, at least partially, replace it with vegetarian sources of protein. Dishes based on legumes (beans, chick-peas, lentils), grains, soya products (tofu, TVP – textured vegetable protein), quinoa and Quorn mycoprotein are all excellent sources of vegetable protein. Plant sources of protein have the added advantage of offering protection by offering other cancer fighters such as fibre, antioxidants and plant hormones.

Animal proteins should ideally be kept to fish sources, which offer the potent breast cancer-fighting omega-3 fats, and meats that are lowest in saturated fats and chemicals, such as skinless organic chicken and game. The importance of non-contaminated sources of meat cannot be over-emphasized in view of possible contamination by oestrogenic compounds which can be found in intensively farmed meat. Ideally, animal sources of protein – meat, fish, fowl, game, eggs and dairy produce – should be used as a condiment to flavour and enhance dishes, rather than as the main ingredient. Instead of a large slab of meat on a plate with a few vegetables, meals which reflect the cuisine of Eastern or Third World countries are best. This means, for example, bean stews, with a little meat for flavour, or stir-fries with a little seafood as one of several ingredients.

Fermented milk products, such as yoghurt and cottage cheese, should be preferred over other dairy sources such as milk and hard cheese as they are more easily digested, the milk proteins having been partially pre-digested by bacteria. Eggs in moderation – about three or four a week – are fine. Eggs, along with cottage cheese, are a valuable source of sulphur containing amino acids, which aid the liver's detoxification process.

If you are already a vegetarian, or are planning to switch over, it is important not to become a 'bread and cheese' vegetarian. A high intake of cheese, milk and eggs with insufficient vegetables, fruits and pulses to redress the balance, is not much better, from the point of view of breast cancer, than being a fully fledged meat-eater.

It is probably not necessary to become vegetarian if it does not suit you, as the main protective benefits that come from a vegetarian diet are derived from the increased intake of vegetables, fruit, grains and pulses. Increasing these in the diet is more important than cutting out all sources of animal protein, though reducing the amount of animal protein, typical of a Western diet, is advisable.

Antioxidant Armoury

One thing which all authorities consistently agree on is that a diet high in fruits and vegetables is protective against most cancers, including breast cancer. It has also been shown that low antioxidant levels are strongly correlated to cancer mortality.[1] The most likely reason why fruits and vegetables are hugely protective is because they are our main source of antioxidants. In this chapter we will be looking at dietary sources of antioxidants, while vitamin and mineral antioxidant supplements are discussed later.

Most people these days have heard of the term 'antioxidant' as it has been a buzz-word for a few years now. But what are antioxidants, and what do they do?

Antioxidants fight oxidation damage. You can see oxidation when iron rusts, or a sliced apple turns brown on contact with the air. You may notice on some food labels that antioxidants have been added. This is especially the case for fats and fatty foods, as they oxidize easily and go rancid.

When oxidation affects body tissues they are damaged. On the outside, our skin gets tougher and discoloured as we age, and the most obvious signs of accelerated oxidation occur with excessive exposure to the sun. We cannot see what goes on inside us with the naked eye, but destructive oxidation happens there as well. Oxidation damage to internal cells is believed to be responsible for, or contribute significantly to, up to eighty different human diseases, including all the main ones – cardiovascular disease, cancer and diabetes.

When there is cumulative damage to the genetic material of our cells, this is one of the triggers for initiation of cancer. Breathing oxygen and the process of metabolizing our food, both of which are natural processes, are major sources of oxidation damage, and to combat such damage our bodies have many inbuilt mechanisms to deal with the problem. We have to have protection – we can't just stop breathing and eating!

Oxidation damage occurs as a result of free radicals, highly unstable and reactive molecules which thieve electrons from our cells in an attempt to stabilize themselves. They attack lipids (fats), proteins, enzymes and DNA. Electrons like to be paired and if they are not coupled up, will work overtime to find a mate. This sets up a chain reaction, which if left unchecked has a cumulative effect and eventually damages DNA. This process has been directly linked with breast cancer.[2] The oxidation process may also be involved in converting oestrogens into carcinogenic forms of the hormones.[3]

We have an assortment of free radical-quenching enzymes in our bodies which deal with these rogue molecules. But we do not have an infinite ability to deal with them. Therefore we are also dependent on free-radical quenchers that are available from our diet – the antioxidants. They act as sacrificial victims, giving up their molecules to stop the chain reaction of damage caused by the free radicals. In offering themselves up, they spare the molecules in our own body tissue. If levels are kept topped up, the body has many of the antioxidants available in cell membranes and body fluids which can spring into action when needed.

This mechanism seems to work very well, unless there are insufficient back-up antioxidants in the diet, or we overwhelm our bodies with oxidation damage from external sources of free radicals. It has been estimated that these days, each of our cells takes 10,000 free-radical 'hits' a day.

Any combustion process is a source of free radicals, and if we expose ourselves to too many of these, we run the risk of over-loading our systems to the point where our bodies and diets can't cope and we develop diseases, including cancer. Sources of free radicals include sunlight, smoking, car exhausts, radiation, fires, heavy metals, barbecued, burnt or smoked foods, rancid fats, overheated oils, stress, excess sugar and refined carbohydrates and excess exercise (exercise in moderation is beneficial). Stress, sugar, refined carbohydrates and excess exercise are sources of free radicals because they increase the use of oxygen in the body.

Antioxidant sources

Vegetables and fruits are the main sources of antioxidants. They are also rich sources of other protective compounds, including phyto-chemicals, fibre and a range of vitamins and minerals, as well as, generally, being low in fat and calories. If eaten raw, they also provide enzymes which are beneficial for digestion.

The best-known antioxidants are the nutrients vitamins A, C and E, beta-carotene, and the minerals selenium and zinc. As they are essential nutrients for humans, they have been better researched than other antioxidants.

There is also a wide range of non-essential compounds found in foods which have potent antioxidant properties. These include poly-phenols, lignans, isoflavones, curcumins, anthocyanidins, proantho-cyanidins, lycopene, co-enzyme Q10, alpha-lipoic acid and quercitin, amongst many.

We are now in the process of identifying these compounds and understanding their remarkable properties. However, one thing is becoming abundantly clear: the sum total is greater than the parts. The concept of synergy is tremendously important when understanding antioxidants and other plant compounds. Unfortunately this makes research difficult. As Dr Richard Passwater, one of the fathers of antioxi-dant research, says, 'Looking at vitamin E by itself, or any antioxidant by itself, is a waste of time. What needs to be done is to look at the effect of all the antioxidants together. Researchers are now devising antioxidant nutrient indices to accomplish this.'[4] The effects of one or two of these compounds might be good, but the effect of several together can be extraordinary. Indeed, this is the way that food is given to us in its natural form – as a complex source of many com-pounds. Science is finally catching up with the wisdom of Mother Nature.

What is the research available relating to antioxidants and breast cancer?

- Greek women in one study, who had the highest intake of veg-etables, had a 90 per cent lower risk of breast cancer when compared to women with the lowest intakes. A Russian study found the same extraordinary results, though mostly in post-menopausal women, and a Singapore study found similar results.[5]

■ The conclusions of the 1998 report of the World Cancer Research Fund and the American Institute of Cancer Research were that 'There is a strong and consistent pattern showing that diets high in vegetables and fruits decrease the risk of many cancers, and perhaps cancer in general (and) they probably protect against breast cancers.'

■ A study that examined women after surgery for early breast cancer found more favourable prognostic tumour characteristics in those who had previously eaten more fruit and vegetables.[6]

■ European countries such as Greece and Spain, which have a high incidence of tobacco smoking, report a low incidence of cancer, probably due to their high intake of dietary antioxidants contained in the fruits and vegetables which are central to the Mediterranean diet. This does not mean that smoking is OK, but that fruit and vegetables are great.[7]

■ Studies have shown that women with diets high in vitamin A and beta-carotene have a lower risk of breast cancer, though more evidence exists for the protective role of beta-carotene.[8] The Singapore study mentioned above showed an 80 per cent lowering of risk for those with high beta-carotene levels, though it is probable that in this instance those at the bottom of the vegetable and fruit intake were significantly beta-carotene deficient. The same level of variation may not be shown in Western women who, on the whole, are not as beta-carotene deficient.

■ An analysis of around ninety studies on the role of vitamin C in cancer prevention concluded that the majority showed statistically significant protection for a number of cancers, including breast cancer.[9] Another meta-analysis of twelve studies concluded that consuming 380 mg of vitamin C daily (along with other dietary modifications) could reduce breast cancer incidence by 16 per cent in pre-menopausal women and by 24 per cent in post-menopausal women.[10] 380 mg of vitamin C is the amount that you would get from five large oranges, seven kiwi fruit, 450 g/1 lb of strawberries, or 225 g/8 oz of blackcurrants.

■ A British study concluded that vitamin E levels showed a statistical relevance to breast cancer. Those with the lowest dietary vitamin E levels have the highest incidence, with some having five times the risk of breast cancer compared to those with the most vitamin E.[11] Vitamin E is probably best studied not in isolation, but in relation to its partner, selenium.

- Geographical areas in the USA as well as in European countries, which have low selenium levels in the soil – and consequently have lower selenium levels in locally grown and eaten foods – have higher breast cancer rates.[12] Japanese women, who have considerably lower breast cancer incidence, consistently have higher selenium levels – from fish and rice in their diets – and even among Japanese women those who develop breast cancer have lower blood selenium levels than those who remain breast cancer-free. The 1992 Nurses' Study failed to confirm these results; however, they used toe-nail clippings to analyse selenium levels which does not have the same correlation with breast cancer incidence as do serum levels.[13]

- In animal experiments, diets high in Brazil nuts, which are particularly rich sources of the antioxidant mineral selenium, have been shown to decrease chemically induced mammary tumours.[14] Women with higher dietary selenium levels have lower DNA mutations, which reduces the risk of breast cancer.[15]

Roasted Peppers

Peppers are loaded with antioxidants and using them at every opportunity in salads, as purées or in casseroles is a major bonus. Roasting brings out the natural sweetness of these cancer-fighting foods.

Serves 2 as a first course
1 red, yellow or orange pepper
2 tomatoes, roughly chopped
4 spring onions or 8 asparagus spears, chopped
2 garlic cloves, peeled
4 canned or fresh anchovy fillets, roughly chopped
olive oil
2 crusty wholemeal bread rolls

Preheat oven to 180°C/350°F/gas mark 4.

Cut the peppers in half and remove the seeds. Stuff with the other vegetables, garlic and anchovies. Drizzle with olive oil, place on a baking sheet and bake in the oven for 40 minutes. The roasted peppers and the garlic will become sweet and the juices are delicious mopped up with a wholemeal bread roll.

The way forward

A diet high in fruits and vegetables is advised for anyone wishing to reduce their risk of cancer, including breast cancer. The official guidelines state five portions of fruit and vegetables – as in the 'Give Me Five' campaign of the British Dietetic Association. But research is showing that ten portions daily confer even more protection by increasing antioxidant markers in the blood.[16] A portion would be one piece of fruit, such as an apple, a banana or a peach, two kiwi fruit or two plums. Vegetable-wise it would mean an ordinary-sized mug full of vegetables such as broccoli, green beans or cabbage, or half an ordinary mug full of more dense vegetables such as beans or lentils. A portion could also be a glass of fruit juice.

Personally, I like to aim for five as a bare minimum, and to go for more like seven to ten portions a day. If this sounds difficult, then turn to **Your Basic Nutrition Plan** (page 202) for some serving ideas.

There is a group of people with highly sensitive taste perceptions who have been dubbed 'supertasters'. They dislike the bitter taste of some fruits and vegetables and will tend to avoid them.[17] Many of the important cancer-protective flavonoids have a bitter taste, such as naranjenin in grapefruit and sulphoraphanes in broccoli. The danger is that these people – around 25 per cent of women – will either avoid these types of food or will smother them in extra butter, cream, cheese or sugar to disguise the flavour and so increase their overall fat intake. Dr Adam Drewnowski, director of the Human Nutrition Program at Michigan University, USA, says that these compounds have a potential chemo-therapeutic value. Better ways for this group of people to change the overall flavour would be to add sweet-tasting fruits to bitter or sour ones to make 'cocktails', or to modify the taste of healthy foods they find unpleasant with other low-fat flavourings: herbs, spices, lemon juice, balsamic vinegar, small amounts of sesame oil, soya sauce, tomato, garlic, onion, mustard and honey, fruit-flavoured vinegars, salsa, wine and yoghurt.

Antioxidants are not just found in fruits, vegetables and legumes. They are also in olive oil, teas and red wine. Even chocolate has antioxidants that are useful.

Organic Food

Are organic foods important for preventing, or recovering from, breast cancer? I would say, yes.

There has been a growing unease about the chemicals used agriculturally and added to our foods, and people are voting with their shopping baskets. It has taken the farming industry by surprise that there is such a demand for organic food, a demand that domestic producers cannot keep up with – we currently have to import 70 per cent of our organic produce.

It has to be of paramount importance for anyone interested in reducing their risk of breast cancer, and avoiding recurrence, to buy organic produce at every opportunity. There is a substantial amount of information which builds a very ugly picture regarding the hormonal influence of a number of the chemicals which find their way into our foods.

Can't you just wash off the residues? Sadly, not very efficiently, because only about 20 per cent of the chemicals are on the surface of fruits and vegetables, and the remainder is systemic – in the fabric of the plant. A lettuce, or an apple, can be sprayed thirty times during its short life from seed to supermarket, and each spray is of a different compound for a different pest. Many fruits and vegetables are then sealed with a waxy substance to lengthen the life of the produce, but this has the effect of sealing in the chemicals and making them harder to wash off.

Meat and dairy produce not only bear oestrogenic compounds lodged in the fat, but also carry the extra burden of antibiotics (there has been recent legislation to reduce antibiotics but they are still a concern). We really are living in . . .

A sea of chemicals

In the last twenty years, the number of toxic chemicals sprayed on cereal crops has trebled in areas of intensive farming. Around 80 per cent of arable fields are regularly coated with up to thirty-six herbicides, fungicides and insecticides. While the total weight of chemicals has dropped, the overall number has risen. This is more sinister than it sounds because while the effects on health of individual compounds are measured, the cumulative effect of a number of chemicals is little understood. The combined effect is suspected of having a stronger carcinogenic impact than that of single chemicals,[1] in the same way that the combined effect of pesticides and other chemicals is suspected to be a strong contributor to 'Gulf War Syndrome'. Professor Ashford, health adviser to the United Nations, has said, 'It is not a question of a single substance poisoning an organism, but rather a multi-stage process which interferes with the whole system.' The rise in the number of chemicals sprayed has been synonymous with a sharp decline in many species of wild birds. This is partly due to their natural food not being available, the grubs and insects having been killed off, but they are also unable to tolerate the chemical load. And for some reason the authorities who license the use of these chemicals expect us to be able to cope with a chemical burden which is too much for wildlife.

There are many examples in the natural world of species which are being affected by mysterious sex hormone-mimicking chemicals, resulting in abnormal sexual development. On Lake Apopka in Florida, alligators are hatching which are predominantly female, or if they are male, they have abnormally small genitals. Male Texan turtles are being born with ovaries.[2] Ranched minks fed on fish from the Great Lakes fail to reproduce, while those fed on fish from other areas breed as normal. And there is a mysterious rise in polar bears with dual-sex organs – about 4 per cent in a population of 2,000 bears[3] – much higher than can be accounted for by chance.

These suspicious events are not confined to animals living in polluted waters. There has been a steady increase in boys born with very small penises, undescended testicles or indeterminate sex organs, as well as a serious drop in adult male fertility since the 1950s.[4] Because of these environmental and human issues the chemicals in question are being nicknamed 'gender benders'. By stark contrast to what is happening to human fertility, it has been observed that organically reared animals have grown increasingly productive over three generations.

It is not just our external environment which is becoming contaminated, but our homes as well. Chemicals called nonylphenols, used in plastic products such as babies' bottles and water jugs, and chlorine compounds and dioxin, which are used to bleach paper products, detergents, toiletries and even spermicides, are suspected to be contributors to the breast cancer problem. These chemicals, along with agri-chemicals, mimic oestrogens and are called xenoestrogens. Concentrations of toxic compounds can be up to 500 times higher inside the home than outdoors as they are trapped by four walls.

The oestrogenic effect of these artificially manufactured compounds was discovered by accident by Ana Soto, MD, and Carlos Sonnenschein, PhD, at Tufts University in Boston, USA, who noticed that cells stored in plastic flasks had suddenly started to grow as if they were in the presence of oestrogens, whereas in previous experiments there had not been a problem. They identified the offending and mysterious substance as nonylphenol, used to stop plastic from cracking. The chemical was present in the plastic flasks. When they switched to using glass flasks the problem stopped. Not long afterwards, they showed that nonylphenols can also cause breast tissue growth. Other nonylphenols include atrazine, the most common pesticide in the USA, and PCBs (polychlorinated biphenyls).

Studies have measured DDE (the breakdown product of DDT) and PCB levels in serum samples of breast cancer patients and have found that a four-fold increase in the risk of breast cancer is associated with higher levels of these chemicals. The conclusions of one study stated, 'organochlorine residues may be an important etiologic factor in breast cancer', and 'the implications are far-reaching for public health intervention world-wide'.[5] One Danish study showed that Dieldrin and organochlorine were associated with a significant dose-related increase in breast cancer.[6]

The pesticide Lindane is the major organochloride still in use in the UK, and it has come under criticism for a direct link with breast cancer. Interest has been stirred among researchers as to whether Lindane, along with similar chemicals such as DDT, could cause breast cancer.[7] Lindane has been found in 30 per cent of all milk samples and, while the quantities are small, the chemical has the unfortunate habit of being stored in our fat cells, and building up over time. Lindane has also been found in breast tissue samples, and areas of high incidence of breast cancer seem to coincide with areas which boast the most extensive usage of Lindane. In the USA, Lindane has been listed as a probable/possible human carcinogen since the late 1970s, and many countries, including Holland, Sweden, Finland, Denmark, Singapore, Japan and Israel, have banned it. For some reason the UK continues to allow its use.

Lindane is sometimes described on products aimed at agrochemical companies as gamma-HCH. While 80 per cent of Lindane is used in agriculture, it is also used in medicines (for the treatment of scabies and headlice), in veterinary products and to treat timber for pest control. Its use has more than doubled since 1987. One aspect about the use of Lindane which certainly gives me pause for thought is that around a third of its use is for sugar beet, a crop which is grown for sugar production (and I do not consider sugar a necessary component of our food supply), and as a farm animal feed (and we probably eat a surfeit of meat and dairy produce in the UK). Surely the use of a toxic organochlorine cannot really be justified in these circumstances?*

It has been found that women with breast cancer have more pesticide residues in their body tissues than women who do not have breast cancer – up to 40 per cent more chlorinated pesticides in their breast tissue and much higher blood levels of DDE. While DDT has been banned in the UK and USA for quite some time, Third World countries from which we import our food still use it, and while levels are supposed to be checked, there have been notorious problems with certification procedures in those countries. Additionally, in the UK, over 50 per cent of wood pigeons tested in the mid-1990s contained DDT residues, in some cases by up to five times the maximum anticipated residue level, indicating that DDT was still being used illegally ten years after being banned.[8]

As these oestrogenic chemicals are all fat-soluble, they concentrate in the fat cells and milk of animals and humans. By gravitating to fat in the body they also end up in high quantities in breast tissue where

* At the time of going to press the UK government has just banned the use of Lindane on seeds, to protect agricultural workers. This will cut levels by 50 per cent, which is gratifying, but should not lead to complacency. A full ban is still needed.

they probably do the most damage. This is one possible reason why research into diets high in animal fats has shown an increased risk of breast cancer. Interestingly, a paper published in 1990 which followed what happened after Israel banned a number of chemicals in 1978 which were determined to be correlated to breast cancer risk, recorded that incidence of the disease dropped by a massive 30 per cent in younger women under forty-four years of age[9] (younger women's breast tissue is more sensitive to carcinogenic agents), while at the same time incidence continued to rise worldwide.

The lacquers that coat the inside of many food cans pose yet another hazard. It has been found that they leach significant levels of biosphenol-A which exhibits an oestrogenic effect. The leaching is worse in foods which have been packed in oil, such as sardines and pilchards.

Xenoestrogens probably contribute to breast cancer risk in a number of ways:

- They bind with oestrogen receptors and then prompt the breast tissue to grow and multiply in the same way that oestradiol (E2) does.
- They trigger the release of a chemical called 'tumour-growth factor' (the name speaks for itself).
- They can even cause the number of oestrogen receptors to increase on the cell surface, making the cell even more susceptible to influence by oestrogens.

The research is far from conclusive on the issue of xenoestrogens, which begs the question: should we take these concerns seriously, until they are proven? Theo Colborn and her co-authors, in their book *Our Stolen Future*, criticizes the designs of the studies to date: '. . . [they] have several shortcomings that make such inconsistent results not at all surprising. The contribution of synthetic chemicals to oestrogen exposure may come from many different chemicals, some of them exceedingly persistent, such as PCBs, and others that are not persistent and leave no telltale evidence of exposure in blood or fat.' They go on to say, 'Also, studies have usually treated all 209 chemicals in the PCB family as one, even though various members of this chemical family have completely different and in some cases opposite biological

effects.'[10] While human studies are the ideal, we may be [...]
point where they are viable as so many chemicals are now [...]
the human body, and one researcher at Tufts University i[...]
USA, concluded that in-vitro studies (in a test-tube, rather tha[...]
or human experiments) were essential for 'evolving dietary strategies
and tactics against the adverse health effects of environmental chemicals' because *it is impossible to have a chemical-free environment* (my
emphasis).[11]

With important questions being raised about the safety of these
chemicals, it seems to be a dangerous policy for long-term health that
governments have not exercised more caution on the use of the
majority of them. But we live in a world governed by short-term
economics, and it is interesting that much of the research into cancer
is funded by the very companies that produce these xenoestrogen
chemicals. It is probably unwise to wait for legislation to catch up,
and a good move to take measures to minimize exposure to these
chemicals yourself as outlined in the chapter **Lifestyle Choices** (page
183) – you have nothing to lose and everything to gain.

The way forward

The best insurance to protect ourselves and our families from the
possibility of contamination by the many chemicals in our food is to
buy organic produce at every opportunity.

Not only does organic produce taste better because it has a lower
water content than non-organic vegetables and fruit, but it has been
found that nutrient levels in organically produced fruits and vegetables
are superior. Mineral levels are up to 50 per cent higher than in
intensively produced vegetables.

Inevitably, it will be argued that not everybody can eat organic all the
time. It is the availability of inexpensive fruits and vegetables – inexpensive because of intensive farming methods which use pesticides,
insecticides and herbicides – that allows a good and plentiful variety to
be available to many people who would not otherwise have as much
choice. The advice to eat at least five portions of fruit and vegetables
takes precedence over every other bit of advice. Having said this, whilst
the pay-off for increased fruit and vegetable consumption may result

in lower cancer incidence, we may find that the next generation has to pay a hefty price: research is now telling us that vegetarian women, with higher fruit and vegetable intake, are having five times the numbers of boys born with sex organ abnormalities, called hypospadias, which now occurs in one in 100–150 male births. It is suggested that this is because of the oestrogenic chemical burden of the produce they eat. I would counsel anyone who is able to, to make that extra investment in avoiding the chemicals when they can.

Some people simply cannot afford organic produce at present as it is generally more expensive than non-organic – about one-third more. But as more people buy organic produce it is slowly coming more into line with the cost of non-organic foods. However, it may never catch up completely as there is inevitably a lower yield per acre when compared to non-organic food. Some supermarkets are beginning to have an equal-pricing policy, and if you shop around some small suppliers have box schemes, and are making an effort to keep prices competitive. It may be a case of paying more for your family's food now, instead of paying with their health later.

If you mainly buy produce which is in season and become more creative with cooking methods using some of the cheaper produce, most budgets can usually cope. For instance, there are many ways of preparing cabbage, potatoes, carrots, rice and beans. All are inexpensive ingredients and with not too much imagination they can be made into feasts. Cabbage, for instance, high in cancer-fighting compounds, can be made into coleslaw, sauerkraut, Polish cabbage soup or French cabbage soup (*garbure*). And then there are cabbage rolls stuffed with rice, onion, chopped nuts, etc., cabbage and potato fritters, red cabbage, stir-fried cabbage, and more . . . If you are planning to cut back on meat, this alone ensures that a major chunk of the food budget is freed for other less expensive ingredients.

People have differing degrees of anxiety about non-organic produce. Generally, my family eat organic produce at home, and drink distilled water, to keep our exposure to pollutants to a minimum. We also buy cleaning products in the same vein, and keep sprays and cleaning fluids to a minimum. However, if we go out we are certainly not going to take our food with us or refuse what we are offered because it may not be organic.

Phytofacts

You have to marvel when you consider how the human body has adapted to use all the factors in our food to maximum effect. We have known for a while about various vitamins, minerals and essential fats, but we are only just coming to appreciate the full range of compounds in our food that can have a profound effect on physiology and health. One group of natural chemicals, or phytonutrients, that are found in foods are plant hormones.

Plant hormones can have a profound influence on the course of breast cancer by their mild oestrogenic effect,[1] and by modulating sex-steroid binding proteins, which reduces the level of damaging oestrogens circulating in the blood,[2] having a moderating effect on tumour growth factors and protecting DNA.[3]

We have talked about oestrogens having a negative effect on breast cancer by encouraging cell growth. The reason why phytoestrogens are protective, and not damaging as are other oestrogens, is probably because they have an antagonistic effect which works against the harmful oestrogens. The natural, strong, oestrogens which we produce, E1 and E2, the harmful environmental xenoestrogens from chemicals and plastics, and the pharmaceutical oestrogens from the contraceptive pill and HRT can all be moderated by plant, or phyto, oestrogens.

It is believed that they have this beneficial effect because they are considerably less potent than the damaging oestrogens – about 1,000 times less active. This means that while they have the same attraction for oestrogen receptor sites on breast cells, they are too weak to trigger significant cell multiplication in the way that other oestrogens do. And when they occupy these oestrogen receptor sites, they also manage to block the damaging oestrogens latching on to these sites, and thereby limit their negative effects.

It is possible that excess consumption of these oestrogens can have a negative effect – as can too much of any food. The discovery that plants could have an oestrogenic effect came about when it was observed in the 1940s that sheep in Western Australia grazing on red clover became infertile. Several species of animals have since been found to be affected in this way by some types of phytoestrogen. But humans have not shown a similar effect on their reproductive capability when eating moderate levels of phytoestrogens, sourced from the foods suggested below. It has been hypothesized that the reason for this is that plants, and the humans who eat them, share a long evolutionary association, and that over many generations sensitive individuals, who may have become sterile by eating too many plant oestrogens, have been selected out of the gene pool.[4] Whether this is true or not, as a species our fertility is not affected when we include sensible amounts of phytoestrogens in our diet.

Some herbs and foods have been used throughout history to reduce fertility, as a contraceptive measure, or to induce abortions. Members of the fennel family, the pomegranate, mistletoe and the wild carrot (Queen Anne's lace) have been used to this effect. The seeds of the wild carrot contain chemicals that block the pregnancy-promoting hormone, progesterone. If you doubt whether plant hormones can have a significant effect when taken in *excessively* high quantities, think for a minute of men who are prone to drinking an excess of oestrogen-rich beer – it is not uncommon to see these men sporting well-developed breasts, a condition known as gynaecomastia. The hops that are used to make the beer are so potent a source of oestrogens that in the days before mechanized cultivation, it was known that female hop pickers' menstrual cycles would be affected.

However, there is probably an optimal intake for maximum protection without downsides. If you look at the diet in Eastern cultures, the intake of phytoestrogens is around 50–100 mg daily. This range seems to confer a protective effect against breast and prostate cancers, but does not interfere in a negative way with other aspects of health which are related to oestrogens, and this has been supported by animal studies.[5] For instance, it does not negatively affect women's menstruation, sexual maturation or the fertility of women or men. Quite the opposite, as phytoestrogens seem to confer a significant degree of relief from menopausal symptoms in women and considerable protection against prostate cancer in men, and encourage slightly longer intervals between menstruation, which is good as this minimizes exposure to the oestrogens E1 and E2. In a review of twenty-six animal studies using soya, one of the richest sources of phytoestrogens, the majority reported protective effects against cancer, while no studies reported soya intake increasing tumour development.[6]

In praise of soya

Soya is one of the most useful dietary sources of beneficial plant oestrogens and more than 1,000 papers have been published on the subject of soya isoflavones. Soya still has, for some people, connotations left over from the 1960s as being a hippy food of the 'knit your own yoghurt' variety. Certainly the soya products of the day were uninspiring enough to make all but the most determined run straight out for a burger and chips, and only oriental food made the best of this versatile bean. But nowadays we have a range of foods made from soya which are tempting to the Western palate.

Soya has been a staple crop, along with rice, in China for around 5,000 years. Around 200 BC they started to make tofu from curdled soya milk, and it was not long before Japanese Buddhist monks took this technique back home with them. The Japanese now consume more tofu than any other group in the world. The popularity of the soya bean spread slowly throughout Asia, but it was only about 200 years ago that this legume was brought to Europe where, it has to be said, the reception was muted. The road to popularity in the West was initiated by Dr John Harvey Kellogg, a member of the breakfast cereal family, who began to market soya milk and soya meat substitutes. The largely vegetarian Seventh Day Adventists were the only group loyally to consume soya in any quantity until we come to the present day, where its popularity is spurred on by the many scientific analyses that are unearthing strong protective health benefits against breast cancer, osteoporosis, cardiovascular disease and menopausal discomfort.

The soya bean is also one of the best plant sources of protein, with almost all the essential amino acids, except methionine. Soya protein also comes saturated fat-free, and with a fabulous range of phytonutrients. The missing methionine is easily made up by combining the soya bean with grain products – we do this almost without thinking when we have soya milk with cereal, soya mince with spaghetti, tofu stir-fried with rice or a soyburger on a bun. Having said this, it is possible that the missing methionine may be a benefit when dealing with cancer. Rats fed a soya diet alone developed significantly fewer tumours, when exposed to carcinogens, than did those on a soya diet with added methionine.[7]

Soya also exerts a protective effect against many other cancers apart from breast cancer, including colon, liver and lung cancers. There are several mechanisms by which this may work including phytic acid and β-sitosterol, and one that has attracted much interest is the protease inhibitor that soya contains called the Bowman-Birk inhibitor (BBI) which has been shown to prevent cancer induction in animals by between 48 and 100 per cent, depending on the type of cancer.[8] Many other foods also contain protease inhibitors, mainly in the bean, seed and nut families.

It may be wise to vary your intake of soya with other sources of phytoestrogens, because some people develop allergies to soya. In order to avoid this you may want to have a couple of soya-free days a week and not to exceed one or two portions a day. It is also probably a good idea to introduce soya into the diet slowly and build up over a couple of months to allow yourself to acclimatize to it. The Japanese eat soya from childhood and their systems are used to a high level by adulthood. There are also many concerns these days about the effects of genetic engineering on foods, and soya is one of the main targets for this manipulation. It is not known what the long-term effect of this alteration in our food may be, and it is probably prudent to buy products which guarantee that the soya is not modified genetically – these are readily available from health food shops, and any soya product which is produced organically will not be genetically modified.

Phytoestrogens
The phytonutrients in plants consist of hundreds of different naturally occurring substances. These chemicals have been made not for our benefit, but for that of the plant – for their own survival. They may act as hormones, growth regulators, enzymes, pigments, or provide colour, taste and odour. They help to protect the plant against oxidation damage from free radicals, parasites, bacteria, viruses, insects and

injury. The good news is that we have adapted so that these benefits are transferred to us when we eat plant foods.

There are so many tongue-twisting names attached to phytonutrients and phytohormones that it can get quite confusing when reading books or papers on this subject. One major group of phytoestrogens are the isoflavones. There are four main groups of the phytoestrogen isoflavones: those that are present in soya are genistein and daidzein; the other two main groups are called biochanin and formononetin and are found principally in chick-peas, lentils, mung beans and peas. Some of the other phytoestrogens are lignans, coumestrol, equol, glycoside and glycitein. For the purpose of simplicity, I have stuck throughout the book to using the overall term 'phytoestrogens'.

And powerful things they are too: a recent review concluded that 'Phytoestrogens can inhibit carcinogenesis, act as agonists and antagonists of estrogens, inhibit protein tyrosine kinase, inhibit angiogenesis and induce apoptosis.'[9] In other words, they interfere with the development of breast cancer at many different stages.[10] It is recognized that they might even have a similar therapeutic effect to currently used medication – a paper in the *British Journal of Nutrition* commented, 'Like the "anti-oestrogen" Tamoxifen, [phytoestrogen isoflavones] seem to have oestrogenic effects in human subjects in the cardiovascular system and bone.'[11] Phytoestrogens are found in at least 300 different foods, including soya beans, chick-peas lentils, mung beans, aduki beans, nuts, seeds and vegetables.

Linseeds (flax seeds)

Other potent phytoestrogens are the lignans, found in linseeds (also called flax seeds) which have the effect of modulating body oestrogens and seem to exert a protective effect specifically against breast cancer,[12] to inhibit the promotion of breast cancer[13] and to inhibit the production of the enzyme aromatase which increases oestrogen levels.[14] Phytoestrogens from linseeds are acted on by the intestinal micro-flora bacteria to produce active phytoestrogens which are up to 100–800 times more plentiful than those derived from other foods.

The way forward

Some people take readily to using soya and find that eating more oriental dishes, and replacing milk with soya milk, is fine. For others, however, it must be said that when faced with a block of tasteless tofu, they just run out of ideas. It helps to be creative and sneak it into Western-style dishes by the back door. For instance, mashing tofu into casseroles, or puréeing it with vegetables is an easy way to slip in a couple of ounces here and there. The dried beans cook in just the same way as other beans such as flageolet or pinto beans. Using soya milk as a substitute for cow's milk in cooked dishes and for sauces is straightforward – it makes the creamiest porridge imaginable. An excellent, filling breakfast is to use tofu in a morning 'milk' shake, along with fruit, to get your daily dose of phytonutrients (see **Your Basic Nutrition and Supplement Plan** (page 197) for other ideas).

Breakfast-in-a-glass

100 g/4 oz silken tofu (if silken is not available use ordinary tofu)

soya milk to liquefy (adjust depending on how liquid you want the mixture to be)

1 banana

other ripe, soft fruit such as peach, strawberries, kiwi, pear, melon (the fruit needs to be sweet and with a good flavour)

1 tablespoon flax seeds (for lignans and gentle fibre)

2 teaspoons flax oil (optional – useful for Omega-3 fats)

1 teaspoon lecithin (optional – emulsifies the flax oil and helps to metabolize other fats)

Put the ingredients into a blender and whizz until smooth. You can also put the mixture into a small container and leave in the freezer for 1½ hours, to make a delicious frozen dessert. The sweetness depends on the fruit you use; if making the frozen version you can add some raisins or other dried fruit.

I also throw in any morning supplements which come in powdered form, such as vitamin C and acidophilus.

Dr Jeffrey Bland, a pioneer in the field of functional medicine, believes that one day the recommendation to eat 30–40 mg of isoflavones may well be a part of public health programmes. To achieve the protective level of around 50 mg of phytoestrogens a day, which is the lower end of the scale for consumption in the Far East, eat a portion of soya products five days a week, a couple of tablespoons of linseeds daily, and then for maximum protective effect eat from a wide variety of foods which provide all four oestrogenic isoflavones. A varied, plant-based diet will ensure that significant amounts of these breast-cancer fighting chemicals are consumed.

Soya foods which are rich in phytoestrogens include:

		Total isoflavone content
Soya flakes	½ cup*	130 mg
Soya flour	½ cup	85 mg
TVP (soya mince)	½ cup	70 mg
Soya beans, cooked	½ cup	35 mg
Soya beans, sprouted	½ cup	35 mg
Tempeh	½ cup	30 mg
Tofu (full-fat)	100 g/4 oz	30 mg
Tofu (low-fat)	100 g/4 oz	20 mg
Soy yoghurt	100 g/4 oz	15 mg
Soya milk (full-fat)	1 cup	10 mg
Soya milk (low-fat)	1 cup	5 mg
Miso	1 tablespoon	5 mg
Soya cheese	100 g/4 oz	3 mg[15]

The packaging of soya-based bars, supplements and protein powders should state the quantity of isoflavones/phytoestrogens contained in the product.

* ½ cup and 1 cup measurements as per measuring cups available from hardware and kitchen equipment shops.

Foods which have useful amounts of phytoestrogens include:
(insufficient research is available to establish the exact isoflavone content)

Alfalfa sprouts	Flax seeds	Peas
Almonds	Lentils	Pinto beans
Apples	Lima beans	Rye
Barley	Millet	Seaweed
Basmati rice	Mung beans	Sesame seeds
Buckwheat	Mushrooms	Sunflower seeds
Chick-peas	Oats	Wholewheat
Corn	Peanuts	

Herbs

Herbs which have oestrogenic and progestogenic effects are available in supplement form, and have been found by many women to relieve the symptoms of the menopause or to regulate their menstrual cycle.[16] Supplements usually come with a mixture of two or more herbs as they seem to be more effective and synergistic in combination. From the point of view of breast cancer there is no real evidence to support the use of these herbs to reduce risk, and it is always possible that they could have a negative effect as herbal phytoestrogens can be far more potent than food sources of phytoestrogens. Many women do find them extremely useful for regulating their hormonal problems and it is really an individual choice as to whether to take these herbs or not. If you have, or have had, breast cancer it is probably best to consult a qualified medical or Chinese herbalist before including herbal supplements with a hormonal effect in your regime (see **Resources** section). Herbal supplements of any type should not be taken while planning a pregnancy, while pregnant or breast-feeding. Herbs should also not be taken while on any prescribed medication because they can be so effective that they can have a compounding effect on many medicines. Consult a herbalist if you are uncertain.

Herbs which have an oestrogenic effect:

Alfalfa	Licorice	Turmeric
Black cohosh	Red clover	Verbena
Dong quai	Sarsaparilla	
Korean Gingseng	Thyme	

Herbs which have a progestogenic effect:

Damiana	Red clover	Verbena
Licorice	Thyme	
Oregano	Turmeric	

A Little of What You Fancy?

The old adage 'A little of what you fancy does you good' is probably true – otherwise life could become very boring. The problem arises when we indulge in 'a *lot* of what we fancy'. The occasional treat or pick-me-up is not going to lead to breast cancer or, for that matter, limit recovery – and feeling deprived is no fun for anyone.

The picture is completely different if we have a 'habit', be it sugar, caffeine, cigarettes, alcohol or any other stimulants. And it may not be that any one of these in its own right is the problem, it could be a cumulative effect – overloading the system again. A couple of coffees a day, a couple of cigarettes, some sugar in your three teas, a chocolate bar, two or three biscuits and a couple of glasses of wine may not seem over the top for many people, but the cumulative effect is that twelve or more times a day you have taken a 'hit'. Eighty-four times a week. Four thousand, three hundred and eighty times a year. And that is being fairly moderate by most people's standards. Sugar is discussed in the chapter **Keep It Complex** (page 72) but what are the pros and cons of the other stimulants?

Alcohol

Alcohol has had a lot of good press recently as it has been established that a couple of measures a day reduce the risk of cardiovascular disease. Most of the research has been done on men and so it is widely assumed that alcohol also protects women from cardiovascular disease. For women, however, one measure per day has been suggested because of their lower body weight, smaller livers and consequent higher risk of toxicity. In promoting this health benefit, the point is also made that whilst a little is good, a lot is not better. Large quantities of alcohol have many adverse health implications. The reason for the protective effect on the cardiovascular system is not clear. In the case of red wine, it seems reasonable that it is the antioxidants inherent in the red grape that offer protection. However, other alcohol sources, beer, gin, vodka and so on, seem to have a similarly protective effect against heart disease in moderate quantities.

But the effect of alcohol on breast cancer is not a positive one. There is a correlation between alcohol and breast cancer which seems to be straightforward – it boosts the effects of oestrogens. When compared to men, women seem to have reduced amounts of, or lack, the enzyme alcohol dehydrogenase, which may go further to explain some of the negative effects. Alcohol may also increase breast cancer by affecting the permeability of cell membranes in the breast, boosting the liver's production of carcinogens by alcohol-induced enzymes, inhibiting DNA repair or triggering the P450 liver enzymes which process oestradiol (E2) to even more active forms. A review of thirty-eight different studies concluded that the relationship becomes significant when just one unit of alcohol a day is consumed[1] (this was a well conducted meta-analysis and all the necessary 'adjustments' for other risk factors for breast cancer were made). Just one unit a day increases risk by 11 per cent, and two units daily lead to an increased risk of 24 per cent, while three units daily increase risk by 38 per cent. One unit of alcohol a day does not represent a huge increase in risk, but the graph escalates dramatically after that. It is also worth remembering that when we pour drinks out at home, we rarely measure them in the same way that they are measured in a bar. One 'home measure' quite often represents a double in a bar. So you may just drink one alcoholic drink a day at home, but the measure is equal to two drinks – beware!

One unit of alcohol = One small glass of wine (125 ml)
One measure of spirits (25 ml)
Half a pint of beer

It does not appear that red wine, for all its antioxidant properties, is protective against breast cancer, yet it is protective against heart disease. You can, however, get the same antioxidant protection from drinking red grape juice, which is not alcoholic and is therefore risk-free (red grape juice is very sugary and needs to be diluted, and it is best to find an organic supplier as grapes are sprayed liberally with pesticides). All alcohol is extremely dehydrating to the body, as anyone who has woken up the morning after the night before will know. It is wise to drink at least an equal quantity of water alongside your alcohol.

If you are having chemotherapy, it really is best to avoid alcohol totally, even though the hospital may advise that it is OK in moderation (except for some specific regimes). However, during chemotherapy your liver has an enormous amount of work to do detoxifying chemicals, and any amount of alcohol will simply give it more work.

Salt

It has been suggested that a high-salt diet changes the dynamics of all cell membranes and makes the passage of oxygen and nutrients more difficult across the membrane barrier. The environment then becomes ideal for cancer growth.[2]

Our bodies need salt and our cells are mini-seas of saline solution – the human body has been described as 'a hairy bag of salty soup' by Professor Michael Crawford, author of the eye-opening and highly readable *Nutrition and Evolution*. Because of this we have a taste for salt, and even have taste-buds specifically to sense this mineral. However, we do not need huge amounts of salt, or sodium chloride – around 6 g a day is the absolute maximum for healthy people.

Potassium is another mineral that we need, and as its chemical structure is similar to sodium, some of the 'low-salt' substitutes are made from potassium chloride instead of sodium chloride. Our ancestors enjoyed a diet that gave them a much higher quantity of potassium than we have today. Potassium is found in fruits and vegetables which our hunter-gatherer forbears ate in much larger quantities than we do. Because sodium was more scarce than potassium, our kidneys evolved so that they retained as much sodium as possible, and the plentiful potassium was excreted. Now that our diets have changed, the ratio of sodium to potassium has been vastly altered in favour of sodium. This causes water retention problems for many people, as our bodies hang on to the sodium and then accumulate water in order to keep it in solution in our bodies. It is common currency that a high-salt diet is a major contributory factor to high blood pressure, which in turn is one of the strongest risk factors for heart disease, but it may also be wise to view salt with suspicion in relation to cancer.

Government recommendations are that adults consume a

maximum of 6 g of salt a day (two teaspoons), but our average intake is 9 g a day (three teaspoons). Most – 80 per cent – of this is consumed from packaged foods rather than from the salt shaker. Salt is added to manufactured foods because it is addictive and sells more products. Despite the fact that high salt levels have been recognized as dangerous for many years, most manufacturers in this country do nothing to reduce levels, as they have done in other countries for branded products that are still sold in a heavily salted form in the UK.

Salt does not have to be itemized in the list of contents for packaged products, and if it is mentioned at all, it is expressed as sodium on the nutrition panels, rather than sodium chloride, which is the chemical name for salt. To work out the amount of salt in a packaged food, you need to obtain the sodium figure and then multiply it by 2.5. So a sodium content of 1.2 g per serving will be equivalent to 3 g of salt – or one teaspoon, and that is if sodium is mentioned on the package at all. Salt turns up in the strangest places, including sweet-tasting products as a flavour booster – for instance, most brands of cornflakes contain twice as much salt, weight for weight, as most brands of potato crisps. If you are consciously avoiding salt, you might easily avoid the crisps but eat the cornflakes. You can, of course, find low- or no-salt brands, but you usually need to look for them in a health food shop rather than the supermarket.

We do not need to have any added salt in our diet, and this is particularly so when taking the offensive against cancer. Sodium is found in all fruits and vegetables, and in an organic form which our bodies can handle and use effectively, and of course is twinned with the vital potassium which works alongside it.

Coffee

The research on coffee and breast cancer is inconclusive, though there is a possibility that coffee affects cancer in general as it is such a concentrated source of caffeine. Research at the Brigham Young University in the USA found that caffeine may inhibit the apoptosis mechanism which is responsible for cell death – and a cell that does not die is a cancerous cell.

Coffee has a potent effect on the body not only because it contains a large amount of caffeine, but also because it contains the other stimulants theobromine and theophylline. Since caffeine has an impact on breast tissue, especially in fibrocystic disease, one researcher concluded that this 'provides a biological foundation from which to implicate caffeine as a potent modulator of developmental growth of normal, benign and *carcinomatous* breast tissues.'[3]

The three stimulants in coffee act on the central nervous system and overstimulate the adrenal glands, leading to blood sugar swings. In addition they are dehydrating and have to be detoxified via the liver.

Coffee also decreases absorption of nutrients from food by up to 20 per cent, which means that a coffee to round off a meal is not a good idea. Many people find that when they stop drinking coffee, many health issues resolve themselves; for example, headaches, migraines, ulcers, insomnia and skin problems. A high level of consumption has been linked to breast pain. Coffee tends to be a concentrated source of pesticides as it is grown in developing countries where there are more lax regulations regarding organophosphates. The process of giving up coffee will frequently entail a withdrawal period, during which complaints are exacerbated, especially headaches. This is the result of the liver releasing stored toxins, and may also be caused by blood sugar lows as the coffee is no longer triggering adrenaline. The withdrawal symptoms are a clear indication of how the stimulants in coffee are potent and addictive drugs.

For people who are undergoing chemotherapy, coffee is probably not helpful. Chemotherapy is processed and eliminated via the liver, and if that organ is working on coffee, processing and storing its toxic residues, it has less capacity for dealing with the chemotherapy. The same obviously goes for alcohol.

Surprisingly, in some disciplines coffee is used to help the liver detoxify. This works from the other end, in the form of coffee enemas. The thinking behind this is that the coffee enema travels straight to the liver via the portal vein, causing it to speed up the dumping of its load of stored toxins. Some people find this procedure effective and useful, while many – perhaps most – would not dream of having a coffee enema. Either way, it brings new meaning to 'I'm just going for my coffee break', as disciples of regimes such as the Gerson therapy joke.

Tea

By tea I mean black teas, of which there are many varieties. Though tea, like coffee, is high in caffeine, we tend not to make tea as strong as we do coffee, and therefore do not take in as much cup for cup – about 50 per cent less. However, tea has protective benefits with cancer in general, as it is a good source of the antioxidant polyphenols. Caffeine-free tea, preferably naturally decaffeinated, may be a better choice as it still has the antioxidants but not the stimulants. There are many other teas that have high antioxidant quotients, in particular Japanese green tea which has been shown to be highly protective against cancer and contains half as much caffeine as black tea. The red-coloured teas include Rooibos, or South African Red Bush tea, and rosehip tea, which are also rich in antioxidants. Herbal teas can have a number of therapeutic benefits and are discussed in the chapter **Wet Your Whistle** (page 130).

Soda drinks

Any number of carbonated soft drinks are on offer these days. All of them will contain either sugar or artificial sweeteners, most will contain artificial colouring or flavouring agents. Carbon dioxide is toxic to the body and needs to be disarmed, sugar is a pro-oxidant, artificial sweeteners are linked to various types of cancer (though not breast cancer in particular), artificial colourings and flavourings similarly tax the body's elimination channels. In satisfying thirst with a soft drink of this type you will miss the opportunity to drink something which promotes health. Whilst there is no research to show that soda drinks are involved in breast cancer, they are probably best avoided. It is quite easy to substitute fresh fruit juices, diluted with sparkling water if you like the fizz, or to drink mixed vegetable or tomato juices.

Chocolate

True chocolate fans will not wish to be told that their favourite treat is not a good thing! Every time some positive news about any health-giving properties in chocolate is announced, many chocoholics will celebrate with – yes, chocolate. Chocolate is not all bad. It does contain useful amounts of magnesium and phenolic antioxidants. However, the bad news about chocolate is that it is high in caffeine, though in moderation this won't do too much harm as long as you are not compounding it with other caffeine sources such as coffee, tea and colas. In the UK most chocolate consumed is milk chocolate, which is low in chocolate solids and extremely high in sugar (around nine teaspoons in a typical 50 g/2 oz bar). A small amount of good-quality, organic, dark chocolate as a treat is probably OK, and may even be a good thing, but large quantities of sugary, pesticide-loaded milk chocolate means more work for your body to deal with, stabilizing blood-sugar levels and disposing of toxic residues.

The way forward

Anything to which you are 'addicted' involves a release of adrenaline, which in turn raises blood-sugar levels. This is probably why we feel better almost immediately after indulging in our particular fancy. However, adrenaline is an emergency hormone which takes priority over other body functions and has a dramatic effect on them, either stimulating (blood sugar and heart rate) or slowing down/constricting (digestion and abdominal and cutaneous blood vessels). The adrenaline process is also an expensive one, using up nutrients such as vitamin C, magnesium and B vitamins, to the detriment of other body functions which need these nutrients. Because of this, and because many stimulants have a direct effect on breast cancer – in particular tobacco, alcohol and sugar – it is best to limit them overall. Keep them for the occasional treat – if they are used as props to get you through the day, it may be wise to question why they are needed and whether you can find better alternatives.

My suggestions would be:

Alcohol	Keep to a minimum – not more than two or three measures of red wine a week if pre-menopausal, or if post-menopausal and using HRT. If post-menopausal and *not* using HRT, when there is less oestrogen for the alcohol to boost, one measure a day may be of benefit, because of the cardiovascular protective element. Avoid alcohol

totally if undergoing chemotherapy or actively fighting breast cancer.

Salt — Avoid adding salt to food, and minimize packaged foods in order to eliminate as much salt as possible from your diet. Use a range of strong-tasting herbs, fresh or dried, as well as ground seaweed, to add flavour to dishes. Soy sauce and miso are very salty, but as they have such strong flavours, if used very sparingly and salt is avoided at other times, they should be OK.

Coffee — Best to avoid – one or two cups a week maximum as a treat.

Tea — Three or four cups a day, preferably decaffeinated, are probably beneficial. It may be a good idea to find other teas which you find acceptable, such as green or red teas, to keep the caffeine levels down.

Sodas — Best to avoid, especially if laden with chemicals and sweeteners. Read the ingredient lists of those that call themselves 'natural'.

Sugar — Be very moderate – best to use natural sources of sweetness such as fruit spreads and moderate amounts of dried fruit. Use small amounts of fructose instead of sugar if you absolutely have to, but do not use artificial sweeteners, which are all chemicals your body has to get rid of.

Chocolate — Good-quality, organic chocolate as a treat a couple of times a week will probably lift your spirits, and as it is strong-tasting can go a long way if you use it to coat fruit, or grate and sprinkle on dessert dishes.

Wet Your Whistle

Anyone interested in investigating the links between diet and cancer will very quickly have a number of types of drink suggested to them – water, vegetable and fruit juices, assorted teas and what can only be termed as 'special brews'. Let's look at the merits of these different types of drink.

Water

Water is the second most essential nutrient we need. We can only last for around three minutes without air – the most vital nutrient – and we can only live a few days without any water at all. Yet many people do not give water intake, or quality, much thought.

We eliminate, on average, around 1½ litres/2½ pints of water a day through our urine, sweat and on our breath – more in the summer. A significant amount of the water we consume comes from food, and the more watery the food, for instance fruit, the more we take in. But we cannot survive just on water from food and we need to drink liquids as well. Whenever I ask the question of people, 'How much water do you drink?' I am inevitably told 'Not enough' – they know that they would benefit from drinking water, but they still do not do it. Only one in five people drinks the recommended five to seven glasses of pure water a day.

Our bodies are about 70 per cent water, which, apart from hydrating our cells, acting as a solvent and allowing our enzymes to function, is also needed to help to carry toxins out of the body. When people complain that they are having to go to the bathroom more frequently because they are drinking more water, I suggest that instead of being annoyed, they should be pleased that their system is being 'flushed through' more frequently.

The water contained in black teas and coffee does not count towards total water intake, because caffeine has a dehydrating effect, causing the kidneys to excrete more water than has been drunk. And alcohol is even more dehydrating.

Water is a fundamental ingredient for all body processes, so any adult's health regime will benefit from keeping up a water intake of around 1½–2 litres/2½–3 pints a day (unless you have damaged kidneys, in which case you must consult your doctor). This becomes doubly important if you have had any sort of chemotherapy, because you will need to eliminate the chemotherapeutic by-products from the liver, and water will help with this process.

Quality of water is important as well. From the point of view of breast cancer the most recent question to emerge is the issue of chemicals in our water that have an oestrogenic effect (see **A sea of chemicals** (page 106)). It is early days, from a research point of view, but many warning signs are there, and anyone concerned with the risk of breast cancer should really take some early decisions about water quality.

There is an array of water treatment options available and the advantages of one over another is not immediately apparent as they all make extravagant claims. It must be borne in mind that most tests for water systems involve *adding* impurities to the water before removing them – which is not the same as filtering the small, but questionable, impurities that are in tap water.

Filter jugs are the most popular type of home water treatment, and certainly can make water lose the chlorine taste. They need to be cleaned out regularly as bacteria can build up in filters. There are some impurities that are less easily filtered out, including aluminium, lead, cadmium, iron, arsenic and nitrates. The finer the 'sieve', the more impurities will be screened out, and carbon filters come in differing grades – to keep them functioning the least that must be done is to replace the filter regularly. Reverse osmosis systems can be viewed as a more efficient form of filtration, though they still do not handle nitrates well and have many of the same problems as filters.

Distillation is the only method that will leave the majority of impurities behind, and works on the same principle as Mother Nature when water evaporates from the earth and turns into rainwater. Some impurities have the same boiling point as water and will remain in boiled water; however, most of these can then be removed by the filtration cartridge. The perceived disadvantage of distillation is that it also removes nutrient minerals from the water, such as calcium, magnesium and phosphorus, or may even leach nutrients out of the body. However, this is not substantiated and if you are eating a nutrient-rich diet should not be an issue. It is also possible that distilled water encourages the body to release excess toxins stored in the body more effectively than non-distilled water. Water treatment suppliers are listed in the **Resources** section.

Finally, bottled water is a popular choice. There is no information available about the levels of oestrogenic chemicals in bottled waters and their quality varies dramatically. Generally speaking, it may be best to buy 'mineral' instead of 'spring' water, as the former is governed by strict controls, whereas the regulations are more lax for spring water. It is also probably a good idea to buy water in glass rather than plastic bottles.

Juices

A glass of juice counts towards your daily minimum of five portions of fruit and vegetables, but there are many types of shop-bought fruit and vegetable juices, and some are better than others.

There are four main types of juice in supermarket chilling cabinets: freshly squeezed; from concentrate; not from concentrate; and fruit drinks. Freshly squeezed juice is the best option as it contains no added water or other ingredients and has a short shelf-life. 'From concentrate' means reconstituted from dried juice, and very high drying temperatures ensure that there is little life left in the juice. 'Not from concentrate' is pure juice that has been pasteurized and so will have more flavour than 'from concentrate', but questionable nutritional value. The last category, fruit drinks, can mean almost anything and the major ingredient by weight, after water, is usually sugar. If the label says '100 per cent pure' this is also advertising double-speak as four out of five of these juices are made from concentrate.

Vegetable juices are an excellent standby for the 'cocktail hour' if you want to avoid alcohol, but as they are quite often salty, it is a good idea to become familiar with the salt content of different brands so that you can make better choices.

The very best juices are freshly made with a juice extractor, rather than shop-bought. These juices have a strong following among the natural health movement in stacking the odds against cancer. Fresh juices are a concentrated source of bioactive plant compounds such as antioxidants and enzymes, and while good-quality shop-bought juices are a better alternative than additive-loaded squashes and sodas, they still do not have the same properties as freshly made juices. A good visual example of this is shop-bought carrot juice, which is brownish in colour when compared to the fresh option – this is because it has already oxidized, meaning that the full potency of the beta-carotene it carries is unavailable. It is ideal to drink fresh juices immediately when you make them, to get all the benefits.

Juices are easy on the digestion and the nutrients they contain are absorbed very quickly. The enzymes in fresh juices effectively eliminate the body's need to produce its own digestive enzymes. There are many therapeutic uses for juices, which can have potent healing properties, probably because they are a concentrated source of bio-active compounds. You can drink more than you can eat – a juice may contain three carrots, a head of broccoli and a couple of apples – meaning that you get all that goodness concentrated in a glass. As the ingredients are raw, the nutrient levels have not been compromised – and it all tastes good as well. If you are unsure about the benefits of juicing I strongly suggest that you try a home-made juice (see page 206) daily for two weeks to experience the wonderful energy boost that this brings – it is really very noticeable.

Since juices are so easy to digest, they can be a very useful supplement for people who feel unwell, possibly during chemotherapy, and can be helpful for recovery. They are not a substitute for food, however, as they do not contain sufficient calories or protein.

As all the fibre has been removed in the juicing process, the remaining fruit sugar and root vegetable sugar have an overall effect on blood-sugar levels. Whilst this is nowhere near as dramatic as the blood-sugar effect of, say, a chocolate bar, it is best to sip the juice slowly and, ideally, to dilute it half-and-half with water.

Teas and other brews

There are numerous types of tea that have various properties in relation to cancer.

These are the most popular:

Black tea	Cup for cup, tea contains about half the amount of caffeine as coffee. It is a good source of antioxidant polyphenols (though about half the amount found in green tea) which have been shown to be protective against cancers. There are many varieties: Assam, Darjeeling, Ceylon, Lapsang Souchong, and more. Earl Grey contains bergamot which can help with intestinal problems. There are several brands of organic tea available.
Green tea	Made from the unfermented leaves from which black tea is also made. Green tea contains about half the caffeine of black tea. It is the king of teas in cancer prevention, with the highest levels of polyphenols. Studies detail its efficacy in cancer prevention at levels of ten cups a day.
Rooibos	This tea is drunk by the bushmen in the Cape area of South Africa. It is caffeine-free, low-tannin, and contains high levels of antioxidants, as well as vitamin C and minerals. Also called South African Red Bush.
Camomile	Caffeine-free. No therapeutic properties that relate to cancer, but soothing and calming. It is a diuretic if used in large quantities (i.e. ten cups a day), which may make it useful in the case of water retention as a result of hormone therapy.
Peppermint	Caffeine-free. No therapeutic properties that relate to cancer, but good digestive properties and can help settle the stomach after chemotherapy. Fresh leaves can be steeped in boiling water.
Ginger	Caffeine-free. No therapeutic properties that relate to cancer, but excellent anti-sickness properties

which are very useful during chemotherapy. Fresh
ginger root can be grated and steeped in boiling
water. Add a little honey for taste if needed.

Essiac: This herbal infusion is a combination of four herbs in specific combinations and was developed by a Canadian nurse called Renée Caisse (Essiac is Caisse spelt backwards). She claimed that the formula had been given to her in 1922 by a patient whose breast cancer had been cured by a native American Ojibwa healer in Toronto. It has been widely used throughout North America for several decades, but has to be obtained under a special licence as both US and Canadian law prohibits the marketing of compounds that claim 'curative' properties against cancer. The original Essiac formula consists of burdock root, Indian rhubarb, sheep sorrel and inner bark of slippery elm. A later formulation, called Flor-Essence, has added four more ingredients: watercress, blessed thistle, red clover and kelp. Essiac is compatible with conventional cancer therapies, and the Canadian Breast Cancer Research Initiative, started in 1993, has, in 1998, published its preliminary survey of Essiac and concluded that there is enough evidence of beneficial effects to warrant further, properly conducted, full-scale clinical evaluation.[1] Toxicity in animal studies has been reported at extremely concentrated levels of use.

Cat's Claw: Also called Una de Gato or *Uncaria tomentosa*, Cat's Claw has emerged from the tropical rainforest of Peru and is available as supplements as well as a tea, though it is most often drunk as a tea and is even available as tea bags. In research Cat's Claw has been shown to have anti-mutagenic properties, as well as inhibiting cell proliferation and inducing cell death (apoptosis)[2] – all of which bode well in the fight against cancer. It is reported to have antioxidant, anti-viral, anti-tumour and anti-inflammatory properties as well as cardiovascular protective properties. It may also be beneficial in balancing irregularities of the female system. Cat's Claw is not advised during pregnancy or lactation, however. So popular are Essiac and Cat's Claw that they are also now available as a mixture in one product (see **Resources**).

Kombucha: Also called Manchurian tea, Mo-Gu, *Fungus japonicus* and Tea Kvass, and referred to as a mushroom tea, it is more accurately a mixture of a yeast and bacteria, and is frankly an acquired taste. Brewed from a live culture in a base of tea and sugar, it is a fermented drink and Kombucha has been popularly touted as a potent anti-cancer, immune-supporting brew. It is also claimed to reduce inflammation, enhance energy and improve digestion and metabolism and to be effective against *Candida albicans* and *Helicobacter pylori*. Its main active ingredient is probably glucuronic acid, which is a major detoxifier made by the human liver, but it may also contain an antibiotic which is effective against resistant strains of bacteria. The pH (acidity) is around 3.0, which may account for some of its antibacterial properties. There has been a degree of concern about the use of Kombucha tea which stems from the fact that two women in Iowa, USA suffered severe acidosis after drinking the tea, and one later died. They had probably drunk from the same batch, and it is assumed that their drink was in some way contaminated. As Kombucha tea is brewed with black tea and sugar this is an invitation for most micro-organisms to flourish, and it could be this that makes it a questionable drink. While many people swear by its efficacy, and many fermented products such as miso and yoghurt confer impressive health benefits, the drink has an alcohol content of around 0.5 per cent and significant amounts of caffeine and sugar which may be undesirable. If you decide to try Kombucha, make sure you use completely sterile equipment, follow the instructions closely and that the cloth that covers the brewing jar is kept scrupulously clean.

Anti-Breast Cancer Superfoods

It is too easy for nutritionists to find themselves saying 'Don't eat this and don't do that.' It is therefore a pleasure to talk about foods which have been shown to lower risk of breast cancer, with no reservations. Even if you did not cut back on any other foods, but included the following in your diet on a regular basis, you would be doing a lot to reduce your risk of developing the disease, as many of these foods have been shown to have chemopreventive properties.[1]

By including some of these foods you are likely to cut back on some of the less positive aspects of your diet, simply because you do not have room for them, and this, in itself, is beneficial. Moreover, if you eat foods which have a profound anti-breast cancer effect, not only do you have less room for fattier and more sugary foods, and not only do they deliver vitamins, minerals and fibre, but they also give you a range of cancer-fighting nutrients: flavonoids, quercetin, kaempferol, allium compounds, dithiolthiones, isothiocyanates, terpenoids, isoflavones, protease inhibitors, phytic acid, polyphenols, glucosinolates, indoles, plant sterols, saponins and coumarins, to name a few. These nutrients and the foods which contain them are now the subject of cutting-edge research.

Alfalfa
This is one of the most studied plants, containing important substances which include saponins, sterols, flavonoids, coumarins and alkaloids as well as vitamins and minerals. It is protein-rich (around 25 per cent by weight) and is one of the most nutritious foods known. Alfalfa can be bought as sprouted seeds, or you can buy seeds and sprout them yourself. As well as containing protective phytoestrogens, alfalfa has a general anti-tumour effect.[2] Protective against radiation damage,[3] it is also rich in fibre which binds to carcinogens.[4]

Almonds

Originally thought to be cancer-preventive because of their relationship to apricot pits which provide laetrile (once thought of as a possible cancer treatment), it is now known that almonds are rich in a number of anti-cancer factors. The protease inhibitors found in many such nuts and legumes were previously thought to be harmful, but it is now considered that protease inhibitors can inhibit tumour growth.[5] Almonds are good sources of phytate, genistein, lignans and benzaldehyde – all cancer foes. Make sure your almonds are fresh (see **Nuts and seeds** on page 143).

Apples

These common fruits have uncommon powers. Chlorogenic and caffeic acids, which are abundant in apples, have anti-cancer properties. Raw, cooked or juiced, or even in the form of unpasteurized cider vinegar or fresh-pressed apple cider – there are many ways to benefit from apples.

Broccoli, cabbage and other brassicas

These familiar vegetables are proving to be the anti-cancer vegetables of the moment, with everyone, including the most staid and conservative of cancer specialists, acknowledging their importance. Broccoli, cauliflower, cabbage, Brussels sprouts, collards, kale, bok choy, kohlrabi, arugula, horseradish, radishes, swede (rutabaga), turnip – all belong to the family called brassica.[6] They contain several potentially anti-carcinogenic, bioactive micronutrients, including dithiolthiones, isothiocyanates, glucosinolates and indole-3-carbinol. Indole-3-carbinol is of particular interest as, in human studies, it encourages oestrogens to be deactivated,[7] while in animal studies it reduces mammary cancers,[8] is associated with hormonal factors that reduce breast cancer risk,[9] and in one study it prevented breast cancer by a massive 65 per cent and was recommended as a 'good candidate for chemoprevention of breast cancer'.[10]

The sulphurophanes found in broccoli, which are responsible for its slightly bitter taste, have in particular been found to improve the performance of the glutathione-S-transferase M1 enzyme,[11] which is produced by the liver and is responsible for some of its major detoxification and antioxidant activities. Levels of this vital enzyme are generally found to be low in women with breast cancer.[12] Broccoli juice, when added to pre-cancerous cells, induced apoptosis (cell suicide) by around 95 per cent.[13]

Cabbage is easiest to digest when lightly cooked or fermented (sauerkraut), and raw it also makes a potent healer for disturbed digestive tracts when juiced (it tastes strong so should be combined with other juices). Too many raw brassica portions may slightly suppress thyroid function, but the cooked vegetables have little such effect, so if you have low thyroid function anyway (not uncommon in women with breast cancer), it may be a good idea not to overdo eating raw vegetables from this family (some will not hurt – it is only excess that causes problems). Equally, do not be tempted to overcook brassicas as excessive heat will destroy a certain amount of the active cancer-fighting compound, indole-3-carbinol.

Another interesting development since broccoli was identified as such an excellent source of chemoprotective sulphoraphanes, has been the discovery that three-day-old sprouted broccoli and cauliflower seeds contain around 10–100 times the quantity of this astounding nutrient as the fully grown vegetables.[14] This means that instead of eating huge quantities of broccoli, you could achieve the same effect with a more modest portion of sprouts. Broccoli and cauliflower sprouting seeds are not yet commercially available, but if you are particularly keen to try them you could buy the seeds from organic seed suppliers and sprout your own.

Burdock root

This is an unfamiliar vegetable to most Westerners, but it is sold in oriental markets as 'gobo'. It has a sweet, rich taste and can be substituted for carrots in many recipes. The compounds it contains include benzaldehyde, phytosterols, glycosides, mokko lactone and arctic acid. These components may help to make burdock root effective in reducing the risk of recurrence of breast cancer. They also reduce sensitivity to radiation-induced cancers which may also make them useful in reducing the effects of radiotherapy. Burdock root is one of the components of Essiac tea (see page 135).[15]

Citrus fruits

Citrus fruits contain coumarins (also found in some vegetables) and D-limonene (specifically found in the oil from the skin of the fruit). Limonene inhibits mammary cancer in both the initiation and pro-motion/progression stages.[16] In animal studies this compound brought advanced mammary cancer to a halt, which is remarkable at this stage. Limonene also enhances liver detoxification enzymes, which helps to remove carcinogens from the body. The flavonoid hesperatin, found in orange juice, has been demonstrated to inhibit breast cancer cells.[17] Naranjenin in grapefruit has a similar, but much weaker, effect. Citrus fruits also contain glutathione, which is a component of the antioxidant enzyme glutathione peroxidase. All citrus fruits – oranges, lemons, grapefruit, limes, tangerines – are great, but make sure they are organic and not waxed if you are going to use the peel. The bitter white pith is a potent source of bioflavonoids which complement the vitamin C found in the fruit and make it even more potent. You can put the pith through a vegetable juicer along with the fleshy part. The zest also makes a delicious tea if you coarsely grate some unwaxed orange or lemon zest into hot water and steep it for a while.

Flax oil

Almost the richest vegetable source of cancer-fighting omega-3 fats (apart from hemp oil, which is not readily available). It is also rich in antioxidants and adversely affects both the initiation and the proliferation stages of breast cancer.[18] It is anti-tumour, anti-viral and anti-mitotic (i.e. slows down cell division). The importance of using fresh, un-rancid flax oil cannot be overstated. This oil is highly bioactive, making it particularly useful for our biochemistry, but also highly susceptible to damage from rancidity. It is vital to buy flax oil in dark, vacuum-sealed, date-stamped bottles; keep them in the freezer or fridge and use them by the best-before date. The oil, which must not be heated, can be used on salads, in shakes, or spread on bread with seasonings. You can also add it to vegetables and baked potatoes which have cooled slightly, instead of a pat of butter.

Garlic

Dracula may not favour garlic, but then neither does cancer. This little vegetable shows remarkable anti-tumour properties and, while it is harmless to normal cells, it is fairly toxic to cancer cells. White blood cells in people who eat garlic were able to kill 139 per cent more tumour cells than were the white blood cells of non-garlic eaters. Garlic is a rich source of selenium[19] and germanium as well as antioxidants, isoflavones and allyl sulfide.[20] The National Cancer Institute in the USA recognizes garlic as a preventive against cancer, and it has been clinically shown to inhibit the growth of breast cancer. One of the mechanisms by which it does this may be because it is rich in sulphur amino acids (as is the legume family) and so limits the metabolism of E1 and E2 oestrogens into carcinogenic catechol oestrogens. Its effectiveness is dose-dependent (i.e. the more you eat the better it works) and is probably most effective if eaten at the same time as exposure to a potential carcinogen. All the allium vegetables such as onions and spring onions, garlic, leeks and chives contain the protective, and smelly, allium compounds, diallyl sulphide and allyl methyl trisulphide.[21] Unfortunately for lovers, raw garlic is much more effective than the cooked vegetable – raw minced garlic is good in salads, or mixed with olive oil and spread on toast, or added at the last minute to fish or vegetable dishes.

Ginger

If this spice is used regularly it has excellent properties in preventing the initiation of breast cancer, even when used in small amounts. Its phytochemicals include antioxidants, gingerol and carotenes, and Japanese scientists have found ginger to be highly effective at blocking mutational changes in DNA. Ginger improves production of gluta-thione-S-transferase, which is one of the key enzymes responsible for detoxifying carcinogens.[22] This tasty root is also extremely useful for reducing nausea induced by chemotherapy. Added to oriental dishes, fish, made into a bracing tea or baked in muffins and cakes, this is a really versatile flavouring. Peel a root and keep it in the freezer to preserve its freshness; it is then ready to be grated into many dishes, or grated and steeped in boiling water to make tea.

Grapes

The traditional gift during illness, but why wait until then to eat grapes? They are rich in antioxidants, trace minerals and ellagic acid, while raisins are also rich in tannins and caffeic acid. Grapes have anti-mutagenic properties and may be particularly good at preventing breast cancers which arise with age. It is wise to buy organic grapes, or to wash ordinary grapes particularly well, as this does tend to be a crop that is sprayed to excess.

Licorice

Not the sweet variety you buy at the candy store, but the spice, which can be added to many dishes. Licorice contains triterpenoids which inhibit oestrogens, slow cell mutation and protect the liver. You can also buy licorice supplements.

Linseeds

Also called flax seeds, these tiny gems have been found in the Egyptian Pyramids and were cultivated by the Babylonians 5,000 years ago. They were prized by these ancient civilizations and are now being scientifically proved to have many health benefits. Depending on type, they contain many times more lignans than do wheat, oats, rye or soya, making them powerful hormone regulators. As well as being rich in this valuable source of fibre, which is beneficial for bowel health and helps to keep oestrogens and toxins moving out of the body, they are also rich in the omega-3 essential fat, alpha-linolenic acid, which is vital for good health. Linseeds have been found to be protective against breast cancer probably by regulating oestrogens,[23] while the oil has been shown to be effective at reducing tumour growth in later stages.[24] They are best bought in the whole form, not 'pre-cracked', and can easily be added to breads, pancakes and muffins as well as sprinkled on cereals, salads, in soups and most other sweet or savoury dishes.

Mushrooms

These delicious vegetables, which we want to eat anyway because of their subtle flavours, turn out to have potent anti-cancer properties as well.[25] Maitake powder, which is rich in beta-glucan, fed to mice in experiments at Kobe Pharmaceutical University in Japan, led to a more than 80 per cent tumour regression rate – not bad when compared to the 45 per cent tumour inhibition rate of the chemotherapy drug Mitomycin C.[26] Extracts of the oriental mushrooms, rei-shi, maitake and shiitake, are proving to work effectively at shrinking, and in some cases eliminating, tumours in animal studies. They are rich in a range of polysaccharides which stimulate the immune system. Shiitake mushrooms boost interferon and interleukin levels. Wild and exotic mushrooms are a true pharmacopeia of anti-cancer compounds: selenium, antioxidants, lignans and adaptogenic compounds. These oriental mushrooms are now available fresh or dried from large supermarkets and can easily be minced and added to soups and other dishes. Other mushrooms to use include puffballs, oyster, straw and tree ear mushrooms – and there are many more.

Nettles

At last a use for those weeds in the garden (as long as you haven't been using weed-killer on them). Stinging nettles made into an infusion are an incredibly rich source of carotenes, chlorophyll, folic acid and selenium. When you pick them, make sure you are wearing protective gloves, and it is best to take young leaves when they are tender in the spring, or to keep the nettles trimmed for a constant supply of new leaves. Just steep the leaves in boiling water for a few minutes before enjoying the tea. You can also make soup or incorporate nettles whenever you might otherwise have greens in a mixed recipe – for instance in Indian bhajis (as recommended by Hugh Fearnley-Whittingstall in his book *A Cook on the Wild Side*).

Nuts and seeds

Fresh, organically grown nuts and seeds are good sources of protease inhibitors, essential fats and antioxidants. The best to choose from are almonds, walnuts, black walnuts, pecans, sunflower, sesame and flax seeds. Care must be taken to buy small packets of very fresh nuts and seeds from suppliers with a high turnover, so that they have not had time to go stale on the shelves, and they should be kept in the fridge. Even better, crack the nuts yourself: rancid nuts, especially roasted ones or those that are sold shelled and broken, can be carcinogenic. Because nuts and seeds are rich sources of omega-6 fats it is best to restrict them to occasional use.

Oily fish

Mackerel, sardines, tuna, salmon, pilchards, anchovies, shark, trout – are all delicious sources of the potent anti-tumour omega-3 fats. Research has shown time and again that we tend to be deficient in the EPA and DHA fats which have been shown to reverse tumour growth in laboratory animals, and which are inversely related to breast cancer incidence in human studies. Three portions a week are recommended.

Olive oil

Rich in antioxidants specific to the olive, this oil is protective against breast cancer. It is best to buy the dark green, richer-tasting cold-pressed extra-virgin oil which is highest in these compounds. Olive oil has the added advantage of not being significantly damaged by cooking, making it safe to use for all dishes.

Orange-/red-/purple-coloured foods

The natural colourings in these foods are potent sources of beta-carotene and proanthocyanidins which are amongst the most power-ful antioxidants known.[27] Beta-carotene, found in orange- and yellow-coloured fruits and vegetables, increases a molecule called MHC II which plays a key role in helping the immune system target and destroy cancer cells. Apricots, cantaloupe melons, carrots, yellow and red peppers, beetroot, squashes, sweet potatoes, red and black berries – a serving of one or two of these fruits and vegetables daily will be highly protective.

Some other notes of interest: beetroot extract has been shown to kill cancer cells in the laboratory. Eating carrots helps tissues to resist radiation damage and carrot broth can help to ease mouth sores caused by chemotherapy. Sweet potatoes are particularly good at reducing the impact of environmental organochlorines, and are also better sources of complex carbohydrates than normal potatoes.

Parsley

This familiar herb, used more often for decoration than for eating, has phytosterols which specifically hinder breast cancer. Parsley is easy to grow, even on a windowsill, and it is a good idea to take every opportunity to include it in dishes. It is high in carotenes, folic acid, chlorophyll, vitamin C and the essential oils terpenes and pinenes. Parsley also contains polyacetylene, which inhibits the carcinogen benzopyrene.

Tabbouli

There aren't many recipes that allow you to have a large amount of parsley at one hit. I like to prepare this in front of the telly, or when talking to friends, because there is a lot of fine chopping to do. It can be made slightly ahead of time for a delicious first course.

a large bunch of parsley, washed, stems removed and leaves
    finely chopped
2 tablespoons bulgar wheat (or use linseeds if you need a
    gluten-free version), soaked for 15 minutes in boiling water,
    drained and patted dry with a clean kitchen cloth
Some, or all, of the following according to taste, washed,
    peeled where appropriate and finely chopped (the finer the
    chopping the better the meld of tastes):
2 large tomatoes, 1/3 cucumber, 1/2 green pepper, 3 spring
    onions, peeled, 1 garlic clove (another option, which is not
    traditional to the recipe, is to add a tablespoon of linseeds to
    the mixture)
olive oil, lemon juice and freshly ground black pepper, to taste

Combine all the ingredients and allow them to marinate for 15 minutes. Scoop up with wholewheat pitta bread, or crisp cos lettuce leaves, for a satisfying light meal.

Pineapple

Rich in a digestive enzyme called bromelain, which can break down up to 1,000 times its own weight of protein, and in protease inhibitors and citric, folic, malic and chlorogenic acids. Bromelain is so potent that workers in canning factories have to wear protective gloves, and this enzyme has been found to help dissolve the glyco-protein shield which tumours throw up around themselves for protection. It has been demonstrated that there is an inhibition of tumour growth with bromelain; with macrophage and phagocytosis (white blood cell) activity being enhanced, neutrophils are stimulated to produce tumour necrosis factor, and anti-metastatic properties exhibited.[28]

Potatoes

As members of the deadly nightshade (belladonna) family, potatoes get bad press for various health problems such as allergies and rheumatoid arthritis. However, all members of this family have a good reputation for effectiveness against cancer. Potato protease inhibitors may be potent against cancer-causing viruses. They are also good sources of chlorogenic acid, a polyphenol that prevents cancer initiation. Potatoes are a valuable source of vitamin C and are best cooked in their skins to preserve the maximum amount of this immune-enhancing nutrient.

Pulses and beans

Dried pulses and beans of all types are excellent for women dealing with breast cancer. Dried beans have cancer-inhibiting enzymes which not only prevent the initiation of breast cancer, but may also help to prevent recurrence. They contain protease inhibitors, lignans, genistein and phytosterols, and stimulate the production of important fatty acids. A daily dose of one cup of cooked pulses and beans is ideal. Some of the choices are: green peas, baked beans, flageolet beans, soya beans, chick-peas (garbanzo), lentils (red, green, brown), split peas, mung beans, kidney beans, fava beans. Lentils have been shown to be capable of reversing cancer and helping to repair DNA.

Rice

Brown rice is the staple in the macrobiotic approach to fighting cancer, and RBS (rice bran saccharide) exhibits anti-tumour properties.[29] There is an inverse relation between rice intake and breast cancer – women who eat the most rice have the lowest incidence. Brown, basmati, wild, short and long – rice has many culinary uses and is a delicious base to cuisines from around the world.[30]

Seaweed

These are real anti-cancer powerhouses,[31] carrying antioxidants, carotenes, selenium, iodine and alginic acid. Alginic acid attaches itself to heavy metals, radioactive isotopes and other chemicals, rendering them harmless and escorting them out of the body. In animal research, a diet with 5 per cent kombu seaweed significantly delayed chemically induced breast cancer, and it could be that the high consumption of seaweed is a major influence on the low rate of breast cancer in Japanese women. Seaweed is one of the richest sources of the all-important mineral iodine which helps to balance thyroid function (often a problem for women with breast cancer). In addition to iodine, seaweeds contain the full range of minerals and trace elements including selenium, calcium, magnesium, potassium and boron. It is also one of our best, and most assimilable, sources of vitamin B12, which is often lacking in women with breast cancer. You can buy powdered kelp or nori flakes which are delicious condiments to add to salads, soups, sauces and other dishes. Seaweeds can be soaked, chopped and added to dishes, toasted and flaked, or nori can be wrapped around sushi or used as an alternative to lettuce leaves, cabbage leaves or vine leaves to wrap parcels of grains, vegetables and spices. Seaweeds to try include: arame, combu, laver bread, nori, dulse, wakame and kelp.

Soya products

Soya has an extraordinary line-up of useful components which puts it into the class of superfood, from many points of view. The isoflavones it contains, genistein and daidzein, are mildly oestrogenic, which is what makes them so useful in the fight against breast cancer. The isoflavones also have an antioxidant effect, as does the phytic acid soya contains. Saponins enhance immune function, have antioxidant properties and help to fight cancer, while protease inhibitors block the activity of cancer-causing enzymes and, in so doing, further help to ward off the disease. The phytosterols that soya gives us have anti-inflammatory properties as well as working against colon and skin cancers. Soya is a source of healthy omega-3 fats, while providing no saturated fat or cholesterol, and it is an almost complete source of protein. Lecithin is another useful component of soya which emulsifies fat, and may help to reduce the incidence of tumours significantly. In test-tubes genistein, one of the main soya phytoestrogens, or isoflavones, has been found to stop the growth of cancer cells, while leaving normal healthy cells to replicate normally. It possibly does this by blocking an enzyme called tyrosine protein kinase which is used by cancer cells during uncontrolled growth and which may also inhibit cell growth by modulating Transforming Growth Factor β1.[32] Another remarkable property of genistein is the ability to inhibit blood vessel formation by malignant tumours[33] – a process called anti-angiogenesis. Blood vessels are created by enlarging tumours to feed themselves and carry away their waste products, so depriving them of this blood supply is a potentially powerful tool in slowing down the development of a tumour. The greatest benefit from soya beans has been shown in pre-menopausal women,[34] but with damage from environmental xenoestrogens becoming more apparent, it may be that post-menopausal women will also benefit from the ability of soya to oppose these unnatural chemicals.

Teas (see also page 130)

Black and green teas have shown excellent anti-cancer properties. Black tea, drunk in normal quantities, interferes with the initiation, promotion and growth stages of breast cancer.[35] Green tea is the strongest antimutagen of any plant yet examined, suppressing solid tumour formation in laboratory mice. It has also been demonstrated in animal studies that green tea, at the equivalent level of only two or three cups a day, reduced new blood vessel formation by tumours by up to 70 per cent, meaning that the tumours are starved to death. The active ingredient responsible for this is epigallocatechin-3-gallate (EGCG). All leaf teas contain differing amounts of antimutagenic tannins, antioxidants and polyphenols. If you find that caffeine is too much of a stimulant for you, green tea has half the caffeine of black tea, and Rooibos (red bush) tea has none at all.

Tomatoes

A member of the same family as potatoes, the tomato is a potent source of antioxidants, flavonoids, lycopene, chlorogenic acid, coumarins, carotenes and carotenoids. Studies have shown tomato consumption to be inversely related to breast cancer incidence. Cooked tomatoes are richer sources of lycopene than raw tomatoes. Lycopene is a stronger antioxidant than beta-carotene and it is anti-mitotic, meaning that it slows down cell division in tumours.

Turmeric

Turmeric is used extensively throughout the Indian subcontinent. The active constituent in turmeric is curcumin, its yellow pigment, which is known to have powerful pharmacological properties including being anti-inflammatory, anti-tumour and antioxidant.[36] Curcumin has been shown to inhibit the growth of oestrogen-positive human breast cancer cells, and is particularly powerful in combination with soya isoflavones. It is also very protective against the xenoestrogen promoters including DDT.[37]

Lentil soup with Lemon and Turmeric

250 g/9 oz split red lentils, picked over and rinsed
1–2 large onions, according to taste, quite finely chopped
olive oil
1 × 400 g/14 oz can tomatoes
vegetable or chicken stock, or water
turmeric, cumin, mild curry powder and freshly ground black pepper
juice of 1 lemon
chopped fresh coriander and lemon wedges, to serve

Steam-fry the onions in a little olive oil and water in a saucepan until opaque. Add the lentils, cover with stock or water and bring to the boil. Allow to simmer for 45 minutes–1 hour, checking to make sure the mixture does not dry out.

Pass the tomatoes through a sieve to remove the seeds, add the spices and lemon juice to taste. The soup should be of a fairly thick consistency. Sprinkle with the coriander and serve with the lemon wedges and crusty wholemeal bread.

Yoghurt

While, superficially, yoghurt seems to be nothing more than fermented milk, the live, active culture can dramatically stimulate and fortify the immune system.[38] Yoghurt is also available as leben, kafir and yakult (though yakult has a lot of sugar in it). In human and animal studies, yoghurt has been shown to triple the production of the potent tumour cells-fighter, interferon, and to raise the production of natural killer cells.[39] One thousand women with breast cancer were matched with a similar group without breast cancer and it was found that the more yoghurt consumed, the lower the risk of breast cancer.[40] Yoghurt is often well tolerated by people with dairy allergies as the bacteria have pre-digested the lactose. Many of the proteins have also been broken down and are usually better tolerated. Home-made yoghurt, cultured for twenty-four hours before refrigeration, is totally lactose-free. It is best to eat organic, live, natural, unflavoured yoghurt, and then to add fruit, instead of eating fruit-flavoured yoghurts which are high in sugar, and non-organic yoghurt which may carry pesticide residues.

Your Supplement Guide

To take supplements or not to take supplements? This is a polarizing question with advocates on both sides of the debate feeling strongly that they are right. The idea of using supplemented micronutrients is sometimes seen as unnecessary and unnatural, and the emergence of the market in vitamin pills is greeted with cynicism by some. There are, however, some very real underlying issues that relate to the environment in which we now find we are living, and how it impacts on our micronutrient status.

On balance I am in favour of having a helping hand to achieve optimum health. Vitamin, mineral, herbal and other supplements will *never* be a substitute for a well-planned diet. However, the evidence that is accumulating about the use of nutritional supplements, for cancer prevention and as an adjunct to conventional treatment, is looking very interesting. There is as yet an insufficient body of research to make these judgments with certainty, but my feeling is that in the long term nutrient therapy will prove to be of significant use in the management of breast cancer. Professor John Smyth, Professor of Oncology at the University of Edinburgh, has said, 'It could be as simple as taking an aspirin every day. We know that some vitamins seem to be able to suppress the malignant tendency. In the future, high-risk cancer candidates may be told, "Your body is biochemically unstable without this particular nutrient or medicine. Take it and you'll put yourself in a different order of risk."'[1]

When a statement such as the following appears in the letters page of *The Times* from a Fellow of the Royal Pharmaceutical Society, Ronald Levin, 'that more than 50 per cent of cancers are diet-related is now widely accepted, as is the finding that fruit, vegetables *and some multi-vitamins appear to increase our defences against cancer*' (my emphasis), it is reasonable to conclude that the importance of diet, *accompanied by the use of supplements*, in the treatment of cancer is now receiving serious consideration in the orthodox community.

It is probably an error of judgment to view something that is not proven as something that does not work. In the eighteenth century it took forty years after the initial treatise that vitamin C was linked to scurvy for the medical establishment to accept this – because it was not proven. And nothing much has changed. Of course, if you are dealing with dangerous medicines all day, it is wise to employ a conservative approach. However, to transfer this attitude to supplements is probably not appropriate.

There is a large body of evidence establishing safe and toxic levels of vitamins, minerals, herbs and other nutritional supplements. Contra-indications have also been established. The list of toxic reactions to excessive doses of vitamins and minerals makes scant reading when compared to the list of side-effects of most drug treatments. If substances are inexpensive (when compared to drug treatment), are known to be safe and have been shown to reduce the risk of cancer in animals, as for instance vitamin C has, then do you really want to wait for ten years for proof positive that they work therapeutically in humans? Especially if you are not sure that you have ten years. The worst that can happen, if it does not work, is that you have wasted some money. The best that can happen is that it is effective.

There is a tantalizing study[2] from Dr Abram Hoffer and Professor Linus Pauling of a profound improvement in the survival of patients. Together these giants of orthomolecular nutritional medicine published a study of women with cancers who received high doses of vitamin C (around 10 g), beta-carotene and vitamin B3 alongside nutritional advice and their hospital oncology treatment. The majority – 80 per cent – lived substantially longer than those women in the other group who did not receive supplementation or dietary advice. The results were particularly impressive for women with cancers of the breast, ovary and fallopian tubes.

Another paper, a review of seventy-eight studies, concluded that vitamins A, C and E and beta-carotene are strong regulatory factors of cancer cell differentiation, regression, membrane structure, DNA and the transformation of pre-cancerous cells into cancer cells, as well as having cytotoxic and cytostatic effects on cancer cells, and strongly suggested that these nutrients have a chemo-preventive and *treatment* role in cancer.[3]

In this chapter I will be putting the, admittedly, pro-lobby case –

along with known contra-indications in certain instances – for the use of supplements. If you are under the care of a physician for treatment of breast cancer, and you plan to use vitamin, mineral or herbal supplements, it is necessary to discuss your plans with them. If you are aiming for prevention, or are post-treatment and interested in avoiding recurrence, here is the information you need to make your own decisions.

Can you get all you need from a balanced diet?

In an ideal world – which you may have noticed we do not live in – we would get everything we need from our diet. But the reality is that there is so much to conspire against our achieving optimal nutrient intake from our food. Take a look at this check-list and decide for yourself if everything is as you would like it to be:

- *Do you eat food that is grown in nutrient-poor soil?* The answer is probably yes, since food production is aimed at producing optimal plants, not optimally nourished people. For instance, the trace minerals zinc, selenium and chromium are not needed by plants and so are not added to the soil. On the other hand, humans need these minerals and a significant number of people are, according to Government figures, deficient.
- *Do you eat non-organic food?* Non-organic produce is about 50 per cent poorer in minerals than organic. Non-organic animal products come with the burden of antibiotics, hormones and pesticides which tax the body's detoxification systems, and therefore require more nutrients to support them.
- *Do you lose nutrients when cooking?* Boiling, deep-frying and intense grilling severely reduce the number of vitamins and minerals in food. Preferred methods of cooking are steaming and baking. Micro-waved food may retain nutrients but has been shown to have a detrimental effect on blood chemistry after a meal (increasing cholesterol and reducing white blood cell counts[4]).
- *Do you feel at all stressed?* The stress response mechanism uses up huge quantities of vitamins B3, B5, B6, C and the minerals magnesium and zinc. It also shuts down the digestive tract by

moving the blood supply away from the intestines to the skeletal muscles – if you are under stress you may not be absorbing all the nutrients from your food properly.

- *Do you eat packaged foods?* Prepared foods are usually depleted of nutrients and many have low-nutrient, inexpensive fillers and bulking agents. Packaged foods are 'enriched' because the manufacturing process has taken out the nutrients in the first place, and while some nutrients are replaced, others are not.
- *Do you take any substances that work as anti-nutrients?* Coffee, tea, alcohol, sugar, cigarettes, the contraceptive pill, antibiotics, painkillers, anti-inflammatory medication and chemotherapy all interfere with the uptake and utilization of nutrients, or can cause nutrients to be excreted in excess.
- *Do you have any digestive problems?* If so, there is a good chance that your absorption of food molecules is less than optimal. This is particularly the case with any inflammatory condition in the digestive tract, where the symptoms are likely to be bloating, wind, constipation, diarrhoea or irritable bowel syndrome.
- *Are you exposed to environmental pollutants?* Food additives, heavy metals from water, an excess of household chemicals, dry-cleaning fluids, farming sprays (carried on the wind and leached into water supplies), car exhausts, or similar, all put an extra load on your body's detoxification systems, meaning that your body needs extra resources.
- *Do you have any diagnosed illness?* If you have breast cancer, or any other condition, and particularly if you are being treated with drugs for any condition, it is quite likely that you have a need for extra nutrient reserves.

If your answer to any of the above is yes, you are not living in the ideal world as far as maximizing the uptake, and utilization, of nutrients from your diet is concerned.

I take a multi-vitamin and mineral supplement, an antioxidant and some extra vitamin C daily. I believe that this minimal supplement programme will help to maintain optimal health when taken alongside a cancer-preventive diet. There are other specific supplements I take as needed – for instance a course of milk thistle to support liver function, L-glutamine for digestive health, or echinacea to support my immune system in the winter.

The following are the most serious dietary nutrient deficiencies that women have, according to the latest available UK Government figures (based on RNIs – reference nutrient intakes)[5]:

Number of women deficient in particular nutrients

Vitamin A	31 per cent	Magnesium	72 per cent
Vitamin B2	21 per cent	Potassium	94 per cent
Vitamin B6	22 per cent	Iodine	32 per cent
Folic Acid	47 per cent	Iron	89 per cent
Vitamin C	34 per cent	Selenium	50 per cent*
Calcium	48 per cent	Zinc	31 per cent

* (approximately – estimate not published)

Is it wise to take supplements?

The RNIs and RDAs (recommended dietary allowances) were established to avoid deficiency diseases. The RNIs are the amounts that it is judged the average person needs to take in from their diet, and these figures superseded the RDAs in the UK. RDAs are still used in other countries, though few countries agree with each other about the correct levels. There are different RDAs and RNIs for men and women.

These average levels are not necessarily the best level for each individual person. Under certain conditions some people need more. This is catered for in some circumstances, for instance there are different RNIs for children, pregnant women and the elderly, but the figures are still generalized.

Research headed up by Dr Emanuel Cheraskin at the University of Alabama, USA, studied 13,500 people over a fifteen-year period to establish a different set of criteria – the SONAs (Suggested Optimum Nutrient Allowances), which had interesting results.[6] The subjects were rated according to their health profile as established by physical and laboratory tests. The results showed that, almost without fail, those who scored highest on health assessments were eating a nutrient-rich diet, compared to calorie intake, *and* taking nutrient supplements. Furthermore, those who were the healthiest were taking nutrient levels that were frequently ten or more times the RDAs.

Simple solutions for complex problems

One of the burdens which nutritional therapy has to bear is that in the complex world in which we live, it seems too simple just to say eat more fruit and vegetables, or take high doses of vitamin C and many problems will be resolved. We are looking for high-tech answers most of the time. And yet researchers are on the verge of establishing that certain nutrients can have a pharmacological effect.

The Government now recommends that a 400 mcg of folic acid supplement is taken by all women pre-conceptually, and for the first three months of a pregnancy, to avoid neural tube defects. Not so many years ago this sort of advice would have been scoffed at, but what we have here is a recommended dose of a nutrient to achieve a particular effect. Widely publicized research is showing that people with heart disease should take the same amount of folic acid, along with vitamins B12 and B6, to lower homocysteine levels – a toxic metabolite which can predispose people to cardiovascular problems – and cereals and other foods are now being fortified with this nutrient.

Widely accepted research at Cambridge University[7] has shown that whilst 'safe intake levels' of vitamin E are estimated at 3 mg/5 ius (international units) per day, levels of 400–800 ius, 100 times this amount or more, reduces the risk of heart attack in those with heart disease by 75 per cent. The same study found only a 25 per cent improvement for aspirin, the most commonly prescribed medication, which also causes bleeding in the digestive tract for a percentage of people. How does this high level of vitamin E correlate to the recommended daily level? Not at all – but it is effective! On the subject of vitamin E one study stated that 'The concentrations needed to suppress the growth of hormone-responsive breast and prostate cancer cells are close to the range that can be reached with dietary supplementation.'[8]

Twenty years from now, it may well be accepted practice for the medical profession to recommend that their patients take vitamins and minerals as a preventive measure against a wide range of diseases, and that this will save the National Health Service a large amount of money. One study worked out that vitamin supplementation of women of child-bearing age and of people over fifty years of age would save $20 billion in the USA alone for the conditions studied (birth defects, low-birth-weight premature births and coronary heart disease).[9] One day someone will work out how much could be saved with supplementation for cancer.

Can supplements be toxic?

Anything can be toxic in excessive quantities. If nutritional supplements are used wisely and safe upper limits are observed, the down-sides of using them are few and far between.[10] People with known kidney or liver damage will need to be more wary, and incrementing doses slowly, under supervision of a doctor and nutritionist, is the best advice in these circumstances. You can have individual reactions to particular supplements, and the common-sense approach is to stop taking any if you think they do not agree with you. You can then reintroduce them to establish whether your response can be repeated or if it was unrelated to the supplement – which I have usually found to be the case with my clients on the very rare occasions that problems have been reported. There are some contra-indications for using specific nutrients with certain medication, including chemotherapy drugs. These contra-indications are outlined in the following pages.

The way forward

Prevention of breast cancer is probably one good reason to take supplements. We already know that antioxidants in food are protective against many cancers, including breast cancer, and it could well be that supplemented antioxidants will also be proved in research to be beneficial. Of course, it must be remembered that the nature of antioxidants is that they work synergistically and trials which do not take this into account are likely to come up with misleading results.

We are also a long way away from confirming whether supplemen-

157

tation, used as an adjunct to chemotherapy, radiotherapy, surgery or hormone treatment, is effective. Sufficient research has not been done, but you can make some fairly good judgments based on existing research that shows a positive relationship, and has served to convince me that there is a place for nutrient therapy alongside orthodox treatment.

One area of concern is that vitamin and mineral supplements taken during chemotherapy will interact with the drugs and reduce their effectiveness. There are hopeful signs that this is not the case, however, and early research is suggesting that supplements will reduce drug toxicity against normal healthy cells, while retaining, or enhancing, toxicity against cancer cells.

The Pauling/Hoffer research, along with newer research from Knud Lockwood and his colleagues from the University of Texas, USA, are lighting the way. These studies which, unusually, focus on administering antioxidants to cancer patients who are undergoing chemotherapy and other treatments, suggest that this course of action has a significant effect on lifespan.

Vitamins

In what follows the daily RNIs (reference nutrient intakes) for women are taken from the 1994 MAFF report. The daily optimum ranges are the amounts generally used in practice by nutritionists who favour the use of supplements.

Vitamin A

Vitamin A is also called retinol, as its first major function to be discovered was its requirement for health of the retina in the eye. It is a fat-soluble vitamin measured in micrograms (mcg) or international units (ius). RNI: 600 mcg/2,000 ius. Optimum range: 2,250–3,000 mcg/7,500–10,000 ius. Excess can cause toxicity as vitamin A is stored in the liver and can build up. Not recommended over 1,800 mcg/6,000 ius for pregnant women or women planning a pregnancy. It is only properly absorbed if taken with some fat.

Food sources: liver, cod-liver oil, egg yolks, full-fat dairy produce, herrings, mackerel.

Uses for breast cancer: One of the key antioxidant vitamins, it protects vitamin C, and is protective against damage to the mucous membranes of the mouth and the intestinal lining from chemotherapy. Studies show that higher levels of vitamin A in the diet correlate to lowered breast cancer risk; however, the evidence is much stronger for beta-carotene (see below).

Beta-carotene

A water-soluble nutrient, not strictly a vitamin, but converts into vitamin A and therefore has vitamin status, measured in ius (international units) and milligrams (mg). RNI: none. Optimum range: 3,000–30,000 mcg (3–30 mg)/5,000–50,000 ius. No toxicity, though excess may cause yellow coloration to skin which is reversible – it does not turn the whites of the eyes yellow, which helps to differentiate between yellow skin coloration from beta-carotene or from illness such as jaundice. Most supplements use synthetic beta-carotene, though natural carotenes, from sea plants and palm oil, are becoming available. Alpha-carotene is a palm-oil derivative which may have similar effects to beta-carotene in its anti-cancer activity, but more studies need to be done to confirm this.

Food sources: Leafy green vegetables such as spinach, kale, beet greens, broccoli, asparagus, and orange-coloured fruit and vegetables such as carrots, sweet potatoes, tomatoes, pumpkins, squash, turnips, cantaloupe melons, mango, papaya, dried apricots, nectarines, prunes, tangerines.

Uses for breast cancer: Beta-carotene may have more potent antioxidant activity for breast cancer when compared to vitamin A. A large case-controlled study (3,500 cancer patients and 9,500 controls) observed that a beta-carotene- and vitamin A-rich diet, along with supplements, confers protection against breast cancer.[1] It is probably most useful to supplement when overt deficiency is apparent, but in any event, as beta-carotene is water-soluble and non-toxic, it is probably useful to supplement some. It is best to use a good-quality natural beta-carotene and to use it with other synergistic antioxidant nutrients.

Vitamin B complex

A water-soluble group of vitamins, easily destroyed by heat, food processing and cooking. Individual B vitamins are best supplemented along with a multiple B-complex. Vitamin B2 will turn your urine bright yellow; this is not harmful and is an indication that the vitamin is being used properly. Vitamin B3 may cause a flushing sensation akin to a hot flush at levels of about 100 mg. Time-release vitamin B3 should not be used as it has been linked to liver damage.

		RNI	Optimum range	
B1	Thiamine	0.8 mg	25–100 mg	Non-toxic
B2	Riboflavin	1.1 mg	25–100 mg	Non-toxic
B3	Niacin or Nicotinamide	13.0 mg	50–150 mg	Non-toxic, may cause temporary skin flushing

B5	Pantothenic acid	No RNI (guide 3–7mg)	50–300 mg	Non-toxic
B6	Pyridoxine	1.2 mg	25–100 mg	Non-toxic, excess may cause reversible neuropathy but unlikely if taken with a B-complex
B12	Cobalamine	1.5 mcg	5–100 mcg	Non-toxic
Folic acid		200 mcg	200–800 mcg	Non-toxic, see notes below re chemotherapy
Biotin		No RNI	50–200 mcg	Non-toxic
Choline		No RNI	25–100 mcg	Non-toxic

Food sources: Whole grains, oatmeal, brewer's yeast, brown rice, legumes, dried yeast, liver, dark green leafy vegetables, egg yolks, crude molasses, yoghurt, lecithin. Fish and meat are good sources of B6 and B12.

Uses for breast cancer: Used for all cellular energy production, so relevant to cell repair. The B vitamins are used to synthesize and repair DNA. Deficiency of B vitamins impairs immune function. Choline helps detoxification by eliminating toxins and drugs from the liver.

Folic acid is the nutrient that the chemotherapy drug Methotrexate deliberately interferes with. It is therefore possible to become very depleted in this nutrient. A special form of folic acid, Leucovorin, is often given alongside Methotrexate, which helps to stop the Methotrexate becoming too toxic. It is unclear if the small amount of folic acid found in multi-supplements (400 mcg) is sufficient to interrupt Methotrexate activity, but this should be discussed with your oncologist. Folic-acid free B-complex supplements are available (see **Appendix**). If you and your oncologist elect to avoid folic acid supplementation during chemotherapy, restoring your levels after treatment is important in order not to exacerbate a deficiency state. Vitamin B6 has been shown to reduce toxicity in intra-hepatic infusion of 5-fluorouracil chemotherapy.[2]

Vitamin C

A water-soluble vitamin, easily destroyed by heat, light and aspirin. Measured in milligrams (mg) or in high doses in grams (g). UK RNI: 40 mg. Optimum range: 500–3,000 mg (½–3 g). Therapeutic range up to 10,000 mg (10 g). As it is water-soluble, high doses of vitamin C should be taken in divided doses throughout the day. Non-toxic but high doses may result in loose bowel movements, in which case lower the dose slightly. High doses of vitamin C may be dangerous for people with haemachromatosis as it increases absorption of iron. There are some reports of kidney stones due to the production of oxalates in a small group of individuals, mostly discounted and unlikely to be a concern, especially if there is no history of the problem. Chewable vitamin C combines sugar and acid and can lead to tooth decay. Non-acidic forms in capsules or powdered form are preferable, such as magnesium ascorbate, potassium ascorbate, Ester-C. There is some possible concern that vitamin C may increase the risk of toxicity of the chemotherapy drug Methotrexate as vitamin C is an organic acid which may inhibit secretion from the kidneys at high doses.[3] In view of this it is advised not to take high doses of vitamin C either twelve hours before, or twelve hours after, Methotrexate administration.

Food sources: Citrus fruit, strawberries, kiwi fruit, green leafy vegetables (spinach, chard, kale, Brussels sprouts), parsley, sweet peppers, potatoes (especially new potatoes), sweet potatoes, bean sprouts, broccoli, cabbage, turnips, cantaloupe melons, liver, currants, cauliflower, sprouted seeds and beans.

Uses for breast cancer: Almost too many to mention! Important for the health of the immune system (anti-viral, anti-bacterial, used for white blood cell formation, detoxifies histamine-reducing allergic responses, increases glutathione levels).[4] Used for collagen building and therefore helps cement cells together, which may interfere with cancer spread, also helps wound healing after surgery. Used and stored by the adrenal glands for the stress reaction. Cancer risks are probably reduced by a higher than normal intake.[5] Increases Natural Killer Cytotoxic activity by 200–400 per cent at levels of 60 mg per kg of body weight (nearly 4 g for a 10-stone/140 lb person).[6] A study by Cameron and Pauling gave terminal cancer patients 10 g of vitamin

C in divided doses and they lived an average of seven months against a similar non-supplemented group who lived one and a half months. The same results were repeated in a follow-up study by the same team (despite the patients being terminal, a couple of them lived for several years after vitamin C treatment).[7] The Mayo Clinic trials which seemed to repudiate the Cameron/Pauling trials have since been heavily criticized.[8] The Cameron/Pauling studies have been confirmed by researchers in Japan.[9] Vitamin C may also neutralize the hyaluronidase enzyme made by cancer cells that helps them to metastasize. Vitamin C is a potent detoxifier of heavy metals, helping to eliminate them. Recent criticism about vitamin C and cancer stemmed from some research showing that the vitamin increased a 'marker' for oxidation stress and DNA damage, 8-oxadenine. The authors of the study cautioned against using vitamin C as a result of this. There was however a concurrent decrease in another marker, 8-oxoguanine, which is a protective conclusion. The authors subsequently withdrew their original recommendations, but not before there was a massive amount of publicity, causing a lot of alarm among people who use high doses of vitamin C. If anything, the study highlights the fact that the effects of vitamin C need to be viewed, as do many dietary and supplemental components, in the light of its total effect and not a single biological effect, and also emphasizes the importance of nutrient synergy since vitamin E, flavonoids and glutathione (a selenium-based enzyme) all serve to protect vitamin C. With hundreds of studies confirming that vitamin C is safe, and many showing that it is effective in protecting against cancer, there is no reason to doubt that its use is beneficial.

Vitamin D

A fat-soluble nutrient measured in international units (ius) and micrograms (mcg), also known as calciferol. Vitamin D3 is made by the skin on exposure to sunlight. Vitamin D3 is converted in the liver to 1,25DHD (1,25 Di-Hydroxy D), which is so active that it is considered a hormone. RNI: none (10 mcg if confined indoors). Optimum range 10–20 mcg/400–800 ius. The lower dose is appropriate if exposed to sunlight regularly, and the higher dose if you are limiting dairy products and get very little sun. Vitamin D is toxic in high doses, so take care not to take a multi-supplement which includes vitamin D alongside cod-liver oil which is naturally very high in vitamin D. Fish oil supplements other than cod liver oil do not usually have vitamin D in them. Sunlight derived vitamin D is self-limiting, so there is no chance of overdose by this route.

Food sources: Sardines, herrings, salmon, tuna, egg yolks, fish oils, dairy produce.

Uses for breast cancer: An interesting dilemma for people wanting to avoid breast cancer is that research shows that despite higher incidences of skin cancer from exposure to sunlight, there is a correspondingly low incidence of breast cancer. Even in the USA incidence is dramatically lower, up to 80 per cent in areas with a lot of sunlight. Other factors do not seem to explain this anomaly and it is put down to vitamin D synthesis in skin from the sun. Breast cancers with high levels of vitamin D receptors have a significantly improved prognosis.[10] Dietary vitamin D does not appear to reduce breast cancer risk, but the vitamin D-rich foods that most people consume are milk, butter and cheese, which may skew the studies. Vitamin D3 supplementation provides the same type of vitamin D that is manufactured by the skin before it goes for processing in the liver, so logic suggests that a sensible range of supplementation may be beneficial if the skin is not regularly exposed to the sun, and studies show that it inhibits breast cancer cell growth.[11] There may be a case for getting out in sunlight to reduce your risk of breast cancer; however, if you are exposed to the sun, ensure that you do not burn. Vitamin D enhances the immune system,[12] encourages apoptosis (cell death) of cancer cells in the laboratory[13] and increases levels of insulin-like growth factor binding proteins,[14] and there may be other ways in which it helps.

Vitamin E

A fat-soluble nutrient measured in international units (ius) or milligrams (mg), also known as tocopherols. The active form is d-alpha-tocopherol and the artificial form, dl-alpha-tocopherol, is not recommended. It is destroyed by heat, freezing, oxygenation and food processing, and works best in conjunction with selenium and vitamin C. RNI: none (3 mg considered adequate). Optimum range 67–

134 mg/100–200 ius. Therapeutic range 268–671 mg/400–1,000 ius. Non-toxic. As vitamin E thins the blood it is useful for cardiovascular problems but, because of its anti-coagulant properties, it should ideally be avoided for ten days before an operation. You should also be cautious about taking vitamin E alongside other blood-thinning medication such as aspirin or Warfarin, and possibly speak to your doctor about slowly reducing medication as you slowly increase vitamin E levels.

Food sources: Wheatgerm, vegetable oils, broccoli, Brussels sprouts, almonds, olive oil, eggs, spinach, soya beans, tomatoes, fresh nuts, fresh seeds, carrots, sunflower seeds, wholegrain cereals, brown rice and rice bran, oatmeal, rye, peanuts.

Uses for breast cancer: Vitamin E is one of the major antioxidants found in cell membranes and protects against lipid peroxidation (damage to the unsaturated fats found in cell membranes). It can help to prevent scarring after operations. Several studies show that blood levels are low in breast cancer patients, usually in conjunction with the compatible antioxidants selenium and/or beta-carotene.[15] Cell-culture experiments show that a commonly found type of vitamin E, d-alpha tocopherol succinate, halts breast cancer cell growth by transforming growth factor-b,[16] and it encourages apoptosis (programmed cell death), in ER-negative breast cancer cells,[17] while another form, tocotrienols, inhibits both hormone status-types of breast cancer cells.[18] It may also discourage angiogenesis, or blood capillary formation by tumours.[19] Some studies have shown vitamin E to be protective against breast cancer.[20] Vitamin E also has a strong protective cardiovascular effect, making it useful for women who are post-menopausal. Vitamin E in high doses (1,000 ius daily) is important to consider to help prevent cardiac toxicity with the chemotherapy drug Adramyecin whilst not affecting its anti-tumour activity.[21] The vitamin can also help to prevent hair loss with other chemotherapy regimes at levels of 1,600 ius daily.[22] There have been some historical concerns about the use of vitamin E supplements with breast cancer which stem from the soya oil they are packed in having an oestrogenic effect. This was in the early days of phytoestrogen research and before the widespread view that phytoestrogens have a protective effect. There was also some concern since vitamin E has a similar, but different, chemical structure to oestrogens. These concerns are now discounted. Leading nutritionist Stephen Terrass says, 'If I had a family member who had breast cancer, I would have no reservations supplementing vitamin E. In fact, I would have greater reservations if their intake of vitamin E was restricted.'

Vitamin K

Fat-soluble and measured in micrograms (mcg). Normally made by intestinal bacteria, but dependent upon the bowel bacteria being in the right balance, and disturbed bowel function may impair vitamin K production. Destroyed by freezing, antibiotics and aspirin. RNI: none. Not normally supplemented, though it is available as a supplement, but not recommended in high doses over 100 mcg.

Food sources: Cauliflower (best source), yoghurt, alfalfa, egg yolks, safflower oil, kelp, fish liver oils, leafy green vegetables, potatoes, milk.

Uses for breast cancer: No specific relationship, though it may have a role in reducing the effects of chemical carcinogens and may help in the prevention of metastasis.[23] Essential for blood-clotting agent prothrombin and useful for bone metabolism (reduces risk of osteoporosis). Vitamin K also enhances the immune system.

Minerals

Calcium

Macro-mineral measured in milligrams (mg). RNI: 700 mg. Optimum range: 500–1,000 mg. Works with magnesium, phosphorus and vitamin D. Excess fats, oxalates (chocolate, rhubarb and spinach), phytates (wheat and other grains) and phosphorus (colas) inhibit absorption. Low vitamin D levels, and medication such as the contraceptive pill and steroids interfere with absorption. Low stomach acid reduces uptake of minerals, but especially calcium, from food. Excess calcium can lead to hypercalcaemia.

Food sources: Dairy produce, soya beans, sardines, salmon, peanuts, sunflower seeds, dried beans, green leafy vegetables, tofu, almonds, sesame seeds, broccoli, eggs, raisins.

Uses for breast cancer: During puberty and adolescence, calcium and vitamin D may inhibit breast carcinogenesis from a high-fat diet.[1] Calcium helps to detoxify the body of the heavy metals: lead, cadmium, aluminium, mercury, arsenic and excess copper.

Chromium

Micro-mineral measured in micrograms (mcg). RNI: none. Optimum range: 50–500 mcg. No known toxicity, however, so effective at regulating blood sugar swings that insulin-dependent diabetics need to introduce it slowly while their doctor monitors medication. Excreted by those on a high-sugar or refined carbohydrate diet, which exacerbates the situation as it is needed for the body's ability to regulate the blood sugar swings that result from eating these foods.

Food sources: Shellfish, chicken, brewer's yeast, brown rice, rye bread, calves' liver, carrots, lettuce, eggs, bananas, cabbage, oranges, green beans, mushrooms, parsnips, apples, strawberries, potatoes, milk, butter.

Uses for breast cancer: Helps to regulate insulin and blood sugar swings. Insulin regulation is important for manufacturing sex-hormone binding globulin, and blood sugar control is important for reducing oxidation damage to tissues. It also helps to curb cravings for sugary foods.

Copper

Micro-mineral measured in milligrams (mg). RNI: 1.2 mg. This mineral has a dual personality. We need it in tiny amounts and it is required for the production of the antioxidant enzyme super-oxide dismutase. However, there are often excessively high blood levels from copper water pipes or a history of contraceptive pill or HRT use. It is rarely supplemented specifically unless high doses of zinc are being used (zinc antagonizes copper). It may be found in small quantities in multi-mineral supplements.

Iodine

Micro-mineral measured in micrograms (mcg). RNI: 140 mcg. Therapeutic level: 200 mcg. No known toxicity, but excess may result in reversible overactive thyroid.

Food sources: Kelp, seaweed, all seafood, vegetables grown in iodine rich soil, iodized salt, meat, milk (milk is an 'accidental' source as milking equipment is treated with iodine antiseptics).

Uses for breast cancer: Essential for proper functioning of the thyroid gland and production of thyroxine. Thyroxine is needed for proper cell metabolism. Thyroid deficiency and iodine deficiency, found in the 'goiter belts', have been linked to increased breast cancer incidence.[2]

Iron

Micro-mineral measured in milligrams (mg). Prefix 'ferric' often used on labels. RNI: 14.8 mg for menstruating women, and 8.7 mg for post-menopausal women. Iron absorption is inhibited by tannins (tea, red wine), oxalates and phytates. Toxic in high amounts and it is also a pro-oxidant,[3] so an excess is not advised. Test for iron deficiency (serum ferritin) before supplementing in high doses. Formulas that should not contribute to constipation are Iron EAP and beetroot extract (iron-rich). Vitamin C-rich foods help the absorption of iron from meat-free meals. Ferric forms of iron destroy vitamin E and are therefore best not used. Excess iron can hinder zinc absorption.

Food sources: Red meat, liver, apricots and peaches (dried fruit are more dense sources), egg yolks, nuts, asparagus, oatmeal, beetroot, blackstrap molasses, seaweed, parsley, figs, cherries, bananas, avocados, brown rice, potatoes, green peas, prunes, sunflower seeds, raisins, walnuts, mushrooms, kale, broccoli.

Uses for breast cancer: Needed for red blood cell formation and for energy production, and also to help metabolize B vitamins. Cancer patients on chemotherapy can become anaemic, as can women who menstruate heavily. Anaemia can easily be checked for with a simple blood test from your doctor. However, if you are not anaemic, supplemented iron should be avoided if you have been diagnosed with cancer, or possibly even if not actually diagnosed, as iron has been shown in research to increase tumour growth.[4] Women with depleted iron levels have a reduced risk of cancer, while high levels have been correlated with higher risks of cancer. Excess 'free' iron (not bound to haemoglobin) acts as a pro-oxidant and as well as being implicated in cancer risk has also been suggested to increase cardiovascular problems. For an iron-free multi-mineral formulation see **Appendix**.

Magnesium

Macro-mineral measured in milligrams (mg). RNI: 270 mg. Optimum range: 375–500 mg. Can be toxic in excess, but this is rare as the intestines normally reject excess (unless kidney damage is present). Magnesium is more commonly deficient, especially after prolonged stress. Works with calcium, and calcium deficiency may actually be due to poor calcium metabolism resulting from magnesium deficiency.

Food sources: All dark green vegetables, soya beans, brewer's yeast, whole grains, seafood, dried fruit, meat, lemons, grapefruit, almonds, seeds, figs, yellow corn, aubergines, raisins, brazil nuts, carrots, mushrooms, crab, tomatoes, garlic, onions, chicken, potatoes.

Uses for breast cancer: Magnesium is necessary for the synthesis of RNA and DNA. It is also essential for the stress response and is usually severely depleted in those under duress for any length of time.

Manganese

Micro-mineral measured in milligrams (mg). RNI: None. Optimum range: 10–50 mg. Toxicity very rare. Manganese is poorly absorbed and readily excreted.

Food sources: Nuts, green leafy vegetables, pulses, peas, root vegetables, beetroot, tropical fruit, egg yolks, wholegrain cereals and bread, black tea.

Uses for breast cancer: Manganese is used for one of the main anti-oxidant enzymes, superoxide dismutase, and it may help to counteract the immune-suppressing stress hormone, cortisol. It is used in the energy cycle of cells and is needed by the thyroid gland (see notes under **Iodine** above).

Potassium

Macro-mineral measured in milligrams (mg). RNI: 3,500 mg. Non-toxic and generally very easily absorbed from vegetables and fruit in the diet. Not usually supplemented though available.

Food sources: Widely available from all fruits and vegetables. In particular bananas, watermelon and potatoes.

Uses for breast cancer: Used for some cancer therapies especially where sodium excess is suspected, the idea being to restore homeostasis (balance) in the cells, but this should ideally be monitored by a doctor or nutritionist.

Selenium

A micro-mineral measured in micrograms (mcg) which is easily destroyed by food processing. The most absorbable forms are sodium selenite and seleno-methionine. RNI: 60 mcg. Optimum range: 100–200 mcg. Selenium can be toxic in very high doses (1,000 mcg or more), so it is best to stick to the optimum range. The first sign of toxicity is loss of thumbnails, which has not been reported from supplement use within the recommended range. European and British intake is falling; a MAFF survey noted a drop from an average intake of 60 mcg, twenty-two years previously, to 34 mcg in 1994. With such low average intake we should probably consider supplementation. All farm animals in the UK have mineral-supplemented feed which has included selenium since 1978 when it was recognized that it helped to prevent a number of diseases – why should we lag behind?

Food sources: Wheatgerm and bran, brown rice, white rice (less than for brown rice), tuna, tomatoes, broccoli, Brazil nuts, seafood, poultry and meat, brewer's yeast.

Uses for breast cancer: One of the most important antioxidant nutrients. Works in conjunction with vitamin E. The key nutrient for the cancer-fighting glutathione peroxidase enzymes which remove hydrogen peroxide and damaging lipid and phospholipid hydroperoxides generated by free radicals and other oxygen-derived species. If not removed, hydroperoxides impair cell membrane structure and function.[5] Low levels of glutathione peroxidase are consistently observed in breast cancer patients. There is an inverse relationship between dietary selenium intake and breast cancer incidence. Selenium also plays an important role in the control of thyroid metabolism by being involved in the conversion of the inactive T4 molecule into the active T3 molecule. Thyroid insufficiency is closely linked to increase in breast cancer risk. Selenium has been shown to reduce nephrotoxicity (toxicity to the kidneys) of cysplatin without reducing the anti-tumour effects of the drug.[6] Selenium is also an effective detoxifier of the heavy metal mercury out of the body. A major multinational £20 million trial involving 52,000 subjects has just been announced, indicating the degree of seriousness attached to selenium and cancer prevention.

Zinc

Micro-mineral measured in milligrams (mg). RNI: 7 mg. Optimum range: 15–20 mg. Can be toxic in very high doses, over 150 mg, but more usually deficient.

Food sources: Meat, liver, oysters, pumpkin seeds, sunflower seeds, wheatgerm, brewer's yeast, sardines, chicken, cucumbers, Brazil nuts, egg yolks, carrots, oats, rye, cauliflower, walnuts, almonds, buckwheat, lettuce, tuna, berries, brown rice.

Uses for breast cancer: Zinc is needed for all protein metabolism and therefore for tissue repair, correct RNA and DNA manufacture and enzyme production. It is a key component of the free radical-fighting enzyme super-oxide-dismutase. Zinc deficiency depresses the immune system, including a reduction in natural killer cells.[7] Detoxifies a number of heavy metals, lead, cadmium, aluminium, mercury, arsenic and excess copper.

Other Useful Supplements

Many nutrients are emerging as having great potential to help in the fight against breast cancer. None are dietary essentials – in other words no deficiency diseases are associated with not having them in the diet (unlike vitamins and minerals) – nevertheless they can have very useful therapeutic effects and you may find it beneficial to add some to your programme. Some of the most interesting ones, which are available in supplement form, are listed here.

It is not always possible to be precise about dosages as much depends upon the manufacturer's ingredients, the intended use and the interaction with other supplements being used. For the most part ranges have been given which are considered safe and effective. If, for instance, you are taking a number of antioxidants, because of the synergistic nature of these nutrients you can probably err on the lower side of the ranges. If you have a particular need for a boost, you may decide to go to the upper part of the range. Herbal supplements should not be taken if you are planning a pregnancy, are pregnant or breast-feeding, and caution should be exercised if on medication.

Acidophilus

This is the generic term for a number of *Lactobacilli* species of 'friendly' bacteria (probiotics) which naturally inhabit healthy intestines. The main species are *L. acidophilus*, *L. bulgaricus* and *L. casei*. Their presence has a number of health benefits: they produce important B vitamins which help to support immune function; they curb or destroy potentially pathogenic bacteria and yeasts, and in so doing free up the immune system for other jobs (such as dealing with cancer); they are an important part of the process of 'activating' lignans and enhancing their phytoestrogenic effect; they help to detoxify, or prevent, the formation of carcinogenic chemicals in the digestive tract. One of the main anti-cancer effects of *Lactobacilli* is to neutralize harmful bile acids.[1]

There are no contra-indications for using any type of probiotics such as acidophilus.

Suggested dosage: 1 g three times daily, ideally for one year at least.

Astragalus

Astragalus root is also called *Astragalus membranaceus* or Huang Qi in Chinese. The Chinese value astragalus as an immune enhancer and as a tonic. Astragalus has been shown significantly to increase natural production of interferon. It also helps to support the immune system during chemotherapy and to reduce some of the side-effects including poor appetite, hair loss and depression. In animal studies astragalus has been shown to be effective at protecting the liver against damage from chemotherapy,[2] as well as improving immune function in cancer patients.[3] No toxicity has been reported for this herb.

Suggested range: One 225-mg capsule two to three times daily.

Chlorella, blue-green algae, 'green foods'

Chlorella is a freshwater, single-cell green alga which has high levels of vitamin A and chlorophyll as well as all the essential amino acids (protein building blocks). In total it contains more than twenty different vitamins. Chlorella is often used in combination with other 'green foods' such as spirulina (a blue-green alga), wheat grass and barley greens, all of which have similar properties. Green drinks may also contain alfalfa (see **Anti-Breast Cancer Superfoods**, page 137) and other grasses such as oat greens.

Suggested range: As these are really 'foods' it is hard to determine a range, and they are very non-toxic. 500–1,500 mg daily should be sufficient to help maintain existing good health.

Co-enzyme Q10

Co-enzyme Q10, also called ubiquinone, CoQ10 or vitamin Q, is a potent, fat-soluble antioxidant. It is used in every cell for energy production and has been described as 'conditionally essential'. It is normally manufactured in the liver from components in our diet; however, if the liver is not functioning well, as it may not be during chemotherapy, it is questionable whether the production of CoQ10 is sufficient. The ability to synthesize CoQ10 also declines dramatically as we age and blood levels are generally lower in cancer patients than for people without cancer.[4]

Early trials on CoQ10 and breast cancer look very interesting. High levels of 390 mg have shown tantalizing effects in reversing breast cancer. The initial study gave thirty-two 'high-risk' breast cancer patients antioxidant, fatty acid and CoQ10 supplements, and the CoQ10 doses ranged from 90–390 mg – these were as an adjunct to their conventional treatment with surgery, chemo- and radio-therapy, and in some cases Tamoxifen. The high doses were justified in the light of the immune-suppressive effects of the powerful chemotherapy drugs that the patients were already receiving. All the patients survived the two years of the study (actuarial data suggests that four of the patients would have died during this time) and six patients had documented remissions of the breast tumours. Morphine doses were reduced, there was no significant weight loss (often associated with late-stage cancer) and no metastases were observed. One woman taking the higher dose had a complete remission after one month, while another case with intraductal cancer showed no evidence of a tumour or metastasis after three months at the high dose.[5] The author of the paper stated that, having treated 200 cases of breast cancer per year for thirty-five years, he 'has never seen a spontaneous complete regression of a 1.5–2.0 cm breast tumour and has never seen a comparable regression on any conventional anti-tumour therapy'. A follow-up study two years later showed similar results.[6]

CoQ10 is known to be cardio-protective and it is found in the heart in higher levels than anywhere else in the body. It can help to reduce cardiac toxicity from the chemotherapy drug Adriamycin.[7] CoQ10 is non-toxic at high doses; however, it is quite an expensive supplement, so supplementing 60–120 mg is more common. It does appear that 100 mg, as part of an overall synergistic antioxidant programme, has definite therapeutic effects. CoQ10 is fat soluble and so best taken with food.

Suggested range: 100–400 mg daily.

Echinacea

This herb has many immune-supportive actions and can be a real bonus when fighting off infections or aiming to restore immune function after illness. Echinacea raises white blood cell counts and increases resistance, as well as stimulating natural killer cells.[8] It is anti-microbial, antiseptic, anti-inflammatory, anti-parasitic, anti-bacterial and has an anti-viral effect.

For maximum effect it is best taken for courses of two months and then not taken for a couple of months before restarting. Taking it continuously creates a 'resistance' to its therapeutic effects. It is also uncertain what the effects of echinacea are likely to be if taken beyond eight weeks while on chemotherapy, and the combination may adversely affect the liver.

Suggested range: 100–200 mg standard extract of echinacea daily. Tinctures contain approximately the equivalent of 285 mg of whole fresh plant, or 65 mg of whole dried plant per 15 drops (0.6 ml). The tincture dose can be taken two to three times daily.

Fish oil capsules

Fish oil is highly protective against breast cancer and eating 100 g/4 oz of oily fish will give you about 2 g of fish oils. Eating oily fish at least three times, or even better five times, a week is likely to be very beneficial.[9]

There may, however, be a case for taking extra fish oil in the form of supplements if, over a long period of time, your diet has been loaded with the 'wrong' type of fats. Sources of the wrong fats would include omega-6 oils that are not cold-pressed (such as corn or sunflower oil, margarines), butter and processed foods such as biscuits, pies and cakes. If this is the case your body tissues will have a high amount of these fats lodged in the cell membranes, and eating more of the 'right' fats can displace these. One way to do this is to increase flax oil in your diet. But another route is to include up to 5 g of fish oil capsules in your programme daily.

Fish oil supplements may also be called EPA/DHA supplements.[10] Generally it is best to avoid cod liver oil as it is also high in vitamins

A and D and this makes it easy to overdose on these fat-soluble nutrients if you are taking multi-vitamin and antioxidant supplements alongside the cod liver oil. Cod liver oil is also more likely to be contaminated with pollutants than are fish oil supplements.

Suggested range: 5 g (5,000 mg) daily in divided doses, which should provide approximately 1,000 mg EPA and 750 mg DHA.

Garlic

Garlic is an age-old remedy for many immune problems. It also appears to have a therapeutic effect against cancer. A review of this humble herb indicates that garlic inhibits the initiation and promotion phases of cancer as well as strengthening the various aspects of the immune system's response to tumours.[11] Garlic may also block the adhesion of cancer cells to the surface of blood vessels and thereby help to prevent metastasis. For more information about garlic see the section **Anti-Breast Cancer Superfoods** (page 137).

Garlic can be taken in supplement form as well as eaten. Many garlic supplements have had the volatile oils, which contain the anti-cancer factors, removed, so it is important not to buy supplements which have been 'deodorized'. Ideally it is best to use 'whole garlic' as it contains allicin, thiosulphinate, alliin and gamma-glutamyl cysteine, which are likely to be beneficial constituents.

Suggested range: 500–1,000 mg daily of whole garlic capsules or 1– 2 mg daily of garlic oil.

L-glutamine

This is an amino acid, or protein building block. It has been termed 'conditionally essential' as, under certain circumstances, such as when immuno-compromised, some people seem to need more than is normally considered sufficient.[12] It is the most abundant amino acid in the body and is used by the lining of the digestive tract as a direct source of energy. The brain is also able to use L-glutamine for energy despite normally being very selective about using glucose. Interestingly it has been shown to improve moods in patients, though this is probably through a different mechanism. Many people report significantly improved energy levels when taking L-glutamine.

L-glutamine is helpful for encouraging liver detoxification. It also has been shown to be extremely effective at reducing damage to the digestive tract from chemotherapy (Methotrexate, 5-fluorouracil and cisplatin). Chemotherapy side-effects which L-glutamine can help to prevent include diarrhoea, mouth ulcers and increased gut permeability. As increased gut permeability can impair the absorption of nutrients from the diet, L-glutamine is likely to maintain the health of the gut sufficiently to avoid nutritional status being compromised during chemotherapy.[13]

There has been some concern from earlier studies that L-glutamine may enhance tumour growth. Tumours have been described as 'glutamine traps' that deplete the individual of glutamine.[14] However, more recent studies, including an overview of all the research available on L-glutamine, have suggested that the benefits to the person outweigh the benefits to tumours, and that L-glutamine actually enhances the ability of the immune system to fight off cancer. The overview concluded, 'Supplemental glutamine does not make tumours grow but in fact results in decreased growth through stimulation of the immune system.'[15] In rats L-glutamine has also been shown to suppress breast cancer growth by lowering prostaglandin PGE2 levels and enhancing natural killer cell activity.[16] In a study in Boston, USA, glutamine-supplemented patients had fewer clinical infections and hospital charges were $21,000 less per patient in the glutamine-supplemented group when compared to the non-supplemented group – the glutamine in that trial cost about £4 per day.[17]

Studies show that L-glutamine significantly enhances the effectiveness of chemotherapy against tumours,[18] while protecting normal body tissues. One review concluded, 'These studies suggest that oral glutamine supplementation is safe in its administration to the tumour-bearing host receiving Methotrexate.'[19] It may be best to discuss the situation with your doctor if you currently have a tumour, despite the fact that the information looks extremely positive regarding using L-glutamine during oncology treatment.

Suggested range: The human trials used between 4 and 30 g daily. The high doses are probably only appropriate during active chemotherapy treatment, with lower doses of 4–15 g being used at other times. It is easier to take in powdered form, stirred into water or juice (it is tasteless), rather than swallowing a number of capsules. Very high doses of L-glutamine can also encourage constipation. Divide the total dose into three and take at three intervals during the day, between meals. Avoid taking it too late at night as it may induce sleeplessness. L-glutamine should not be taken if there is known liver or kidney damage, or if pregnant or breast-feeding.

Lipoic acid

This is a very interesting antioxidant, also referred to as alpha-lipoic acid. It has the fairly unique property of working in both the water- and fat-soluble mediums in the body, as well as in non-aerobic (without oxygen) environments. This means that it can work both inside and outside cells, effectively giving you two-for-the-price-of-one.

Lipoic acid is a powerful antioxidant which can prevent both cell membrane and DNA damage. It has been called the universal antioxidant as other antioxidants, including vitamins A, C and E, work even better when in a lipoic acid-rich environment. As a part of its role in regenerating its partner antioxidants, lipoic acid increases levels of the cancer-fighting enzyme that we produce, called glutathione peroxidase. It also seems to have the ability to regenerate vitamin C, and to be a substitute for vitamins C and E in certain circumstances – for instance, it can reverse scurvy, which is caused by a severe deficiency of vitamin C.

Lipoic acid can help to protect against the initiation of cancer by preventing a complex called Nuclear Factor Kappa-B from activating oncogenes (cancer switch-on genes). Finally, lipoic acid can help to regulate blood sugar levels as it facilitates the conversion of blood sugar into energy. This helps to reduce oxidation damage to body tissues.[20]

Suggested range: Doses in excess of 100 mg daily are most useful, with 500–600 mg showing most effectiveness.

Lycopene

This antioxidant is a member of the carotenoid family and is a more potent antioxidant than beta-carotene.[21] It is found in red-coloured fruits and vegetables, tomatoes and watermelons being the richest sources. Interestingly, more lycopene is available from cooked tomatoes and tomato products such as ketchup and other sauces, because the lycopene is released from the protein bonds by cooking. Supplements are also now widely available. Lycopene has been more closely linked to inhibiting prostate cancer, and men are advised to eat ten portions of tomato products daily. A recent, and large, study of over 7,000 women has indicated that low lycopene blood levels are significantly associated with breast cancer risk.[22] Lycopene may be useful for retarding or inhibiting breast cancer as it exhibits an anti-mitotic (cell division) action.

Suggested range: 30–60 mg daily.

Milk thistle (silymarin)

The botanical name of milk thistle is *Silybum marianum* and its active compounds are silymarin and other flavo-lignans. This herb provides potent antioxidants which are specific to the liver, the organ of detoxification. Most of the research has been done in Germany where it is Government-endorsed as a supportive treatment for chronic inflammatory liver conditions. It helps liver cells to repair and regenerate themselves after they have been damaged, and contains a flavone which protects liver cell organelles (mitochondria and microsomes) against lipid peroxidation damage. As milk thistle is immensely useful as a liver support it can be beneficial to all people on chemotherapy.

Suggested range: 200–600 mg of standardized extract daily.

N-acetyl-cysteine

N-acetyl-cysteine has a fundamental role in the detoxifying enzyme system known as the cytochrome P450 system and is helpful in detoxifying chemotherapy drugs out of the liver. It is a potent antioxidant and may help to protect against the cardio-toxicity of adriamycin.

N-acetyl-cysteine is the precursor (forerunner) for an important anti-oxidant enzyme system, glutathione peroxidase.

Suggested dosage: 500–1,000 mg daily.

Quercitin

There are a number of flavonoids found in our food and all of them have a beneficial effect to one degree or another. For this reason it is important to have a varied diet of flavonoid-containing foods, which are fruits, vegetables, grains and teas. One flavonoid in particular, quercitin, stands out as being of interest for breast cancer prevention, and may be useful to supplement. It appears to exhibit a number of mechanisms by which it is useful against breast cancer, including inhibiting proliferation and increasing glutathione levels.[23] Many combined antioxidant supplement formulas are now including quercitin.

Suggested range: 500 mg daily.

Soya isoflavones

As an alternative to adding soya to the diet it is possible to take soya isoflavone supplements. As these extracts are not used by the body in the same way as dietary sources of isoflavones, and because of the potential to overdose on them, it is probably best advice to stick to dietary sources of soya isoflavones. It is also probable that the effects of soya on cancer prevention are not only influenced by the isoflavones, but by other components in soya foods as well (see **Anti-Breast Cancer Superfoods** (page 137)), and by taking the isoflavones in the form of supplements alone you will be missing out on other useful compounds.[24] One researcher has concluded that soya supplementation should be studied as adjuvant dietary treatment after primary surgery for early breast cancer with the aim of looking for a decrease in secondary occurrence of tumours[25] and we may see more supporting research in coming years – the times they are a-changing. Two food sources of 'supplements' which could provide the answer for those who prefer to supplement rather than change their cooking habits, are soya-rich snack bars, or the addition of ⅕ cup of soya flakes to a variety of dishes.

If you do choose to take the isoflavone supplements, two to four capsules a day, depending on the brand, are equivalent to the intake of soya phytoestrogens recommended in studies of 50–60 mg. Phytoestrogen supplements should not be taken while planning a pregnancy, pregnant or breast-feeding.

Suggested dosage: Not more than 50 mg of isoflavones daily, but food sources are preferred over supplementation.

Health warning

I mean what I say – 'health warning' as opposed to 'ill-health warning'. As a result of supporting yourself nutritionally, you may feel really well. You will probably have more energy, better moods, better sleep patterns, minor complaints may clear up, even major ones may do so . . .

Paradoxically, in the West, we tend to be over-fed, but under-nourished at the same time. Addressing the causes of this can create a revolution in health. Be prepared to feel well.

And if you do feel well when combining nutrition with medical treatment, this leads to another word of warning: many people feel so well, unexpectedly, that they take advantage of the situation and do too much. Part of the healing process is to conserve energy to allow your body's systems to do their jobs and fight off the cancer – as well as the effects of the hospital treatment. Do not be tempted to over-tax yourself or do too much, even if you feel fine. It is not so much a question of treating yourself as an invalid, as of treating yourself well.

Lifestyle Choices

Apart from diet and supplements there are other lifestyle factors which can have a significant impact on breast health.

Tobacco

Smoking has no place at all in the regime of anybody interested in their health. In particular definite links have been established between smoking tobacco and breast cancer in the (up to) 50 per cent of women who have a mutation on the NAT2 gene. This mutation means that these women do not break down carcinogens very effectively. Smoking for such women can lead to a four-fold increase of risk. If that is not enough to put you off, consider the fact that cigarettes are an overwhelming source of free radicals, and also introduce toxins into your body which are extremely difficult to eliminate – and of course the connection between cigarettes and lung cancer is well established. It is best to avoid passive smoking as well.

No more couch potato

Lack of exercise or physical activity increases the risk of breast cancer and research is showing us that women who do four hours or more of exercise a week have a 37 per cent reduction in risk.[1] The effect is slightly more pronounced in pre-menopausal women than post-menopausal women,[2] but the message is that all women benefit. The exercise could be walking, swimming, tennis, jogging or aerobics – anything that causes an increase in heart rate. Even two hours a week give increased protection. If you have a physically active job this will also benefit you.[3] The positive effect is attributed to exercise lowering the levels of circulating oestrogens, deemed to be more significant than reducing excess body fat. So, along with the known benefits of lowering risk of osteoporosis, heart disease and diabetes, breast cancer risk is also improved. Unfortunately, this message is not getting through at the moment as only a third of women in the UK take regular exercise.

Starting slowly and building up at a steady pace are always advised. If you have not exercised for many years, suspect that you have a heart condition or suffer from osteoporosis, you will need to consult your doctor first.

Excess exercise

Though a moderate amount of exercise is good, this does not mean that going over the top is better. Defining what is 'excess' is not an exact science, and is age-related. However, doing more than an hour of cardiovascular exercise a day is excess in terms of impact on the body. At this level of intensity exercise stresses body tissues, which have to be repaired, uses up proteins in muscle repair and, most important of all, increases oxidation damage and suppresses the immune system. If you are hooked on exercise or if it is part of your job – for example, if you are a dancer, aerobic instructor or athlete – you may be well advised to take antioxidant supplements to reduce the worst of the oxidation damage before doing your turn around the block.[4]

The way forward

If the very idea of exercising makes you reach for the television remote control, remember that any activity is good and that benefits can be cumulative throughout the day. So if a stretch of half an hour to an hour is too much to start off with, you could break it up into manageable portions. A fifteen-minute walk in the morning, some gardening in the afternoon and a short bike ride in the evening will have the same benefit as a single longer stint. On the other hand, it is easier for some people to do it all in one go and 'get it out of the way' – resolve may flag as the day wears on.

Gentle forms of exercise are a good place to start, such as walking or gently bouncing on a mini-trampoline. Using opportunities for exercise such as walking upstairs instead of using lifts, or walking a mile instead of taking the car, can all help. Eventually you should get to the point where you exercise for half an hour or more at a level where you are increasing your heart rate but can still hold a conversation and are not completely breathless. Exercise also increases levels of endorphins in the brain – our feel-good brain chemicals – so it can help to keep your spirits up if you exercise regularly.

It is important to set realistic goals and to understand your constraints. Being unfit, having a bad knee or hip, or needing to find childcare can all make taking exercise that bit harder. On the other hand, finding a friend to exercise with or setting positive goals, such as learning a new sport, make it all the easier. Find activities which you enjoy – there is no point slogging it out if you hate what you are doing. Also, if you decide to swim or join a gym, remember that travelling for more than fifteen minutes from home or work usually condemns the initiative to failure. My personal favourites are working out at home – I just turn up the music and dance until my heart rate is up and I manage a light sweat (sorry, ladies, glow!). My other standby is an inexpensive mini-trampoline, called a rebounder, which is ideal for the odd ten minutes here and there. It has the added advantage of improving lymph flow to help cleansing and to support the immune system. Beginners on a rebounder can go as gently as they like without even letting their feet leave the tarpaulin, and this makes it very safe for people with joint or osteoporosis problems. If you do invest in a rebounder, buy one with six legs as this type is more stable than those with fewer legs. Another inexpensive and weather-proof option, though much harder work, is to use a skipping rope indoors, but build up slowly as this is quite a hefty work-out.

Weigh-in

Excess body fat is an added risk factor for breast cancer, especially for women who put on weight on their upper body, around the torso, breasts and arms, and particularly when this is post-menopausally.[5] The shift for many women in later years from a gynoid (female) shape to an android (male) body shape, where weight is put on around the waist and above, is associated with a one-and-a-half times increase in risk for breast cancer. The main reason for this is probably because fat both produces and stores oestrogens. Because of this, if you are overweight and post-menopausal, or nearly post-menopausal, a policy of gradual fat reduction, over time, is probably a good idea.

There are three major caveats to this. If you are currently under a lot of stress, with a diagnosis of breast cancer or treatment, the last thing you need is the added stress of worrying about excess weight. It may not be the right time for you to go on a weight-loss diet, but if you are increasing your overall consumption of fruits, vegetables and pulses, concentrating on eating healthy fats and reducing harmful fats, and gently increasing exercise, you may surprise yourself and find that you are losing weight slowly at the same time, without consciously dieting to lose weight. It is also possible that you are having chemotherapy or are on Tamoxifen, which is having a temporary effect of increasing your body weight. In this case you may want to keep your weight under control, but you should not become panicked about it as you will probably return to your usual weight when you stop these treatments.

Finally, it is absolutely not a good idea to go on a calorie-restricted crash diet and attempt to lose large amounts of weight in a short timespan if you currently have breast cancer. First of all, you need a highly nutritious diet while dealing with breast cancer, and severely calorie-restricted diets cannot accomplish this. Second, crash-dieting raises oxidation damage of tissues, and one of the key aims of an anti-breast cancer regime is to keep oxidation damage to a minimum in order to avoid overburdening the immune system. So if you do need to lose excess fat, it is a good idea to do it in a relaxed way over time, and not to do it too quickly or let it become the cause of anxiety.

Curbing chemicals

Our exposure to harmful oestrogens from chemicals in the environment, called xenoestrogens, is on the increase, and to a large degree is unquantifiable. Despite the fact that the situation is escalating and seems to be difficult to control, there are a number of measures that we can take to reduce our risk of exposure from foods and in our homes. The following steps to avoid sources of xenoestrogens could have far-reaching, beneficial effects for your health.

- Minimize your use of plastics coming into contact with food, in particular soft pliable plastics such as food-wrap. Plastics are a source of oestrogenic nonylphenols which leach into fatty foods and, to a lesser degree, into water. Use ceramic or glass storage jars and PVC-free clingfilm to store food. You can wrap food for the freezer in greaseproof paper surrounded by a layer of aluminium foil (it may not be a good idea to let aluminium foil get into contact with food). Buy and store water in glass bottles, or in very rigid plastic containers.
- Filter your water, use a water distiller or buy bottled mineral water in glass bottles – spring water is not necessarily a good source, as the term 'spring water' can include well water from agricultural areas.
- Restrict your intake of animal fats. Oestrogen-mimicking chemicals include pesticides and insecticides and these are stored in animal fats and dissolved in vegetable oils. Trim visible fat off meat and reduce or cut out fatty dairy products, such as cream, butter, full- or half-fat milk.
- Eat organic food as far as possible, as this produce has not been directly exposed to environmental chemicals which have an oes-trogenic action. Meat, dairy produce and eggs which are organically produced will have a minimum amount of xenoestrogens stored in the fat. Organic vegetables, juices, wines, canned foods, baking products, teas, snacks, prepared desserts and many other products are all available. See the **Resources** section for how to find infor-mation about organic suppliers.
- Include as many phytoestrogen-rich foods, such as soya, linseeds, chick-peas, legumes, grains and vegetables, in your diet as possible, as well as adding in the spice turmeric. These help to antagonize environmental oestrogens, presumably by competing at cell recep-tor sites, thus reducing their negative effects.[6]
- Restrict canned foods as the linings of the tin cans are usually lacquered with an oestrogen-leaching compound. The worst offenders are likely to be foods packed in oil, so choose fish which is packed in brine or spring water.
- Keep your exposure to household chemicals, many of which are xenoestrogens, to a bare minimum. Do not use herbicides or

pesticides in the garden. Use paper products that are unbleached –
bathroom paper, kitchen roll, coffee filters (if you still have a coffee
habit after reading this book!) and stationery. Use chlorine-free
tampons and sanitary towels – chlorine-free alternatives to bleach
are also available. Aerosol propellants are best avoided, including
cosmetic aerosols like hair spray and anti-perspirants. If you have
any dry-cleaned garments make sure that they are well aired before
bringing them into the house.

■ Use a barrier method of birth control, or work with your cycle,
instead of using the contraceptive pill. Consider using natural
methods to control menopausal symptoms instead of using HRT.
If you are concerned about post-menopausal problems such as
increased risk of cardiovascular disease or osteoporosis, investigate
whether natural progesterone, along with dietary changes, would
be appropriate for you instead of HRT (for more information see
Managing your menopause naturally, page 261, in the chapter
Harmonizing Hormones).

How far do you take all this? It depends on your mindset and your
habits. I was once asked by a nutrition student if avoiding chlorinated
products also meant avoiding swimming pools. This is a perfect
example of how we must get the balance right. It is obvious that the
benefits of exercise are huge, and to avoid something as pleasurable
as swimming would be a great shame. We cannot possibly do it all –
no doubt some people may find the perfect solution to all problems,
but in the real world it is probably best to do what you can to reduce
xenoestrogens in your environment, especially if you have a great
deal of exposure, and then relax about the rest.

Popping the pill

The contraceptive pill was probably one of the major facilitators of
the social changes which came about from the 1960s onwards. For
the first time in history women had the ability to control their fertility
easily and effectively. But there is always a price to pay for privileges
– there is no such thing as a free lunch. The speed with which the
contraceptive pill became available has been widely criticized, and it

was viewed by many as a huge, uncontrolled, experiment at the expense of millions of unsuspecting women. Of course, the perceived benefits are extremely attractive to young women who do not wish to start a family, and by the end of the 1970s nine out of ten young women in the UK had taken the pill. Looking at the difference in influences on breast cancer between industrialized Japan, and the UK and the USA, it is interesting to note that the contraceptive pill is still banned in Japan.

Recent research in 1998 from the Royal College of General Practitioners concluded that ten years after stopping the contraceptive pill women had no greater risk of some cancers or heart disease than those that did not take the pill (though there is increased risk whilst taking it and just after). However it did acknowledge that there was still a slightly increased risk of breast cancer.

Length of time on the pill also affects risk – if you have been on the pill for a relatively short time, the risk of breast cancer is fairly small, but using the pill for four or more years before a first pregnancy is associated with increased risk.[7]

Any woman trying to decide whether to take the contraceptive pill needs to weigh up the issues. Specifically, are the risks of unwanted pregnancies greater than the risks associated with breast cancer, especially among younger women before they have had their first pregnancy? On a large-scale population basis, this may be rated as important when considering the increase in teenage pregnancies, since adopting less convenient forms of contraception can be unreliable. However, it is still a question that every woman – teenager or adult – should answer for herself. What are the alternatives to the contraceptive pill and how can they be used within the context of the individual woman's reproductive and personal life? This is often not even considered as prescriptions for the pill are handed out without debate. Other options for controlling pregnancy include the coil (which can result in heavy bleeding in some women, and some coils can raise body copper levels), barrier methods such as the cap and the condom, and timing intercourse for infertile periods, as in the Billings method (see **Resources** section).

Another point to take on board about the pill is that it depletes nutrients in the body, in particular B vitamins and magnesium. It also

189

increases copper to high levels and copper competes and interferes with zinc in the body – zinc is required for healthy cell division. In cases where the pill is being prescribed to control pre-menstrual problems, or excessive bleeding during menstruation, or sometimes even to control acne, it must be questioned whether it is appropriate to suppress these symptoms with a drug which has possible serious consequences. It would seem more appropriate to seek to discover causative factors for these symptoms which could include diet, lifestyle and environmental factors.

Any woman who has had breast cancer, or who is over thirty-five (when the risk of breast cancer begins to rise), or who smokes heavily (when there is an increased risk of thrombosis) is usually denied the pill by her GP. Personally, I think it undesirable to wait for these increased risks to manifest themselves, and recommend working out other ways to control fertility.

One group of women who definitely should not take the pill, but who are most likely to, are the under-twenty year age group. Twenty thousand young girls under the age of sixteen – lower than the age of consent per year – consult their doctors or family planning associations to seek contraception, and a large proportion of them will be given the pill. However, women who start to take the pill before the age of twenty have a massive 50 per cent increased risk of developing breast cancer subsequently. This increased risk was first noted by Dr Malcolm Pike in the *Lancet* in 1983; he was savagely criticized for scare-mongering, and the study was dismissed as flawed. Since then studies have confirmed Dr Pike's original observations, but there has still been no directive to doctors to change their prescribing habits for this vulnerable group of young women.[8]

Forever young

HRT increases the risk of breast cancer. A recent meta-study based on fifty-one separate studies worldwide[9] concluded that an extra two women per 1,000 would develop breast cancer if HRT were taken for five years, six per 1,000 if taken for ten years, and twelve per 1,000 if taken for fifteen years. As prescriptions for HRT have increased two and a half times from around 2½ million per year in 1989 to 6½ million in 1997,[10] this means we are probably sitting on a time-bomb.

It seems fairly clear that the increased risk is associated with prolonged exposure to oestrogens, but it is also probable that there is a negative impact from the synthetic progestogens included in the preparation. It is argued by supporters of HRT that this increased risk must be weighed in the balance against its purported benefits.

It is also argued that whilst there might be an increased risk of breast cancer associated with long-term use of HRT, the mortality rates appear no higher. This is not fully confirmed but, in the meantime, do you really need the increased risk of developing breast cancer with all the implications of treatment, and worry to you and your family, which such a diagnosis would imply? The problem with statistics is that they are also real people.

It is easy to view HRT as a fountain of youth. Yet you very rarely hear mentioned that an early menopause is protective against breast cancer because, once again, there is a reduction in oestrogen levels from exposure to menstrual cycles.

The many claimed benefits of HRT are very appealing indeed – the ability to avoid the changes to a woman's body that comes with the pre-menopausal phase such as hot flushes and dry vagina, protection from osteoporosis (the crumbling bone disease) and lowered risk of cardiovascular disease. But any drug has its downside, a price to pay.

In the short term, HRT does not always suit all women, who may find that they have significant symptoms such as weight gain, bloating and headaches – half of all women give up HRT within six months of starting to take it. But more interestingly, in relation to its longer-term, well-advertised benefits, it would appear on closer scrutiny that HRT does not necessarily confer the benefits promoted so heavily by the manufacturers of these drugs, who have a huge financial interest in the sale of these medications.

We are also falling into a trap of viewing the menopause as a deficiency disease, rather than a natural step in a woman's life cycle. Suppressing the symptoms of menopause rather than looking at what the underlying causes might be is a highly questionable process. Japanese women, about whom you have heard much in this book, experience far fewer menopausal symptoms when compared to Western women, and there is no word for hot flushes in the Japanese language.

There are more natural ways of managing the process. A diet high in plant hormones has been shown to help reduce the symptoms associated with the pre-menopausal transition phase, and several supplements – vitamins, essential fats and herbs – have been shown to have a tremendous impact on these symptoms. Osteoporosis incidence is very low in societies with diets which are high in vegetables and fruits and low in dairy produce, meat, salt and alcohol, and where smoking is low and physical work high – in other words, the opposite of a typical Western lifestyle and diet. Heart disease is hugely influenced by lifestyle and diet – stress, salt, fats, smoking and vegetable and fruit intake all influence the progress of cardiovascular problems.

So why not approach these post-menopausal problems from a preventive point of view? Obviously, changes in lifestyle and diet are not as easy as taking a pill once a day, or wearing a patch, and it takes time to see the effects.

Questions have also been raised about the supposed protective effects of HRT. The retrospective studies which showed a protective effect of HRT against cardiovascular disease did not allow for the possibility that women who have taken HRT are more likely to be in the higher socio-economic groups (what the advertisers call an ABC profile) and, statistically, are more likely to have a diet which is protective against cardiovascular problems. These studies are, by and large, financed by the pharmaceutical industry, and it is in the interest of pharmaceutical companies to avoid considering these questions. When the HRT users in the higher socio-economic groups are compared with the non-HRT users, who are more likely to be in lower socio-economic groups, with diets more conducive to cardiovascular problems, it seems extraordinary that such major factors as diet and lifestyle are not taken into consideration.

Osteoporosis is a dangerous condition which manifests itself in broken hips or crushed vertebrae and kills many people, both women and men, every year. Oestrogen in HRT slows down the process. But again, it is important to look at the details. Oestrogen does not build bone, but it does stop the degeneration process by slowing down bone loss. While this is helpful, it is nowhere near as useful as encouraging deposition of minerals in bones to increase bone density. Progesterone (not the progestogens found in HRT) is one of the hormones which helps to increase bone density. Most women do not stay on HRT for more than ten years as they usually do not want to continue experiencing breast tenderness and bleeding into their sixties and seventies. But when HRT is stopped, the bone loss is accelerated, and by the age of eighty there is little difference in hip and wrist fractures between HRT and non-HRT users. A study in the *New England Journal of Medicine* showed that women who had never taken HRT would expect to lose 30 per cent of their bone density by age eighty, while women who had taken HRT for ten years lost 27 per cent of bone density by the same age. They concluded that '[HRT] may have little residual effect on bone density among women seventy-five years of age or older, who have the highest risk of fracture'.[11] It is around this age that bone fractures are likely to occur, so it is not of much use to someone to maintain their bone density up to the age of sixty-five or seventy, only to find that they have no benefit at the age of eighty, which is when it would count. For more information see **Managing your menopause naturally** (page 261).

Benign breast lump solutions

Apart from the subjects of avoiding and recovering from breast cancer, a few points need to be made about benign breast problems – the lumps, bumps and discomforts which we would all rather live without. Twice as many women have some form of benign breast disease as have breast cancer – one in five versus one in eleven. Remember, however, that if you have a lump that remains suspicious you *must* have it checked out by your doctor.

The cause of benign breast disease is probably linked to oestrogen and progesterone balance, since benign conditions do not generally appear before menstruation or after menopause.

If you suffer in any way from such problems there are a number of possible solutions:

- If you have cyclical pain and discomfort linked to your periods, the obvious answer is to aim to balance your hormones. Women are sometimes put on the contraceptive pill to ease the situation, but this measure only masks the problem and does not address why it is occurring in the first place. And, of course, the hormones in the pill are probably detrimental to long-term health. The strategies that have the best effect on balancing pre-menstrual problems, including swollen and uncomfortable breasts, are:

– Balancing blood-sugar levels as the hormones that regulate blood-sugar balance also have an impact on female hormone (oestrogen and progesterone) balance. See **Blood-sugar balance** in the chapter **Harmonizing Hormones**, page 246).
– Avoiding wheat, and sometimes other gluten grains. To do this avoid all bread, pasta, biscuits, pastry and cakes for at least two months to see if this has an effect on your pre-menstrual breast symptoms.
– Magnesium levels often need to be boosted to reduce any water retention problems – take a dose of around 400 mg daily for two or three months to see if this is effective. Dietary sources of magnesium are green leafy vegetables, fresh seeds and nuts.
– Vitamin B6 can also ease pre-menstrual symptoms significantly. 100–150 mg daily can be very effective, though it is best to take a B-complex supplement alongside the B6.
– The Chinese herb Dong Quai has a balancing effect on female hormones and can help to regulate pre-menstrual swings. Take it for at least two or three cycles to decide if the herb is having an effect.

■ A high intake of caffeine has been specifically linked to breast pain and to fibrocystic disease. Cutting out all sources of caffeine for three months can be very useful for some women to determine if caffeine is related to their problem. Caffeine is found in coffee, black tea, green tea, chocolate, colas and some pain-killers and cold remedies.

■ Evening primrose oil is often found to be helpful, and is even available on prescription from your doctor. However, the doses prescribed are usually on the low side and you may need to make up the amount from supplements you buy. One gram of evening primrose oil gives 100 mg of GLA, the active compound. 100–200 mg of GLA is the level which seems to help most people. You can also get more concentrated sources of GLA from star flower, borage oil and raspberry seed oil. Very rarely some people find that their symptoms get worse using evening primrose oil and this is likely to mean that they already have a surfeit of the omega-6 fats, causing increased inflammation. It is then necessary to balance this out by having more omega-3 fats from oily fish or flax oil.

- Another supplement to experiment with in the case of benign breast disease, which is helpful for some women, is vitamin E. A dosage of 800 ius for three months may help. If this dose is found effective, then you can experiment with cutting back to half this level after three months as a maintenance dose. It is not known exactly how vitamin E might have a beneficial effect but it alters levels of various hormones including adrenal androgens and the gonadotrophins and this may help to explain its action. Do not take vitamin E in high doses if you are using blood-thinning medication such as Warfarin (see **Vitamins** (page 159) and **Minerals** (page 167)). Trials testing vitamin E for benign breast disease have had mixed results, and it may be that it is more effective if taken alongside the other antioxidant vitamins (vitamins A, C and beta-carotene), especially since vitamin A has been shown to have a therapeutic effect on benign breast problems.

Other help can be found through massage and detoxification:

- A remarkable method, which helped me personally after suffering two years of discomfort after surgery, is called the breast congestion technique. It is unclear how or why this works, but I can vouch that it did for me. It involves the therapist massaging lymphatic points on the outer legs which relate to the breast area and, in so doing, helping to dissolve lumpy breast tissue. It is imperative that this technique is not used to attempt to deal with breast cancer lumps, but once a lump is known to be benign, this form of massage can be used safely. It seems to work in more than half of cases, and is therefore worth trying. You may want to ensure that the therapist you see is female as it also involves light touch, though not massage, to the area of the breast that is lumpy, congested or painful. To find a therapist see the **Resources** section.
- Most natural therapists would view benign breast disease as being related to hormone balance, as above, and to an excess of toxins

building up in the breast tissue. Detoxification is discussed in the chapter **Detox Your System** (see page 282) and deals with all aspects, including diet and improving lymph flow with manual lymphatic drainage, skin-brushing and rebounding. All these measures are appropriate for benign breast problems and usually bring tremendous relief.

Close companions

And now a word about our breasts' closest companion – the brassière.

The type of bra that a woman chooses is likely to be governed by questions of fashion and appearance, as well as comfort. About 70 to 80 per cent of bras purchased are badly fitted or not fitted at all. This may suggest interest solely in the fashionable aspect of underwear, or that many women are too shy to be fitted properly or simply do not have the time or consider it important. Most good department stores or specialized lingerie shops are happy to give a proper fitting – just ask.

From the perspective of breast cancer or benign breast disease, when you take into account that the lymph system is responsible for keeping the breast tissue cleansed, by dealing with unfriendly organisms, it follows that it is a good idea to allow the lymph to flow freely in order to perform its functions to the optimum. For this reason, I would suggest that a well-fitting bra is essential and one that does not constrict or press into the tissue surrounding the breasts is ideal. This automatically precludes underwired bras. The bras which constrict the least are those with wide support straps and cups that support well and do not 'dig in' underneath. Ideally, they should be made from elasticized cotton, which allows the skin to breathe, rather than man-made fabrics which do not. If the breasts are of radically different sizes, it is the larger breast that needs to be accommodated, and some light padding can be added to the cup for the smaller breast.

Special bras for women who have had mastectomies are readily available. See the **Resources** section for addresses.

Part 3 **Your Basic Nutrition and Supplement Plan**

If you are eager to incorporate protective measures against breast cancer into your diet, you may have skipped straight from the introduction to these pages. They set out the most important changes to make to your diet, with details about how to achieve them efficiently. If you have not done so already, you can refer back to Part II for the explanations which may make the transitions easier to understand.

The following measures are the basic platform from which to create your action plan. They are appropriate for everyone interested in minimizing their risk of developing breast cancer, and for moving towards recovery. These first steps are the bedrock and, once secured, you can go on to tailor your plan individually by identifying which of the **Five Pillars of Health** (page 235) apply to you, and decide whether you want to incorporate the information regarding supplements.

Making Changes

We all live with entrenched habits. We have ways of doing things that are comfortingly familiar and make life easy by not having to think about how to go about a particular task or activity. Changes in life happen, but they happen at different speeds for different people. Some are naturally motivated individuals, or have been motivated by circumstances – for instance, being diagnosed with breast cancer. Some are less so, or feel the idea of moving into new spheres is destabilizing.

It may not be an easy matter to change your diet. Often we have been eating in a particular way for our entire lives, possibly in much the same way as our parents and grandparents did. It could be that consciously or unconsciously we feel we are fixed into a particular routine which dictates certain eating patterns – perhaps you work shifts, or late nights, or in an office with no preparation facilities, or on a site with a works canteen and not much choice? Eating habits may also be dictated by the whole family's likes and dislikes. All of these are real problems which cannot be swept under the carpet, but creative ways can be found to move forward. Some people are adventurous and flexible in their dietary choices, but for many, the idea of not having their coffee and doughnut when they get into the office may be quite upsetting.

If changes are necessary, clearly it is much easier to make them at a pace which you find comfortable. If it causes stress to alter eating habits it will not be as successful as if you enjoy the process.

So there is the first tip – enjoy the process. Put food higher up the agenda than it may have been previously, and make more time to shop for new ingredients and learn how to prepare them. This includes making your food look attractive – we eat with all our senses, including our eyes.

To avoid any sense of pressure, make one change at a time instead of overwhelming yourself. Make this the week that you test different herbal teas, next week experiment with soya products, increase oily fish in your diet the week after. And so on.

You may need to think through the practicalities of eating in a new way. If, for instance, you have decided to switch to brown rice, but your family insist on white, cooking a meal is inevitably going to be more time-consuming. You could, for instance, make brown rice and freeze it, so that you can take out a portion for yourself whenever you need it. Of course, persuading the rest of the family to eat brown rice can only be healthy for them, but sometimes it just isn't worth the long faces, and it may be better to lead by example.

There are many ways to solve the problems of dietary changes and you may need to be creative. Certainly, making good use of your freezer is an important tactic. Fish freezes well, as do individual portions of beans and pulses. Having a ready selection of meals that you made at quieter times ensures that you have healthy options available for periods when you are too busy to cook, though a good store cupboard means that you can usually throw together a fifteen-minute meal which is delicious and full of nutrients.

Your Basic Nutrition Plan

The first, and the majority, of the following measures are expressed in positive terms – in other words, how to add more 'good' things into your regime. The theory behind this is that, if you do these things, you will automatically crowd out the negative factors, as there is less room or time for them. Inevitably there will be a few 'don'ts' as well as 'do's', but my hope is that by the time you get to the 'don'ts' you will find that you have, at the very least, reduced them in number and significance. It is difficult to find an order of priority as all the measures will have a synergistic effect, raising your level of health and fitness, and helping you to avoid or recover from breast cancer.

It is probably asking a bit much of yourself to become an overnight convert to new eating habits, and you will find some measures easier than others. I suggest that you tick the ones you are taking already, and then aim to introduce one new measure every so often until you have worked through the list. You may need to re-read this section at intervals as a sort of stock-check to make sure that you are not slipping back into old habits. If you find the changes stressful or complicated, re-examine how you are tackling them. Are you trying to do too much in one go? Are you well prepared and organized – for example, with your store cupboard, shopping and food preparation? Do you have the support of your family? Is your work environment conducive to adopting these measures, and if not how can you overcome the drawbacks?

If you do not like a particular measure – you may hate fish or tofu – I have given ideas on how to compensate by putting in alternatives and easy tips. Good luck with making these positive changes, and enjoy the process!

Travels with my kitchen

We've had over-the-top PC (politically correct) and we may be in danger of a new hazard: over-the-top DC (dietarily correct), but this need not be the case. It may have seemed in the past that the diet police insisted that eating healthily also meant unexciting and tasteless meals. Not long ago standard supermarket items, such as sun-dried tomatoes and kiwi fruit, would have seemed impossibly exotic. Now they are almost staples. Increased world-wide travel has exposed us to a variety of culinary experiences and these can give us an insight into how to get the best out of ingredients which we know are healthy:

- In India, vegetables, pulses, rice and spices are at the heart of the delicious dishes the Indians create.
- The Middle East is the source of tasty delights focusing on legumes, fish, nuts, seeds and salads.
- Japan is famous for its fish- and soya-based, low-fat meals.
- In the Mediterranean, maximum use is made of fruit, vegetables, olive oil, herbs and fish.
- Mexico is the home of low-fat tortillas, bean and fish dishes.
- Many cultures eat mezze or hors-d'oeuvre-type meals featuring pulses, fish and vegetables and offering infinite variety.

Preparation methods in other cultures also emphasize healthier cooking methods such as steaming, baking and stir-frying, which use a minimum of fats and retain maximum nutrients.

Choosing the best ingredients and the healthiest eating habits and cooking methods from around the globe can give us the best opportunity to avoid breast cancer. Here, in a nutshell, are twelve basic steps which you can incorporate into your meal planning – starting today.

Step 1. Eat a minimum of five portions of fruits and vegetables daily

This is the most basic anti-cancer advice, on which all authorities agree. In an ideal world, it is even better to aim for more – perhaps seven to ten portions a day. All fruits and vegetables count, but potatoes, pulses, nuts, seeds and grains are not included. The minimum of five portions should total 400 g/14 oz in weight, which means that a portion of fruit is usually a whole piece or equivalent weighing around 80 g/3 oz – 1 orange, 1 apple, 1 peach, 1 banana, 2 plums, 2 kiwi fruits, ½ grapefruit, 2 tangerines, a large slice of melon. For vegetables this would mean a cup (a standard-sized mug) of densely packed vegetables. A wine glassful of vegetable or fruit juice also counts as a portion.

The most useful fruits and vegetables in antioxidant terms are the purple, red, orange and yellow ones. In colour terms this could mean:

Purple	Aubergine, red onions, beetroot, plums, blackberries, cherries, blueberries, red grapes
Red	Red peppers, tomatoes, strawberries, raspberries, pink grapefruit, watermelon
Orange	Carrots, sweet potatoes, cantaloupe melons, apricots, oranges, mangoes
Yellow	Yellow peppers, sweetcorn, squashes

The most potent anti-cancer fighters are members of the cruciferous family: broccoli, cabbage, kale, Brussels sprouts, cauliflower, collards, kale, bok choy, arugula, horseradish, radishes, swede (rutabaga), turnips, kohlrabi, and having a portion or two of these a day is highly protective.

I find it most useful to front-load my day with fruits at breakfast-time and as snacks in the morning. This means that whatever happens with the rest of the day, I know I have fulfilled my 'Give me five' commitment. Fruit is the perfect fast food, so if you are having breakfast on the run you might take three pieces of fruit to munch in the car or on the train, while dropping the children off at school or going into work. If you have more time, you can make a large fruit salad to enjoy with live yoghurt, or a breakfast-in-a-glass (see page 118), have a piece of fruit chopped up with porridge or other cereal along with freshly squeezed juice, or make up a fruit plate with cottage cheese. Mid-morning, you could have another piece of fruit as a snack. Lunch could be a kitchen-sink salad (salad with at least seven to ten different ingredients, see page 78); some hummus; roasted red peppers (see page 103) and other vegetables; baked potato with fresh coleslaw made with yoghurt; lentil soup or an avocado, tomato, basil and balsamic vinegar sandwich. All these lunches are quick and light, and are vegetable-based. The rest of the day can then pretty much take care of itself.

Juices

Getting in the juicing habit is a bonus on many levels. Juices are a concentrated source of antioxidants, chlorophyll and other phyto-nutrients, they are terrific cleansers and energy boosters – and the very act of making them makes you feel that you are nurturing yourself.

There are four types of juicing machine. The first is the citrus juicer which many homes are likely to have already. This is only suitable for oranges, lemons, grapefruits and other citrus fruits. Next comes the blender which, again, many homes will have. You can put in all kinds of soft fruits, such as ripe pears, peaches, grapes, bananas or strawberries, and whizz them up with water, crushed ice, milk, soya milk, yoghurt or soya ice-cream for a liquid 'full fruit' drink that has all the fibre of the original fruit (you will need to peel some fruits before blending in this way).

The other two types of juicer separate juice from the whole fruit or vegetable – to take carrot as an example, they extract juice from the root. The two types of extractor are centrifugal and non-centrifugal machines. The centrifugal types are fairly inexpensive, are made by all the main electrical goods manufacturers and are available from most department stores. They shred the ingredients and then spin them at high speed to extract the juice. While fairly efficient, this type does not extract the juice from unbroken cell-wall matter, meaning that you do not get the full benefit from the fruit or vegetable. Never-theless, for most people embarking on juicing for the first time, this less expensive option is a reasonable one.

The non-centrifugal type is much more expensive and is available from speciality suppliers (see the **Resources** section). Its merits over the centrifugal type are that it breaks down the cell walls of the plant matter and therefore liberates all the nutrients and enzymes that are intrinsic to the vegetable or fruit. Special nutrition-based cancer therapies, such as the Gerson therapy, insist on using this type of juicer, along with a special press which improves the performance further. For real juice devotees this more high-powered type of juicer is a sound investment as it is likely to last a lifetime.

Juicing is quick and easy to do. You do not even need to peel many fruits or vegetables or deseed them, though you do need to wash them thoroughly, especially if they are not organic. The only minor irritation is washing the machine parts, and a good tip is to soak them in a sinkful of water within moments of making the juice. It is also a good idea to bear this in mind when you buy your machine. Take it apart to see how easy it is to disassemble and if there are any little 'nooks' that will be hard to clean.

Carrots and apples are good bases for juices and you can add in a myriad of other ingredients depending on your needs or whims.

Some therapeutic juices to try are:

Liver detoxifiers: The following vegetable juices are renowned for encouraging the liver to work efficiently. Mix them in any combination you like, three to four vegetables in each drink, according to taste, about 150–225 ml/5–8 fl oz of each juice unless otherwise stated. You can also include apples in the juice. If you are on drug treatment, you may want to take this juice daily:

Carrot, beetroot, celery, cucumber, spinach, parsley (50 ml/2 fl oz), artichoke (50 ml/2 fl oz), dandelion (50 ml/2 fl oz), asparagus (75 ml/3 fl oz), watercress (50 ml/2 fl oz), lemon or lime juice (50 ml/2 fl oz), grapes, peach.

Digestive restorers: These vegetables and fruits have therapeutic properties for healing the digestive tract, restoring bacterial balance and easing digestion. You can also add in some plain live yoghurt for the beneficial bacteria, and ground linseeds. Use carrot or apple as a base and add in two to three of the following, about 150–225 ml/5–8 fl oz juice of each unless otherwise stated:

Green cabbage, raw potato, beetroot, tomatoes, nettle (50 ml/2 fl oz), garlic (1–2 cloves), lettuce (75 ml/3 fl oz), endive (75 ml/3 fl oz), radish (50 ml/2 fl oz), water from a coconut, papaya, pineapple, pear.

Energy boosters: The carrot and apple base will give a quick 'hit' of blood sugar, without the negative impact of a sugary snack. Add in

150–225 ml/5–8 fl oz juice of any of the following unless otherwise stated:

Beetroot, parsnip, watercress (50 ml/2 fl oz), lettuce (75 ml/3 fl oz), spinach (75 ml/3 fl oz), lemon, orange, raspberries, strawberries, ginger (1 cm/½ in cube).

Step 2. Eat at least three portions of oily fish a week

The omega-3 fats contained in oily fish have potent anti-cancer properties and are delicious as well. Fish freezes particularly well and is best cooked in a short time to retain its succulent flavours. So if you buy really fresh fish and then freeze it quickly in portion sizes, it makes the perfect fast food.

Canned fish is an excellent store-cupboard standby. The valuable fish oils are not significantly altered by the canning process; this is done under vacuum conditions, which means that oxygen, and oxidation damage, do not alter the oils. The only exception to this rule is tuna, where the fish oil content is significantly lower than in the fresh fish. The cans do leach some oestrogenic compounds into the vegetable oils used to pack the fish, so it is advisable to buy canned fish which is packed in spring water, or in brine, and then to run off as much of the salt water as you can. In any event the vegetable oils used to pack the fish are best avoided as they are high sources of omega-6 fats and add excess calories.

Fish with the most omega-3 oils (1.5–3.5 g oils per 100 g/4 oz portion) are:

Tuna, mackerel (NB smoked mackerel has over 6 g omega-3 oils per 100 g/4 oz), sardines (fresh or canned), herrings, pink trout, sprats, sturgeon, eel, anchovies, pilchards, kippers, salmon (fresh or canned), mullet, bream

Fish with medium amounts of omega-3 oils (0.5–1.5 g oils per 100 g/ 4 oz portion) are:

Halibut, bass, smelt, shark, oyster, swordfish, trout

Fish with the least omega-3 oils (less than 0.5 g oils per 100 g/4 oz portion) are:

Tuna (canned, vegetable oil drained), cod, carp, coley, prawns, mussels, haddock

Fish is easy to incorporate into the diet – added to salads (salad Niçoise, tonno e fagiole (see page 248), etc.), sandwiches (salmon, sardines, anchovies), as fillings for baked potatoes, rice dishes (kedgeree, fish curry), or in omelettes.

Smoked foods pose a bit of a dilemma for the ardent anti-cancer fighter. The process of smoking food results in carcinogens which are best avoided. So any chargrilled, barbecued or smoked foods should, theoretically, be eliminated or cut back to a bare minimum. Many fish dishes are enjoyed by people precisely because they are smoked: smoked salmon, kippers, smoked herrings, smoked mackerel. In view of the valuable oils they contain, there may be a case for relaxing here occasionally as long as you don't over-expose yourself to other sources of carcinogens from smoked foods, such as bacon. The balanced advice might be to ensure that lots of antioxidant-rich fruits and vegetables are eaten alongside the smoked fish to give your body a defence shield.

Instant Mackerel Pâté

½ a 100 g/4 oz tub of cottage cheese makes the pâté more fishy, and the whole tub makes it more 'creamy' and lower in fat. An even more breast-cancer correct version is to substitute silken tofu for some or all of the cottage cheese, in which case the pâté needs a touch more lemon, according to taste.

1 smoked mackerel fillet, all bones removed
50–100 g/2–4 oz low-fat cottage cheese or silken tofu
juice of ½ lemon
chopped parsley

Put all the ingredients into a blender and whizz up until smooth. Spread on rye crackers or hot wholemeal bread and enjoy with a tomato, basil and balsamic vinegar salad or a grilled red, yellow and orange pepper salad dressed with balsamic vinegar. The pâté will keep well in the fridge for two to three days.

Some people simply do not like fish, no matter how good it is for them, or they may be vegetarians or vegans. The oils provided by fish have been shown to be the most beneficial, but the family of fats known as the omega-3 fats also include the fats found in cold-pressed flax oil and pumpkin seeds. An alternative option to eating fish might be to take some fish oil capsules and/or to have a tablespoon of cold-pressed flax oil daily. The essential fat in flax oil, alpha-linolenic acid, converts into the EPA/DHA fats in the body at the ratio of about 10 to 1 and it has not been determined if this process is as useful as getting EPA/DHA directly from fish in terms of its effect on cancer. However, it does appear to have beneficial effects in its own right on late-stage breast tumours, and there are many other health benefits associated with this level of flax oil being taken daily, including improving skin quality and liver function. Some people find that taking a whole tablespoon of oil in one go is too much of a strain on their liver, and it can make them nauseous. If this happens, either divide the dose, or start small and build up slowly to one or even two tablespoons. It also may be best to take your antioxidant supplement alongside the oil to protect against lipid (fat) peroxidation.

Step 3. Eat a portion of beans or other pulses daily

A cup of pulses a day, around 200 g/7 oz, provides about 12 g/½ oz of fibre, a significant part of which will be lignans which have potent anti-breast cancer properties. Pulses also come loaded with protease inhibitors which have similarly beneficial effects.

In some countries beans are eaten as a regular part of the diet, and it is often the most economically deprived countries that have this healthy habit. Beans, pulses, lentils – all legumes – are just about the cheapest foods around, and they have the advantage of being very filling and are a good substitute for grains for people who are wheat or grain sensitive.

Cooking beans to get rid of the 'flatulence factor' is quite easy. First soak them, in accordance with the instructions on the packet, but change the water two or three times. You will notice bubbles rising to the top of the water, and these are some of the gases you want to get rid of. When you cook the beans, change the water a further couple of times, using freshly boiled water each time. This helps to get rid of more of the gases. It is always best to soak and cook pulses in filtered or distilled water because as they absorb the water, its quality is important to overall health. Frequently people experience gas problems because the bacterial balance in their bowels is not optimal (see the chapter **Healthy Digestion**, page 267). The best way to redress the balance is to eat a fibre-rich diet which includes lots of pulses. Canned beans are often tolerated better than freshly cooked beans, as they have been cooked that much more thoroughly. Cans make a good store-cupboard standby, but remember, if you eat too many canned foods, you will be exposing yourself to more of the oestrogens which leak from the lining of the cans. I limit myself to one or two canned foods a week – oily fish, beans or tomatoes. Freshly cooked beans, while they take some time to prepare, can be frozen in portion sizes, which equals the convenience of canned beans.

Types of pulses to stock up on could include:

Red, yellow, brown or Puy lentils, spilt peas, kidney beans, soya beans, flageolet beans, butter beans, chick-peas (garbanzo), black-eye beans, green peas, fava beans, baked beans, aduki beans, cannelini beans

Serving ideas to get your hill-o'-beans each day:

- Green peas, frozen or fresh
- Lentil soup (see page 149)
- Tonno e fagiole salad (see page 248)
- Mexican re-fried beans and tacos
- Mildly curried lentils or chick-peas – excellent with fish
- Chick-pea soup
- Hummus
- Falafel
- Baked beans, canned (salt-free, organic) or home-made
- Lentil or chick-pea curry
- Red kidney beans added to shepherd's pie or chilli (vegetarian or meat-based)
- Lamb with flageolet beans, as traditionally eaten in France
- Cooked beans added to salads

- Ful medames (Middle Eastern fava bean dip)
- Beans tossed in an olive oil and garlic-based vinaigrette as a first course or side vegetable dish
- A few handfuls of beans added to vegetable soups or stews

Step 4. Use olive oil and flax oil as your sources of added fats

Throw margarines, which are full of trans-fats, in the bin and keep butter for high days and holidays. The Mediterranean diet focuses on olive oil, and Mediterranean countries enjoy many health benefits including a strong degree of protection from breast cancer. Cold-pressed extra-virgin olive oil is rich in antioxidants and is quite stable when used for cooking, meaning that harmful trans-fats and free radicals are not so readily created. Olive oil is not, however, a good source of essential fatty acids, so this is where the flax oil comes in. Ideally, use cold-pressed flax oil on salads, or use a little as a topping on vegetables where once you might have used butter. Do not be tempted to cook with flax oil, or to use it on piping hot vegetables, as the useful essential fatty acids can be destroyed quite readily. Flax oil needs to be very fresh and is subject to rancidity if not kept properly. Buy it in dark bottles, use it by the sell-by date, keep it in the fridge and consume the oil within six weeks of opening the bottle. All oils should be stored in the fridge to keep them fresh.

If you want to use other oils such as sesame, sunflower, safflower or walnut, it is important to buy them cold-pressed as all other extraction processes are damaging to the oils – and therefore damaging to you. It is also important to buy them in small portions and to keep them refrigerated. Use them after cooking, as flavouring, rather than to cook with, as this also destroys the essential fatty acids. Unfortunately, it is difficult to use up these oils in the short period of time which does not allow them to go rancid, and since an excess of the fats that these oils contain – the omega-6 fats – has been linked to an increased risk of breast cancer (though possibly this comes more from margarines and packaged foods), I believe it is best to stick to olive oil and flax oil – this makes life simple and safe.

Step 5. Eat a portion of soya products five days a week, along with other phytoestrogen-rich foods

One serving of soya food most days of the week is probably sufficient to confer important protective benefits against breast cancer.[1] One serving would be 125 g/4–5 oz of tofu or ¼ cup/2 oz of soya flour or soya flakes to give 40–50 mg of the phytoestrogen isoflavones. (See the chart of phytoestrogen-rich soya foods in the **Phytofacts** chapter, page 119.) Persuading the average teenager, husband or partner to eat soya with you can be an uphill task, but as this food also confers protection against prostate cancer and is probably particularly useful against breast cancer when consumed in younger years, you may want to add it as an ingredient to many dishes without significantly changing your cooking habits.

Other phytoestrogen-rich foods include chick-peas, aduki beans, lentils, mung beans, fresh nuts and seeds, whole grains and vegetables.

Here is how to get soya, an almost tailor-made breast cancer-fighting food, into your and your family's diet:

Whole soya beans: Dried soya beans can be found in most health food and Asian shops, and come in yellow, brown and black versions. They can be stored in an airtight container for many months, making them a good store cupboard standby. Soya beans cook in exactly the same way as kidney beans, flageolet beans and chick-peas. Soak them in water for several hours, then simmer in plenty of water until they are tender (do not add salt to the water as this will toughen them and prevent them from cooking properly). Soya beans have a rich, nutty flavour and lend themselves to most dishes you would make with other beans, such as curries, soups, stews and Mexican dishes. Once cooked, they can be frozen for convenience. Soya beans can also be sprouted, in the same way as mung beans and other sprouted seeds, lentils, grains and beans. They are delicious as a snack on their own, added to salads, as a side vegetable, or stir-fried.

Soya mince: Also called, uninspiringly, TVP (textured soya protein). Made from soya flour and formed into mince-like shapes, TVP is dehydrated and needs to be reconstituted with boiling water. It can then be added to any number of meat dishes, to bulk them out, reduce the amount of meat in the dish, and provide the benefits of a vegetable and, of course, of soya beans. It can also be used as a complete meat replacement in a number of dishes. Ideas could include: hamburgers, shepherd's pie, 'sloppy joes', bolognese sauce and chilli with or without carne (see page 96).

Soya milk: Soya milk is making such an impact these days that it is no longer just a health food shop item, but is found in all major supermarkets. Soya milk can be used almost totally as an alternative to milk – on cereals, as a drink or in most recipes. Many brands now fortify the soya milk with nutrients such as calcium and vitamin D, to match it more closely to some of the benefits of dairy milk. If you add it to a drink and find that it curdles (it does this with coffee and some coffee substitutes such as dandelion coffee) the trick is to add the hot drink to the soya milk – this stops it from curdling.

Soya yoghurt: Never was there a more painless way of eating soya. The appearance, taste and texture of fruit-flavoured soya yoghurts are like those of any other fruit yoghurt; these yoghurts make a great dessert, and can easily be taken to work for a snack. The only downside is that they usually have added sugar, but as an occasional treat they are terrific. You can also blend plain soya yoghurt with fruit for a delicious snack, and you can get many brands of live 'bio' soya yoghurts which are helpful for regulating bowel bacteria.

Tofu: Also called bean curd, tofu is fairly tasteless but takes on the flavour of the dishes in which it is prepared, and is ideal for both savoury and dessert dishes. Three types are commonly found: firm tofu which is useful for kebabs, grills or stir-frying; soft tofu which lends itself to mashing or blending with other ingredients; and silken tofu, which has a creamy texture, making it good for purées, 'ice-creams' and 'milk' shakes. Many products have calcium added, making them a good alternative to cheese, yoghurt or milk in some dishes.

Soya flour: Soya flour is made from the whole beans and can replace a certain amount of wheat flour in many recipes, including breads, pastries and cakes (all wholemeal, of course!). Soya flour is best stored in the fridge.

Soya flakes: These can easily be added to a wide variety of foods to boost their phytoestrogen content, without significantly altering the basic dish, and adding a nutty, crunchy taste and texture. Add them to baked products, such as bread, cakes, muffins, crumbles, pies and biscuits, mix them into soups and stews, add them to minced meat dishes or sprinkle them on salads or cereals.

'Meat' products: An extensive variety of vegetarian sausages, burgers and other imitation-meat products are produced these days, and they are available from supermarkets as well as health food shops. Some people wonder why vegetarians want to be reminded of meat by these imitations, but they certainly sell well – maybe to non-vegetarians who want to increase their soya intake. Many products are high in hydrogenated fats, so it may be advisable to check the label.

Soya snacks: Soya-based 'health bars' are now available; they are similar to muesli bars and make excellent energy snacks while you are on the go – one bar can give you your daily quota of 50 mg of phytoestrogens. Roasted soya nuts resemble peanuts and can be found in good health food shops alongside nuts in the nibbles section. You can also find soya chips which are extremely more-ish.

Miso: This is a fermented soya product made from soya beans, grains, salt and beneficial bacteria. It is a smooth paste and makes a great stock or soup base. It is very high in salt, so a little goes a long way.

Step 6. Eat at least 25 g of fibre daily

Fibre in the diet is undoubtedly related to a lower incidence of breast cancer. The average person in the UK gets around 9 g of fibre daily, while the Government recommends 18 g. Research shows that a level of 25–35 g is most protective against breast cancer, and some cultures get considerably more than this.

Fibre in foods

Most packaged foods will give the fibre content in 100 g/4 oz of the product, from which you can work out the amount of fibre in a portion

214

size. Listed below are fibre values for common fresh or cooked dried foods:[2]

	Portion size	Grams of dietary fibre		Portion size	Grams of dietary fibre
Almonds	10 g/⅓ oz	1.4	Lentils, cooked	50 g/2 oz	2.0
Apples	1 medium	2.0	Lettuce	25 g/1 oz	0.3
Apricots, dried	15 g/½ oz	3.6	Linseeds	1 tablespoon	2.0
Apricots, fresh	2 medium	1.0	Melons	50 g/2 oz	0.5
Asparagus	50 g/2 oz	0.5	Muesli	25 g/1 oz	2.0
Avocado	½ medium	2.0	Mushrooms	15 g/½ oz	0.5
Bananas	1 medium	2.0	Oatmeal, uncooked	25 g/1 oz	1.7
Barley, cooked	50 g/2 oz	1.0	Okra	25 g/1.0 oz	0.5
Beans, butter, cooked	50 g/2 oz	2.5	Oranges	1 medium	2.0
Beans, French	25 g/1 oz	0.7	Parsnips	50 g/2 oz	2.0
Beans, haricot, cooked	50 g/2 oz	3.5	Peaches	1 medium	2.3
Beetroot, raw	25 g/1 oz	1.5	Peanuts	15 g/½ oz	1.4
Blackberries	15 g/½ oz	1.0	Pears	1 medium	2.0
Blackcurrants	15 g/½ oz	1.5	Peas	25 g/1 oz	1.3
Bread, white	25 g/1 oz	1.0	Pineapple	50 g/2 oz	0.5
Bread, wholemeal	25 g/1 oz	2.0	Plantain	25 g/1 oz	2.0
Broccoli	25 g/1 oz	1.0	Plums	1 medium	1.0
Brussels sprouts	25 g/1 oz	1.0	Potatoes, whole	100 g/4 oz	2.0
Buckwheat (kasha),			Prunes, dried	15 g/½ oz	2.6
cooked	50 g/2 oz	3.0	Raisins	15 g/½ oz	1.2
Cabbage	25 g/1 oz	0.7	Raspberries	25 g/1 oz	2.0
Carrots	25 g/1 oz	0.7	Rhubarb	50 g/2 oz	1.0
Cauliflower	25 g/1 oz	0.5	Rice, brown, cooked	100 g/4 oz	1.7
Celery	25 g/1 oz	0.5	Rice, white, cooked	100 g/4 oz	1.0
Cherries	25 g/1 oz	0.5	Soya flour	100 g/4 oz	11.0
Chestnuts	15 g/½ oz	1.1	Spaghetti, brown,		
Chick-peas, cooked	50 g/2 oz	3.0	cooked	100 g/4 oz	4.0
Coconut, fresh	15 g/½ oz	2.3	Spaghetti, white,		
Corn on the cob	1 medium	5.0	cooked	100 g/4 oz	2.0
Currants	10 g/⅓ oz	0.7	Spinach, cooked	25 g/1 oz	1.5
Dates, dried	15 g/½ oz	1.5	Strawberries	25 g/1 oz	0.5
Figs, dried	15 g/½ oz	3.1	Sunflower seeds	15 g/½ oz	1.2
Figs, fresh	25 g/1 oz	0.7	Swedes	50 g/2 oz	1.5
Flour, rye	100 g/4 oz	6.0	Tofu	100 g/4 oz	0.4
Flour, white	100 g/4 oz	3.0	Tomatoes	50 g/2 oz	0.7
Flour, wholemeal	100 g/4 oz	9.0	Walnuts	15 g/½ oz	0.8
Laverbread	25 g/1 oz	0.7	Yam	50 g/2 oz	2.0
Leeks	50 g/2 oz	1.5			

We need a mixture of different types of fibre from a full range of fruits, vegetables, pulses, grains, nuts and seeds. If you are currently eating a low level of fibre, and especially if you tend to be constipated, it is wise to add fibre into your diet slowly and build up by 5 g a week or every two weeks, in order not to put your digestive tract under pressure – it has been out of training for a while and needs time to tone up. It is also inadvisable to buy packets of wheat-bran and to sprinkle this on your food every day. It is far too harsh and can irritate the gut wall, and some people are particularly sensitive to large amounts of wheat products. A more balanced approach is needed, and 25–35 g can be obtained daily as follows:

Breakfast:	1 bowl of porridge or muesli, with 2 tablespoons linseeds
Lunch:	2 slices of wholemeal or rye bread
Evening:	1 serving brown rice
	1 serving legumes
	2 servings vegetables
Snacks:	4 pieces of fruit

Following the dietary recommendations in this book should ensure that you reach this target, but it may help to keep a food diary for a few days to work out if you are achieving 25 g daily. Use the chart to keep a tally.

Step 7. Add two tablespoons of linseeds to your food each day

You can buy either golden or brown linseeds, and it is always advisable to buy organic varieties, which are easy to find in health food shops. One tablespoon of linseeds gives about 2 g of fibre, which is a welcome contribution to your overall total.

Whole cracked linseeds are available. The whole seeds have the advantage of being rich in the omega-3 and omega-6 essential fatty acids which are so beneficial. To get the maximum fibre benefit from them, and therefore the maximum phytoestrogen benefit from the lignans, it is best to grind them up in your now redundant(!) coffee-grinder – not absolutely essential, but the ideal method. The other option is to buy the seeds already cracked – this is more convenient but you run the risk of the fats they contain being rancid. I prefer to use organic whole uncracked linseeds.

If you tend to have irregular bowel habits, either constipation or diarrhoea, you will find that linseeds can help to regulate the problem. However, if you are usually constipated you should add the linseeds slowly to your diet – start with half a tablespoon and build up slowly over two or three weeks to two tablespoons.

Linseeds have a nutty taste and are very versatile. They can be added to soups, baked products, juices and shakes, salads, cereals, stews, desserts and yoghurt. If you do not get the opportunity to add them to a meal, you can be heroic and soak them in water and then drink them down. They are completely tasteless when consumed this way, though they have the consistency of frog spawn! After including your linseeds in a meal, drink an extra glass of water to ensure that they swell up in the digestive tract and are able to do their job efficiently.

Flour made from linseeds is now being added to some brands of bread, dubbed 'ladies' bread' because of its phytoestrogen benefits. The resulting taste is delicious and nutty with an excellent texture.

Step 8. Buy organic food

I am not going to labour this point too much as it is covered in detail in the chapter on **Organic Food** (page 106), but this is a most important measure. If cost is an issue, examine ways in which you can bring the overall cost of your shopping basket down. Substitute bean, rice and potato dishes for meat-based meals. Use less expensive fish, such as mackerel and sardines, instead of more expensive fish. Buy produce in season and freeze it for use at other times of the year. Become more creative with cheaper vegetables and pulses – discover the recipes of the Mediterranean and the Middle and Far East for inexpensive vegetable- and bean-based dishes. Become less dependent on packaged foods and plan ahead by cooking and freezing meals which are then available when you are in a hurry (when you come back from work, for instance). If convenience is an issue, subscribe to a box scheme – nothing could be more convenient as they deliver to your door each week. Organic meat, and now fish as well, can be ordered by mail, as can a wide range of dried and bottled goods – shopping by telephone, or even the Internet, is probably here to stay.

By hook or by crook, make sure that most of your food is organic to avoid potentially harmful xenoestrogens and other chemicals, and to get a better nutritional return from your food.

Step 9. Treat meat as a condiment, not the main event, and keep dairy products to a minimum

It is best to keep meat intake to around 100 g/4 oz (uncooked weight) a day. Meat includes red meat, poultry, minced meat, meat products such as sausages (I spell this out because often I will find that people forget about minced meat or poultry, for instance, as being part of their total). If this looks a bit meagre on your plate you can stretch it out by making more dishes where chopped or shredded meat is part of a greater whole – savoury rice dishes, pasta sauces, baked potato filling, stews – 50 g/2 oz of meat in these dishes can go a long way. Cut off all visible fat and remove the skin from chicken and other fowl. Where possible eat fish, chicken breast and game as preferred sources of meat, and increase the number of vegetarian dishes you eat during the week. When you do eat meat avoid over-cooking or chargrilling as this can increase your exposure to carcinogenic compounds.

The other main source of animal protein, and animal fat, is dairy products. Cheese is really best avoided where possible as it is high in saturated fats – the occasional gratiné dish for a special occasion is not the end of the world, but avoid keeping cheese in your fridge. Soya milk is easily substituted for milk and serves the greater cause of increasing soya in the diet. Preferred sources of dairy products are yoghurt, which is a potent cancer-fighter, and cottage cheese with its useful detoxifying sulphur amino acids. Many people are dairy-intolerant and this measure will help to resolve quite a few health problems for a number of people. If you are dairy intolerant you may still be able to have the occasional treat of goat's or sheep's cheese as these are better tolerated than cow's milk cheese. If you are concerned about calcium for healthy bones, a diet which emphasizes green leafy vegetables and fresh seeds, along with yoghurt, calcium-enriched soya products and bony fish such as sardines and salmon, will provide ample calcium in a more healthy form.

Step 10. Drink at least 1.5 litres/2½ pints of filtered water daily

All our body processes are dependent on water – the enzymes which govern every single function are water-dependent. This means that thousands of chemical reactions will not occur effectively if you are dehydrated. Drinking sufficient water is probably the single most important health measure anyone can make. And it is (virtually) free. Virtually, because we need to concern ourselves with water quality – for more information on this see the chapter **Wet Your Whistle** (page 130).

Do not wait until you feel thirsty before you reach for your water glass. By the time your body is signalling thirst, you are already severely dehydrated.

1.5 litres/2½ pints of water is six large glasses of water. If I were given £1 for every time somebody told me that they could not drink six glasses of water a day, although they drink six glasses of other, dehydrating, liquids, I would be very rich indeed. The point is that we do usually drink sufficient liquid, but not in a form that the body can use – caffeinated drinks and sugary sodas are dehydrating.

There are several ways to go about ensuring sufficient water intake:

- Fill a 1.5 or 2 litre bottle with filtered water and make sure that by the end of the day you have drunk the whole bottle. Flavour it with some freshly squeezed lemon or orange juice, fresh ginger, or some mint leaves.
- At work, keep a glass of water on your desk topped up and sip from it all day.
- Make a schedule to drink your six glasses during the day – say one every two hours.
- If you prefer hot drinks and are already in the habit of putting on the kettle at certain times, switch to fruit or different types of herbal tea as these will count towards your water total.

Step 11. Reduce intake of fats to less than 30 per cent of calories

The average moderately active woman needs around 2,000 calories a day. There are 9 calories per gram of fat, therefore if she is seeking to eat no more than 30 per cent of her 2,000 daily calories from fat, she needs to have no more than 65 g of fat per day.

- The average Western diet contains around 40–45 per cent of calories from fat.
- A low-fat Western diet contains about 30 per cent of calories from fat.
- A low-fat Eastern diet contains about 20–25 per cent of calories from fat.

The Fat Content chart below[3] gives various foods and the quantities which provide a 'block' of 5 g of fat. It also gives a rough guide to what a 'block' of that food looks like visually, so that you do not have to consult the kitchen scales before you dare to eat anything!

- 40 per cent of calories from fat = 800 calories = 90 g of fat = 18 fat 'blocks' or servings
- 30 per cent of calories from fat = 600 calories = 65 g of fat = 15 fat 'blocks' or servings
- 25 per cent of calories from fat = 500 calories = 55 g of fat = 11 fat 'blocks' or servings
- 20 per cent of calories from fat = 400 calories = 45 g of fat = 9 fat 'blocks' or servings

It is not healthy, or desirable, to cut out all fats, and favouring healthy fats is vital. Cutting back on overall fat intake, while ensuring that the fats you do eat come from healthy selections (marked * in the chart opposite) is likely to have a significant impact on breast cancer risk. If you find it difficult to cut back on overall fat intake, concentrate on eating the foods marked * which provide healthy fats. This is probably the first priority and likely to have the most significant impact.

Fat content chart

Food	Serving to give 1 'block' of 5 g of fat	
	Weight	Approx. serving
Avocado*	25 g/1 oz	⅙ small
Bread, wholemeal	200 g/7 oz	8 slices
Butter	6 g/⅕ oz	1 level teaspoon
Cheese, cottage	125 g/4–5 oz	1 small tub
Cheese, cream	10 g/⅓ oz	2 teaspoons
Cheese (cheddar, stilton)	14 g/½ oz	1 cm/½ in square
Cheese (feta, Edam, camembert)	22 g/¾ oz	1.5–2 cm/¾ in sq
Egg yolks (whites are protein)	½ of 1 yolk	½ of 1 yolk
Fish, oily*, mackerel, raw	31 g/1 generous oz	⅓ medium fillet
Fish, oily*, mackerel, smoked	17 g/½ oz	⅙ medium fillet
Fish, oily*, salmon, raw	41 g/1½ oz	5 × 2 × 3 cm/2 × ¾ × 1 in
Fish, oily*, sardines, canned	43 g/1½ oz	⅓ can
Fish, oily*, tuna, canned in brine	830 g/33 oz	4 cans
Fish, prawns, cooked and shelled	275 g/9 oz	1½ cups
Fish, crab, lobster	150 g/5 oz	2½ cups
Fish, white (raw, with bones)*	800 g/32 oz	5-cm/2-in fillet
Ice-cream	50 g/2 oz	1 scoop
Legumes, soya beans*	27 g/1 oz	1 heaped tablespoon
Legumes, chick-peas*	100 g/4 oz	½ cup
Legumes, most beans and lentils*	300 g/10 oz	1½ cups
Legumes, peas*	500 g/18 oz	3¼ cups
Linseeds*	12 g/½ oz	2 level teaspoons
Mayonnaise	7 g/¼ oz	1 tsp
Meat, beef, raw	108 g/4 oz	1.5 × 10 × 8 cm/¾ × 4 × 3 in
Meat, lamb or pork, raw	62 g/2¼ oz	1.5 × 10 × 4 cm/¾ × 4 × 1½ in
Meat, chicken breast, no skin, raw	155 g/4 oz	1 medium breast
Meat, chicken leg, no skin, raw	91 g/1¾ oz	1 thigh or 2 drumsticks
Milk, full-fat	125 ml/4 fl oz	½ cup
Milk, semi-skimmed	310 ml/10 fl oz	1¼ cups
Milk, fully skimmed	negligible fat content	
Milk, soya*	260 ml/9 fl oz	1 cup
Muesli	80 g/3 oz (variable)	1¼ cups
Nuts (most varieties)†	10 g/⅓ oz	e.g. about 5 almonds
Nuts, chestnuts	185 g/6½ oz	about 24
Nuts and seed butters	9 g	1 teaspoon
Oils (olive, flax)*	5 g	1 teaspoon
Oils (all other)	5 g	1 teaspoon
Olives, pitted*	45 g/1½ oz	15 medium
Seeds*	9 g	2 teaspoons
Tofu*	120 g/4½ oz	1¼ cups
Yoghurt, low-fat	negligible fat content	
Yoghurt, Greek strained	55 g/2 oz	2 tablespoons
Yoghurt, whole-milk	165 g/6 oz	9 tablespoons

NB: Most fruits, vegetables and grains are virtually fat-free.
*Denotes source of healthy fats. We need these fats!
†Peanuts are not really nuts but are legumes. As they are frequently contaminated with aflatoxins they may be best avoided.

Packaged foods give the information on the nutrition panel and state the number of grams of fat in 100 g/4 oz of product, and you can work out from that how many grams of that particular food you can eat to get one 5-g 'block' of fat.

When choosing foods, beware of products that are labelled 'reduced fat' as these often have high amounts of sugar to compensate for the lack of flavour. Sugar, if it is not needed immediately for energy, can be metabolized into fat after it is eaten. This type of fat does not have the ability to function as the healthy fats do.

You will probably be surprised, initially, at how awkward it is on a traditional Western diet to get below 30 per cent of calories from fat. It helps to become a bit more creative with strong-tasting condiments. It is amazing how a squeeze of lemon juice on vegetables livens them up and negates the need for butter and salt. Possible low-, or no-fat, sauce ideas could include:

- A sprinkling of soy sauce
- A dash of balsamic vinegar
- Salsa, a vegetable dip available from most supermarkets
- A squeeze of fresh lemon
- Grain mustard and honey is a delicious coating for skinless chicken
- Sesame oil has a strong taste and a little goes a long way – you can sprinkle a tiny amount for a delicious taste and few calories
- Low-fat yoghurt for salads or to make creamy sauces for cooking
- Canned tomatoes with wine and garlic
- Strong-tasting herbs which include: mint, rosemary, coriander, French tarragon, basil, sage
- Strong-tasting spices which include: cumin, cloves, coriander, ginger, turmeric, cinnamon

Step 12. Foods to avoid

Avoid alcohol

This should probably come with point number three or four as there is such a close correlation between alcohol intake and breast cancer, but as I promised to give the positive steps first, this item has been relegated towards the end.

If you are at very increased risk because of elevated oestrogen levels from HRT, alcohol should be avoided or restricted severely (see **Managing your menopause naturally** in the chapter **Harmonizing Hormones**, page 260).

Here are some tips to help break the alcohol habit. If you are in the habit of drinking daily, especially if it is habitual – for example always with your evening meal, or first thing when you get home – it is as well to break the habit. Apart from anything else, there is probably an element of propping up your blood sugar and this spiral is perpetuated by such a habit. Initially you may find it easier to limit yourself to drinking on alternate days – tomorrow comes around soon enough! Other people find it easier just to stop 'cold turkey'. If you are a weekend drinker, drinking nothing during the week but heavily at weekends – perhaps enough to make up for a whole week of consumption – experiment with diluting your weekend drinks to half-strength. You may also find it easier to give up partially or totally if you switch to a different type of drink from your usual favourite. And finally, there are other drinks to have socially which look the part, so that you are not left out of the party: tomato juice, mineral water with a slice of lemon or lime, and herbal 'infusions' designed as non-alcoholic cocktails.

Avoid sugar and refined grain products

Sugar has been described as 'sweet, white and deadly' and I do not think that I can come up with a better description. No sugar is good – although significant numbers of people believe that brown sugar is somehow healthier than white, it isn't. Honey has the same effect on blood chemistry as sugar, and is probably no better, but if you buy honey that is not heat-treated (from small suppliers) you stand a better chance of getting some therapeutic value out of it. If you have a sweet tooth, eating a piece of fruit can satisfy the craving, and having a savoury snack instead of a sweet one can also serve to change your craving over time.

White bread, white pasta, white rice and pastries, pies and biscuits made with refined wheat are poor cousins of the wholegrain varieties.

If you can, make a straight switch to wholemeal bread, wholemeal pasta, brown rice, whole porridge oats, muesli, buckwheat, quinoa and other whole grains. Some people find the taste difficult to get used to if they have been eating processed foods for a long time, but this is a very important change to make. You may find that you need to be creative if your family prefer not to make the switch with you, in which case you could:

- Keep wholemeal bread, sliced previously, in the freezer and take out the amount you need to defrost or pop straight into the toaster.
- Make a batch of brown rice and freeze in portion sizes. Defrost your portion beforehand and 'refresh' in a sieve with boiling water – no need to cook it each time.
- Persuade your family to change habits gradually. For instance, you can make rice 75 per cent white and 25 per cent brown and slowly change the ratios over time. Their long-term health can only benefit.

Avoid coffee, excess caffeinated tea and over-the-counter drugs
No easy way round these steps, you just have to get on with them.

Giving up coffee may result in a number of health benefits which make you wonder why you carried on drinking it for so long – better sleep, fewer headaches, better digestion, better blood sugar balance or better skin, for instance. If you give up in one go, be warned that you may well have headaches, sometimes quite severe, for up to five days. It should not go on longer than this, and the worst thing to do is to go back to the coffee in desperation. Believe it or not, the headaches are a good sign, indicating that your liver now has the chance to throw off stored toxins.

Excess tea means more than three or four cups a day. Helpful ways to avoid going overboard include introducing fruit or herbal teas, drinking more water, or water and juice mixtures, and making weaker cups of tea – all these can help the process.

Reading the lists of side-effects for even the most common over-the-counter medications is a stark reminder of the impact that regular use of these drugs can have on health. Far better to work out the cause of your discomfort rather than simply mask the symptoms. These drugs have to be detoxified by your liver, which means that it is unable to deal effectively with other jobs including protecting you from breast cancer, and they interfere with the uptake and utilization of a number of vitamins and minerals, meaning that these are not then available for other vital body processes. Complaints such as headaches, indigestion, bowel problems, arthritis and skin problems often have a nutritional basis, or at the very least dietary habits are a contributory factor. You may find that following the advice in this book eliminates a number of minor complaints, which enables you to reduce or cut out over-the-counter medication. Any prescribed medication must not be stopped without first discussing the options with your doctor.

Daily Menu Suggestions

When working with clients to make positive changes to their regimes, I quickly learned that changes to dietary habits have to be simple and accessible. The next few pages prove that making valuable dietary changes can be quite easy, and with almost no effort you can have a diet which is healthy.

Included are three one-week menu plans to suit specific requirements: for non-vegetarians, vegetarians, and for those with a gluten sensitivity. The way most of us eat, on a day-to-day basis, is fairly straightforward, and you will notice that the menu plans and the recipe suggestions are designed for the average person, not the average master chef! They also take the following daily recommendations into account:

Fat	No more than 25–30 per cent of the daily intake of calories is from fat, mostly from the beneficial fats.
Fibre	25–35 g/1–1¼ oz of fibre is included.
Fruit and vegetables	At least seven portions are included.
Brassica vegetables	Within the seven portions of fruit and vegetables, at least one is a brassica.
Soya	Soya has been included on five out of seven days.
Linseeds	Although not listed, it is assumed that two tablespoons of linseeds are included each day, usually at breakfast, but it could be later in the day.

For some people a menu plan makes life easier. For others, sticking to a rigid plan does not – you will know which category you belong to. Whichever it is, the ideas are here – use them as they are, or adapt them to suit you. Ideally, if you do mix and match the menus, keep in mind the daily recommendations above.

You will find the recipes for many of the meal suggestions through-out the book (see the **Recipe Index**). For the suggestions that don't have a recipe in the book, your own familiar recipe books are likely to have a version. You may have to adapt ingredients slightly to fit in with the dietary recommendations but this should be fairly easy when you get the hang of the basic principles. It is a case of just giving it a go.

In one of my recipe books at home I have a favourite recipe for wild mushroom risotto. I adapt it to fit in with my preferred eating plan by using brown rice instead of white arborio (brown rice takes twenty to thirty minutes longer to cook); I add broccoli florets in the last five minutes; I use a small amount of olive oil instead of butter, steam-fry the onions and keep the parmesan to the barest minimum. It's excellent!

Meals such as the kitchen-sink salad (see page 78), in its many guises, can rely on basic ingredients which are kept in the fridge or store cupboard, so it is just a case of choosing a selection of these, and a little bit of chopping, just minutes before eating. Many meals can be eaten as leftovers for lunch the next day with just the addition of a few fresh vegetables.

The menu plans do not list snacks or dessert ideas for each day, but the best option is always fruit, the more often the better – the infinite variety means that there is no chance of getting bored. You may occasionally want something more exotic, and an interesting fresh fruit salad can fit the bill. I often add chopped dried fruit, chopped fresh nuts and apple juice and top it with yoghurt to make it a bit more special. Here are some more ideas:

Desserts
– Baked apple stuffed with dates or prunes and served with yoghurt
– Banana baked in a little orange juice and topped with yoghurt and cinnamon
– Frozen soya dessert with raisins – see breakfast-in-a-glass recipe (page 118)
– Stewed fruit with oat crumble and honey topping
– Cottage cheese with figs, or goat's cheese with pears

– Strawberries with a tablespoon of kirsch, topped with yoghurt
– Orange slices, and orange zest, soaked in a little orange liqueur

Snacks
– Home-made popcorn
– Rye or rice crackers or oatcakes with a variety of spreads
– Pumpernickel bread with toppings
– Soya yoghurt
– Olives, pickles and crudités with salsa and tzatziki
– Soya and linseed snack bar
– Tomato juice

Non-vegetarian

	Day 1	Day 2	Day 3	Day 4	Day 5	Day 6	Day 7
Breakfast	Orange juice Porridge with grated apple and soya milk Fruit	Wholemeal toast with 100 per cent fruit jam or sesame spread Fruit	Carrot juice Bran flakes with live yoghurt and berries (fresh or frozen) Fruit	Breakfast rice (page 285) with soya milk, dried fruit and coconut flakes Fruit	Tomato juice Cornflakes (organic) with soya milk Fruit	Soya breakfast-in-a-glass (page 118) Fruit	Apple juice Pumpernickel toast with mashed banana topping Fruit
Lunch	Salmon e fagiole (see tonno e fagiole page 248) Green salad Wholemeal roll	Huge tomato, avocado, spring onion and hummus sandwich Coleslaw	Gazpacho soup with canellini beans Crudités with yoghurt dip	Savoury rice with cruciferous vegetables	Corn pasta salad with chick-peas (see kitchen-sink salad, page 78)	Poached eggs on spinach tossed with minced garlic	Grilled chicken and tofu kebabs Stir-fried vegetables
Evening	Baked aubergines and peppers with tofu and feta cheese cubes Bok choy salad	Omelette with oriental mushrooms and leeks (page 249) Green salad	Pasta with soya mince bolognaise	Chilli made with soya protein and kidney beans Baked potato	Falafel with rye toast or wholemeal pitta pockets, with alfalfa sprouts and cucumber salad	Fish pie with green peas and mashed swede topping Broccoli	Wholemeal pizza with goat's cheese, tuna, anchovies and olives

Vegetarian

	Day 1	Day 2	Day 3	Day 4	Day 5	Day 6	Day 7
Breakfast	Vegetable juice Oat muesli with grated apple in soya milk Fruit	Oatcakes with cottage cheese and tomato slices Fruit	Orange juice Wholegrain puffed rice cereal with linseeds and soya milk Fruit	Soya breakfast-in-a-glass (page 118) Fruit	Apple and pear juice Breakfast rice (page 285) Fruit	Baked beans (sugar-free) on wholemeal toast Fruit	Carrot juice Grilled tomatoes and mushrooms with potato pancakes Fruit
Lunch	Baked potato with hummus and coleslaw Tomato salad	Pitta pocket stuffed with goat's cheese, sun-dried tomatoes, alfalfa sprouts and basil leaves	Rice salad with black-eyed beans, marinated tofu chunks and broccoli	Lentil soup with lemon and turmeric (page 149) wholemeal roll	Kitchen-sink salad (page 78) with soya beans in garlic dressing and cauliflower	Soya burger on a wholemeal bun with red cabbage and a green salad	Cous-cous with Moroccan vegetable tajine (to include swedes and turnips)
Evening	Wholemeal or buckwheat pasta with tomato, onion, garlic and black olive sauce Mixed leaf salad	Marinated tofu kebabs with rainbow vegetables and broccoli florets	Spanish omelette made with potato, peas, peppers and onions (page 249) Salad	Brown rice risotto with wild mushrooms and broccoli or leeks	Chick-pea and spinach curry served with wholegrain rice Cucumber and yoghurt raita	Tortillas with Mexican re-fried beans, avocado strips, tomato slices, spring onions and yoghurt Crunchy spring vegetable salad	Home-made vegetable and bean soup served with a wholemeal roll

Gluten-free

	Day 1	Day 2	Day 3	Day 4	Day 5	Day 6	Day 7
Breakfast	Orange juice Millet porridge made with soya milk and figs, chopped dates or raisins Fruit	Wholegrain rice cereal with sliced banana and soya milk Fruit	Gluten-free muesli soaked in apple juice topped with yoghurt Fruit	Soya breakfast-in-a-glass (page 118) Fruit	Cornflakes (organic) with berries and soya milk Fruit	Tomato juice Poached or boiled eggs with gluten-free toast Fruit	Carrot juice Buckwheat pancakes (blinis) (page 277) with apple sauce or berries, topped with Greek yoghurt Fruit
Lunch	Rice and bean salad with marinated tofu Watercress salad	Baked potato with sweetcorn and bean salad Tzatziki	Mackerel pâté (page 208) on rice crackers Tomato and red onion salad	Buckwheat pancake (blini) (page 277) 'tortilla' sandwich with spicy bean and spring vegetable filling	Quinoa-based kitchen-sink salad (page 78) with feta cheese and nutty-tasting soya flakes	Corn pasta salad (see kitchen-sink salad, page 78) with arugula leaves	Roast pheasant with roasted root vegetables (including swedes or turnips) and red cabbage
Evening	Fish poached in wine, garlic and herbs Steamed cabbage and onion sprinkled with lemon juice	Quinoa with vegetable, tofu and broccoli curry Dhal with garlic	Oriental salmon (with spring onions, ginger and soya sauce) Stir-fried vegetables with Chinese leaves	Grilled vegetables Baked sweet potato Grilled polenta	Wholegrain rice kedgeree made with haddock Cauliflower with white sauce (made with soya milk and soya flour)	Japanese Udon noodles with vegetables and soya cubes in miso broth	Peppers (stuffed with brown rice, onion, garlic and pine nuts) Baked fennel

Your Basic Supplement Plan

Everyone has a different attitude towards supplementation even if they are generally in favour. Some people may be happy to take one or two capsules a day, while others will line up the bottles on their kitchen counter and take a whole array of supplements.

If you are of the former persuasion, and are generally healthy, I would suggest a minimum supplement regime of one multi-vitamin/mineral formula, one antioxidant formula (usually contains vitamins A, C, E, beta-carotene and the mineral selenium), and a couple of grams of vitamin C daily.

If you prefer to take a whole array of supplements, you can take as many of those mentioned as you wish, as long as you do not exceed the maximum safe dosages for individual nutrients, which are described under **Vitamins** and **Minerals** (pages 159 and 167).

The majority of people want a supplement regime that is manageable and reasonable in terms of numbers of capsules/pills/powders. The following regimes are best taken in divided doses of two lots a day. While this is the ideal because it means that doses are spread out over a twenty-four-hour period, if you find this difficult and you want to take the supplements all in one go in the morning, that is fine. The exception is vitamin C which, as it is water-soluble, really is ideally taken in divided doses throughout the day.

Daily plan for supplementation aimed at breast cancer prevention

- Multi-vitamin and mineral – low iron (5 mg) – and giving 50 mg B vitamins
- Antioxidant supplement giving 200 mcg selenium total, 200 ius vitamin E total, 10 mg beta-carotene total (totals should allow for any selenium in the multi-vitamin/mineral).

– Buffered vitamin C with flavonoids 2 g each dose twice daily
  (4 g total)
– CoQ10 100 mg (50 mg each dose)

Other favourite supplements
– Fish oil 5 g daily (if you have been on a low oily fish diet for
  several years)
– Linseed oil ½–1 tablespoon daily
– Garlic 500–1,000 mg daily
– Acidophilus two capsules daily

Daily plan for supplementation for those in remission from breast cancer

– Multi-vitamin and mineral – no iron – and giving 50 mg
  B vitamins
– Antioxidant supplements giving 200 mcg selenium total, 200 ius
  vitamin E total, 15 mg beta-carotene total (totals should allow
  for any selenium and vitamin E in the multi-vitamin/mineral)
– Buffered vitamin C with flavonoids 2 g each dose three times
  daily (6 g total)
– CoQ10 100 mg (50 mg each dose)

Other favourite supplements
– Fish oil 5 g daily (if you have been on a low oily fish diet for
  several years)
– Garlic 500–1,000 mg daily
– Acidophilus two capsules daily
– Lipoic acid 200 mg daily
– Mixed flavonoids and carotenes including quercitin and
  lycopene

For a six-month period following chemotherapy
– Folic acid 400–800 mg daily if you have been avoiding it
– L-Glutamine 10–15 g daily in two or three divided doses
– Milk thistle 600 mg daily in two or three divided doses

Daily plan for supplementation while actively being treated for breast cancer
(*all these should be checked with your doctor*)

- Multi-vitamin and mineral – no iron – and giving 50 mg
  B vitamins (avoid folic acid if on Methotrexate chemotherapy)
- Antioxidant supplements giving 200 mcg selenium total,
  200 ius vitamin E total, and 15 mg beta-carotene total (totals
  should allow for any selenium and vitamin E in the
  multi-vitamin/mineral)
- Buffered vitamin C with flavonoids 3 g each dose three times
  daily (9 g total)
- CoQ10 200 mg (100 mg each dose)
- Lipoic acid 300 mg

Other favourite supplements
- Milk thistle 600 mg daily in two or three divided doses
- L-glutamine 20 g daily in three divided doses
- Fish oils 5 g daily
- Mixed flavonoids and carotenes including quercitin and
  lycopene

See other suggestions in the **Surgery Radiotherapy** and **Chemotherapy** chapters (pages 310, 320 and 330).

Part 4 **The Five Pillars of Health**

If all that you do after reading this book, is to follow the advice within the Basic Nutrition Plan, you will have done a massive amount to reduce your risk of, or the risk of recurrence of, breast cancer. Looking at overall health from a personal and individual perspective, as we will do now, takes the effectiveness several steps further.

Imagine you are a boat floating on the water. Cargo is then added. That cargo could comprise things that belong to or have happened in the past: a particular genetic make-up, risk factors such as early onset of periods, the contraceptive pill, exposure to oestrogen-mimicking chemicals in your environment. To this cargo load you may then add other lifestyle factors: perhaps you don't do much exercise, drink a few glasses of wine each week, have a sweet tooth, eat on the run without much time for fruit and vegetables, don't like fish so tend to eat more meat and cheese. Then add to this some symptoms, or health changes, which have been building up for a while: tender breasts pre-menstrually for several years, or perhaps you have taken HRT to ward off unpleasant menopausal symptoms, have a tendency to be more constipated than in the past, and have noticed that if there is a bug going round you catch it and find it hard to shake off. None of these, individually, necessarily means that you will develop a major disease. However, by the time all this cargo has been loaded on to the boat – you – it is easy to see how it can become overloaded and sink. For you, when the crisis happens, it may take the form of breast cancer. Others may be predisposed to heart disease, or diabetes, or chronic rheumatoid arthritis – their boat is loaded up differently.

Now imagine that you can unload some cargo – quite a lot of it, as much as you are able to return you to full health.

The Five Pillars of Health will help you to rebalance your body's chemistry to optimize your health:

- **Building powerful immunity**
- **Harmonizing hormones**
- **Healthy digestion**
- **Detoxing your system**
- **Reducing your stress load**

You will very quickly work out which chapters are most important to you, from the **Five Pillars of Health Check-list** (page 24). If you have not already done so, take some time to go through it now.

All these aspects of health are important, to a greater or lesser extent, for most people. Once again, do not try to do too much all in one go as you may find that you are overwhelmed with things to do. You may also find that dealing with one area of your health will impact on other aspects, meaning that the check-lists become shorter, or even disappear!

Building Powerful Immunity

The immune system is often described as our army, constantly patrolling and defending our territory against foreign invaders. It comprises our bone marrow, various organs and glands, our lymph system and the white immune cells in our blood.

Its job is to identify micro-organisms, such as bacteria, viruses, parasites, allergy-causing antigens (such as pollen for hayfever sufferers) and improperly digested proteins. When it recognizes them as being invaders, it neutralizes or destroys them, and then disposes of them. Your immune system works incredibly hard to do this. It is astounding to think that within only one minute, your body is capable of producing one million 'strait-jackets' (antibodies) to disarm invaders.

Another vital job of the immune system is to identify cells which are 'non-self', i.e. cells which have mutated into pre-cancerous cells, cells which are old or have been damaged in some way.

The immune system is well equipped to do this under normal circumstances. However, there are many circumstances when it does not work effectively, and we take it for granted at our peril.

- It could be overloaded with too much work to do. For instance, if we are exposed to large amounts of free radicals, which damage cells, the immune system has a harder task to neutralize these damaged cells and mop up the debris. One way to approach the problem of overload is to reduce the damage to cells in the first place.
- It could be that the building blocks and ammunition which are needed when an immune defence needs to be mounted are simply not there. In order to produce the millions of white blood cells at high speed there have to be adequate amounts of vitamin C, B vitamins and zinc to create them.
- It is possible that the immune system is damaged. After undergoing a course of chemotherapy, bone marrow which produces white blood cells may be compromised.

A number of factors can impact on the action of the immune system – factors over which we have control. No one aspect of our lifestyle or diet is likely to be the sole culprit, or answer, as many factors have a cumulative effect and they all affect each other. We can stand the stress of any one of the following factors for a while, but if it goes on for too long, the numbers of immune cells decrease. As a result, the immune system is unable to fulfil its tasks.

Immune Infusion

This brew is good for supporting your immune system, especially through the dark, damp winter months. It is warming and comforting and also gives an anti-bug boost. You can even add a few drops of liquid echinacea to your toddy for extra insurance.

6 dried shiitake mushrooms
7½ cm/3 in piece of fresh ginger root, thinly sliced
4 garlic cloves
4 teaspoons miso
2 litres/3½ pints distilled or filtered water

Let the mushrooms soak in ½ litre/18 fl oz of the water for 30 minutes, then drain and reserve the water. Bring the remaining water to the boil and add all the ingredients, except the miso, reducing the heat so that the infusion simmers. Mix a little of the hot water with the miso to make a smooth paste and add it and the mushroom soaking water to the pot. Simmer for 30 minutes, strain and drink while hot. The infusion can be kept in the fridge for a couple of days.

The following can suppress the immune system and impair its performance:

- Stimulants, including smoking, excess alcohol, coffee, and excess tea, all impact on the ability of the immune system to perform at its peak.
- Sugar radically lowers immune function by suppressing white blood cell counts.
- Stress, or more accurately dis-stress, also impairs immune function.

Mental stress takes many forms – overwork, anxiety, depression, feelings of helplessness, emotional shock – and if any of these are in your picture, it is necessary to address them. If this is a problem for you, read the chapter **Reducing Your Stress Load** (page 290).

■ Taking antibiotics on a regular basis taxes the immune system by wiping out protective bacterial colonies and allowing space for harmful bacteria, or yeasts, to get a foothold. The toxins which these bacteria, or yeast infections, produce reduce the effectiveness of the immune system. Consider using natural antibiotics, such as citrus seed extract, echinacea and garlic, and do not over-use antibiotics. They are powerful medication which should be kept for times when it is really needed. If you are on chemotherapy your doctor may advise you to take antibiotics if he or she thinks that you are at risk of infection. There may be other circumstances when they are important, but frequently antibiotic prescriptions are superfluous to need. If you find that you have to take a course of antibiotics, it is wise to ensure that they are followed by a course of pro-biotics which, as the name implies, help your system to 'stock up' on the beneficial bacteria. You can buy acidophilus bacteria (make sure they are refrigerated and within their sell-by date) from good health food shops. Eating live yoghurt can also be helpful, but after a course of antibiotics you may find a harder-hitting dose of combined pro-biotics to be more effective. For suppliers see the **Resources** section.

■ Chemotherapy, radiotherapy, and surgery all have a negative effect on the immune system, and redressing the balance with the measures set out in the section above becomes more important than ever. In particular, taking high doses of vitamin C is highly protective – see **Supporting Your Medical Treatment Choices with Nutrition** (page 301).

■ Food allergies and sensitivities can tax the immune system. Poor digestion and an increase in permeability of the digestive tract can lead to food allergies or insensitivities. These add to the total load that your immune system must deal with. (See the chapter **Healthy Digestion**, page 267.)

■ Allergies, the more classic sort, and related problems overtax the system. Problems such as hayfever, asthma, eczema and psoriasis are all related to the immune process. They can suppress the immune system, but in turn they can be alleviated by enhancing the immune system's capabilities and, if appropriate, identifying foods that are contributing to the problem.

- Pollutants in the environment serve to over-tax the immune system. It is quite common, in areas of high pollution, for the incidence of immune problems, such as asthma, to be elevated.
- Infections can exacerbate the problem of reduced immunity. Generally, if our immune systems are working efficiently, infections do not have the chance to set in, but if they are compromised we become open to a variety of pathogens. Louis Pasteur, the father of the germ theory, amended his ideas (on his deathbed as the story goes) and is quoted as saying, 'The germ is nothing, the terrain is everything.'
- It is well established that malnutrition will lead to an increase in immune problems, and this is particularly evident in people from countries where there are food supply problems, and in the elderly in our own country. However, as we have already discussed, the general population is deficient in at least some nutrients from dietary intake, and we are suffering a problem of excess calories, with insufficient nutrients. While the signs of overt malnourishment are recognized, this more subtle form of under-nourishment also compromises optimal immune function.

Boosting the immune army

By giving the immune system the building blocks it needs, reducing oxidation damage to lighten the load, and by eating foods which have cancer-fighting properties, we can reduce the impact on the immune system, build it up, and allow it to work to its full potential.

Supporting your immune system is the first step in preventing cancer in the first place. Using the appropriate nutritional tools from your kit-bag you can optimize your chances of building the healthiest possible immune system.

These measures can improve immune system performance. Use this list to check where you can make changes to support your immune health:

- Eat a diet high in antioxidants. These foods include at least five portions of fruit and vegetables a day, and preferably seven to ten, and also olive oil and black and green teas. It is the antioxidants that disarm the free radicals which damage cells. They also help to protect against allergies and to repair body tissues.
- Reduce stimulants, in particular sugar, to a minimum as they all have an immuno-suppressive effect if taken to excess.
- If stress is a feature in your life, work out ways to reduce the levels you are experiencing. See **Reducing Your Stress Load** (page 290).
- If you have any allergies, address the likely causes as a priority. It is quite possible that foods play a significant part in many allergies as well as other symptoms, and the first foods to suspect are wheat and dairy products. See the information in **Healthy Digestion** (page 267) for how to tackle food intolerances.
- Specific foods seem to have an immune-modulating effect, in particular garlic, live yoghurt, oriental mushrooms and soya. See **Anti-Breast Cancer Superfoods** (page 137) for other foods which can help.
- Certain herbs have powerful immune-modulating effects, increasing white blood cell count, improving natural killer cell activity, or acting directly as anti-viral, anti-bacterial or anti-parasitic agents. These include echinacea, curcumin, astragalus and ginger.
- The immune system does not function effectively without vitamin C, and taking moderately high doses of 1–3 g on a daily basis is a tremendous preventive measure against lowered immunity.
- Other nutrients for immune health which can be supplemented include zinc (15 mg), selenium (200 mcg), magnesium (300 mg) and the B vitamins (100 mg). Look at the information under **Vitamins** (page 159) and **Minerals** (page 167) to find food sources of these nutrients, and consider supplementing them.
- Laughter has been shown, without question, to improve immune function. Of course, going around and grinning like our simian cousins is not going to make you well in a trice, but it will help, especially if you make a resolution to do things that you really enjoy – watch your favourite comedy show, spend time with people you enjoy being with, read a light-hearted novel . . .

Roasted Vegetables

Aubergine chunks, thickish slices of courgettes, quartered onions (red onions are best), several whole garlic cloves (unpeeled if you wish), red and yellow peppers, chunks of butternut squash: all are delicious sources of immune-boosting antioxidants, and this recipe is an easy way to add them to your diet.

Cut all the vegetables about the same size and put them into a large baking tin. Drizzle with olive oil, place in the middle of the oven preheated to 180°C/350°F/gas mark 4 and bake for 20–30 minutes. Take out and turn the vegetables lightly – they should be caramelizing slightly (not burning!). Add in quartered tomatoes and black olives, and return to the oven for a further 10–15 minutes.

Serve with grilled polenta slices. This dish is delicious as an accompaniment for fish or chicken, or as a topping for baked potatoes, cous-cous, quinoa or pasta (try wheat-free varieties of pasta such as corn pasta shapes or buckwheat noodles).

Harmonizing Hormones

We are complex beings, and it is balancing the total dance of the hormones that is likely to bring maximum effect in avoiding breast cancer. Avoiding environmental sources of damaging oestrogens is probably critical, and modulating the effects of oestrogens in the body will undoubtedly bring huge benefits. But what about all the other hormones in the picture?

Hormones interplay subtly with each other. Progesterone is the hormone which works in direct opposition to oestrogen, and high oestrogen levels may be due, in part, to low progesterone levels. Thyroxin (the hormone that is secreted from the thyroid gland and principally governs our metabolic rate) impacts upon how the liver handles oestrogen and whether 'good' – benign – oestrogens or 'bad' – pro-carcinogenic – oestrogens are made.

Insulin is the hormone which is responsible for blood-sugar regulation, but also has a profound impact upon the quantity of free-circulating oestrogens. The stress hormone, adrenaline, affects insulin levels by triggering another hormone, glucagon. Yet another stress hormone, cortisol, competes with progesterone at cell receptor sites, reducing its positive effect on breast tissue.

Complex interactions like these suggest that the 'whole body' approach is the one which offers the best chance of success. Oestrogen management with Tamoxifen, the oestrogen-modulating drug, or with dietary sources of oestrogen modulators, offers improved chances of survival, but dealing with related hormone issues at the same time probably reduces risk further and provides an improved climate for recovery.

The hormone, or endocrine, system behaves like an orchestra. If one instrument is out of tune, all the rest seem to be so as well, as each instrument influences the performance of the whole. So when we talk about the oestrogens it is really impossible to divorce them from the actions of other hormones – especially those in the same section of the orchestra. There are four main hormones to think about, in addition to oestrogens:

– Insulin (and blood-sugar balance)
– Progesterone
– Thyroid hormones
– Stress hormones (supporting the adrenal glands which produce our stress hormones will be discussed in the chapter **Reducing Your Stress Load**, page 290).

While it is best to use diet, exercise and relaxation methods to resolve hormonal balance problems, for some women these imbalances have been going on for so long that a helping hand is needed. In many cases, it may be necessary to use nutritional supplements or natural forms of hormones to achieve the desired result. It is possible that if you have a non-hormonal breast cancer this section is not relevant to you; however, it may be worth reading it for other tips, for instance how to plan for a natural menopause.

Blood-sugar balance

Over 10 per cent of the National Health budget is devoted to diabetes-related problems, a major factor in the health of the nation. But only one in ten people who exhibit signs of blood-sugar imbalance will go on to develop diabetes. The remaining nine out of ten will never get that far. But in the meantime they may suffer from a series of symptoms including sugar cravings, excess fatigue or drowsiness, the need for stimulants, weight problems and others.

We eat so many refined carbohydrate and sugary products that a vast number of people with health problems are suffering from blood-sugar balance problems. Sugars and refined carbohydrates trigger insulin, and if too much is triggered, too quickly, the body goes into a mini-crisis and has to bring the insulin level down – quickly. However, we can over-compensate and bring insulin down too far – this leads to a blood-sugar low. Blood-sugar lows on a regular basis can lead to a number of symptoms including low energy, drowsiness and the need for a pick-me-up.

Blood-sugar swings can also encourage mental symptoms such as tiredness, dizziness, headaches, anxiety and mood swings, which result from the brain being starved of glucose, its chief source of fuel, during the blood-sugar dips.

Another related problem, frequently encountered, is that of insulin resistance. Insulin resistance can result after many years on a high-sugar or refined-carbohydrate diet, usually accompanied by a high-fat diet. Cells become damaged – oxidized – by the glucose load with which they have to deal. The level of insulin is kept high in the blood because of high levels of glucose in the blood. In the meantime the damaged cells do not respond to the insulin and do not absorb the glucose from the blood. This is relevant to breast cancer because raised insulin level encourages free oestrogens to circulate in the body, making them more available to latch on to breast tissue cells.[1]

It is also common for oestrogen imbalance problems, in particular pre-menstrual symptoms, to be alleviated wholly or in part by dealing with blood-sugar balance. Most of the dietary measures discussed in this book are designed to balance blood sugar. This is a summary of the key points, along with information about some supplements and herbs which can give a helping hand:

- Increase fibre in the diet, especially from wholegrains, beans and pulses. They release their energy into the bloodstream slowly, meaning that blood-sugar peaks and troughs are avoided.
- Reduce or cut out sugar, honey and refined carbohydrates.
- Dilute fruit juices by at least half. Moderate your intake of dried fruit or eat them with a protein food.
- Reduce or cut out stimulants such as coffee, tea, alcohol and smoking.
- Moderate exercise – half to one hour daily – helps to keep blood-sugar levels stable.
- The minerals chromium and magnesium, along with the B vitamins, help to keep blood sugar balanced. Between 200 and 500 mcg of chromium, and 200–300 mg magnesium, along with a 50 mg B-complex can make a difference. All these supplements are safe, although an insulin-dependent diabetic should introduce chromium very slowly – in increments of

100 mcg – as it can have such a profound effect on insulin that a reduced insulin dose may be needed – consult your doctor.
- The herb licorice root (DGL) (deglycyrrhizinated) helps to stabilize blood-sugar swings.
- L-glutamine, the amino acid, helps to reduce blood-sugar swings by providing alternative fuel for the brain.
- The antioxidant lipoic acid helps to stabilize blood sugar, though high doses of around 300 mg are needed.

Store-cupboard quick meals

You get home exhausted and desperately hungry. What can you eat that takes less than five minutes to prepare and really fills the gap? A good store cupboard will avoid the need to call the pizza delivery and keep you on track with your anti-breast cancer eating plan. All these quick meals will help to maintain blood-sugar balance.

If you have the following in your store cupboard, you will never be short of a quick, filling and healthy meal: canned tuna, salmon, pilchards, sardines, anchovies, all types of canned beans, lentils and chick-peas, canned tomatoes, sun-dried tomatoes, capers, wholewheat or 'other grain' pasta shapes, cous-cous, black and green olives, small pickled cucumbers, dried herbs, spices. Fresh ingredients which last a reasonable amount of time in the fridge: eggs, yoghurt, lemons, potatoes, onions, garlic.

Tonno e Fagiole

Put some canned flageolet or cannelini beans into a sieve and hold under running cold water to get rid of the brine. Chop up an onion (a red onion is best) and mix these ingredients with some olive oil and lemon dressing. Flake some canned tuna on top and serve with a crusty wholewheat bread roll. For a deluxe version you can flake some fresh cooked salmon instead of tuna (I always cook more than I need and have some left over in the fridge for the next day – I like salmon better cold than warm).

Perfect Pasta

Cook some pasta shapes, either wholewheat or corn, rice or buckwheat. While the pasta is cooking, chop up lots of sun-dried tomatoes, capers, black olives and anchovies. If you have time, steam-fry some onions, garlic and any other vegetables you have around and add to the previous ingredients. At the last minute stir in the pasta to meld all the flavours. Instead of pasta you could also use leftover brown rice, quinoa or steamed cous-cous.

Mild Chick-Pea Curry

Steam-fry some onion and garlic until translucent. Add in a half or whole teaspoon (according to taste) each of cumin, turmeric, garam masala and mild curry powder. Stir over a low heat for a few minutes. Add a drained and rinsed can of chick-peas or lentils and warm up until all the flavours meld. If you have any spinach in the fridge this is nice wilted into the curry. I keep a jar of 'fresh' coriander in the fridge to add at the last minute, though real fresh coriander is best. Serve on top of leftover brown rice, or cous-cous which only takes 10 minutes to steam. This quick curry also works as a delicious side dish to steamed or baked fish.

Omelettes

Eggs are the ultimate store-cupboard standby. To lower the fat content omelettes can be made with one egg and two egg whites (per person). Anything can be added to the omelette from the store cupboard, though I like to get some fresh vegetables in. Steaming takes much less time than any other form of cooking and you can steam some leeks, onions, and mushrooms in minutes. Spanish omelettes are terrific with cubed steamed potato, red peppers (canned if no fresh peppers are available), frozen peas and lots of herbs. If you are really organized you can keep some organic blanched vegetables in the freezer in portion sizes, ready for instant steaming. Steam your vegetables, then put them into the pan with a little olive oil, add the eggs, and flip over when set.

The power of progesterone

While there are several types of oestrogen which we produce naturally, there is only one progesterone. Women produce progesterone in the ovaries and the adrenal glands, and men produce a lesser amount in the testes.

Simply put, the main function of progesterone is to PRO-long GEST-ation, hence its name. When a fertilized egg starts its life, this hormone is responsible for ensuring that conditions in the womb are optimal for the egg to implant, develop and mature. During pregnancy progesterone is produced by the corpus luteum of the ejected egg, and eventually by the placenta. If, however, fertilization has not taken place, progesterone levels drop dramatically, until triggered again half-way through the next cycle.

Following the menopause, a woman's progesterone production only takes place in the adrenal glands. This abrupt drop in levels has led to the idea that progesterone is not an important consideration post-menopausally.

A simplified explanation of progesterone's primary job fails to make clear its important function in breast cancer management. Progesterone is also critical for maintaining a woman's hormone balance. It does this in two ways. First, it is the first step on the ladder – or precursor hormone – for a number of other hormones which are made from progesterone. These 'daughter' hormones include oestrogen, testosterone and the cortico-steroid hormones. The second, hugely important, job is to counterbalance the effects of oestrogen, which from the point of view of breast cancer management is of key interest.

The general assumption is that progesterone drops at menopause because, apart from not being needed to promote pregnancy, there is a concurrent drop in oestrogen levels to around 25 per cent of full capacity, meaning that progesterone no longer has to work in opposition to oestrogen in order to maintain a woman's health. But this was before we had hundreds of man-made chemicals in our environment which exert a damaging xenoestrogenic effect, and this thinking may now be outmoded. Additionally, after the age of about thirty-five, women are statistically more likely to have a number of 'anovulatory' cycles. These are cycles when everything appears to function normally, but she does not produce an egg. The implication of this is that the woman will continue to produce oestrogen in ever-increasing amounts during her cycle, but will not produce any progesterone to counter-balance it.[2] This leads to an increasing oestrogen load.

The majority of breast cancers are detected post-menopausally, but you will recall that the average time taken to develop a detectable breast cancer tumour is around ten years. This means that a large number of breast cancers are probably initiated during this phase of high, unopposed, oestrogen levels prior to the menopause.[3]

Progesterone is of interest for women with breast cancer, or with a risk of breast cancer, because it has the opposite effect to oestrogen on breast tissue – it slows down cell division.[4] The slower the cell division, the more chance there is that cells will be produced intact and undamaged. A study of over 1,000 women, at Johns Hopkins University, showed that women who had low levels of progesterone, sufficient to interfere with fertility, had over five times the normal risk of developing breast cancer. Even more alarmingly, they had a ten-fold higher death rate from all malignancies.[5] One interesting study noted that women tracked for a twenty-eight-year period, who had given birth to twins, were 29 per cent less likely to go on to contract breast cancer. The researchers suggested that the higher hor-mone levels which occur with twin pregnancies might be responsible for this protection. The hormones which are being produced in double dose, from two placentas, are progesterone and the breast cancer-protective oestriol (E3). Two genes are important in the process of apoptosis, or natural cell death, which occurs when healthy cells die in order to be replaced. The p53 gene prevents cancer by signalling that the cell is ready to die, and p53 is turned on by progesterone. The Bcl-2 gene triggers cancer by preventing the cell from dying. Bcl-2 is turned on by oestrogens.[6]

Oestrogen dominance

The condition of excess oestrogens, combined with exposure to highly damaging environmental oestrogens, has been termed oestrogen dominance by Dr John Lee, author of *Natural Progesterone: The Multiple Roles of a Remarkable Hormone*. Dr Lee has spent his career working with progesterone and observing its effects on a variety of predominantly female problems, including breast cancer. His books on the subject[7] have revolutionized thinking in this area and he is of the opinion that natural progesterone 'should be used by all patients who either have or had breast cancer, or are at risk of breast cancer . . . The effect of progesterone is to prevent breast cancer, late recurrences and metastasis.' Dr Lee also cites the work of clinical biochemist Dr David Zava who has examined thousands of breast cancer tissue biopsies and found, without exception, that oestrogen dominance is present.[8] Breast cancer surgery at times of oestrogen dominance may increase the likelihood of recurrence.[9]

Signs of oestrogen dominance can include:

– Water retention
– Pre-menstrual problems
– Breast swelling and discomfort
– Fibrocystic breasts
– Blood-sugar swings
– Polycystic ovaries
– Uterine fibroids
– Increased risk of breast, endometrial and cervical cancers
– Reduced thyroid hormone effectiveness.

Artificial progestogens

Early on, the pharmaceutical industry became aware of the impact of unopposed oestrogens, when their first attempts at producing oestrogen-only contraceptive pills met with an alarming increase in a number of complaints, including thrombosis and hormone-triggered cancers. The next strategy adopted was to add some progestogens to the pill and to HRT preparations. Progestogens (progestins in the USA) are artificially manufactured progesterone near-clones. Sure enough, the risks decreased somewhat, but not as much as would be hoped. Progestogens do not have exactly the same advantages as the natural progesterone molecule, and may actually enhance the risk of breast cancer from the oestrogens in HRT,[10] whereas progesterone may have the opposite effect and actually reduce breast cancer risk from HRT.[11] A natural approach to the menopause is discussed later in this chapter.

Progestogens, of which there are many, are synthetically designed and frequently made from horses' urine: the unfortunate pregnant mares are tethered in stalls, as well as being kept thirsty to increase the concentration of oestrogen in their urine. The reason why progestogens vary slightly from the progesterone which is made in the body is that any product made from chemicals which can be found in nature is not patentable. This means that profit margins are lamentably small for an industry used to bigger stuff. Progestogens *are* patentable and, of course, the contraceptive pill and HRT, using artificial progestogens, are very big business indeed. So these artificial progestogens are perhaps produced more for the benefit of the pharmaceutical companies than for the long-term benefit of the women taking them.

It might appear that they are helpful to women taking the hormones, especially if you listen to the catalogue of benefits which are loudly proclaimed, such as preventing osteoporosis and heart disease, but, on closer scrutiny these claims do not necessarily hold up (see **Forever young** (page 190) in the chapter **Lifestyle Choices**).

Natural progesterone versus Mexican yam

The term 'natural progesterone' can be slightly misleading, because it is not technically natural and is actually a manufactured product. It is created in the laboratory from diosgenin, an extract of the Mexican wild yam. However, the resultant progesterone can accurately be described as natural since it is identical to the hormone which is produced by our bodies and therefore has identical functions to our naturally produced hormone.

Natural progesterone is available as a cream which is rubbed into the skin, rotating the patches of skin on which you rub it for best effect. It is absorbed into the fat under the skin and is then taken up by the blood supply.

You will also find that there are other similar products available, Mexican wild yam creams or capsules. A degree of confusion exists about the differences between natural progesterone cream and Mexican wild yam creams. The first key difference is that natural progesterone cream is only available on prescription from a GP, while Mexican wild yam cream is available over the counter. The former is much more potent than the latter. Mexican wild yam products contain diosgenin, which cannot be converted directly by the body into progesterone (this can only be achieved in the laboratory as described above). Mexican wild yam products do have their uses, particularly for menopausal symptoms as they have a phytoestrogenic effect and a mild progestogenic effect, but they are not as potent as natural progesterone.

Either of these products, natural progesterone or Mexican wild yam, is well worth trying. Mexican wild yam is appropriate if you want a slower, more subtle solution to your hormone problems, and natural progesterone if you exhibit more severe symptoms of oestrogen dominance.

Tests

The most useful test for progesterone levels when testing for the effectiveness of natural progesterone products is not a blood test but a saliva test. This is because plasma levels (taken from blood) do not show relevant levels of this fat-soluble hormone. Criticism of trials that have drawn negative conclusions on the effectiveness of natural progesterone (such as the King's College Hospital trial reported in the *Lancet* in 1997) has centred on the fact that they have used plasma tests instead of saliva tests. Saliva tests can only be done privately and the sample is sent off to the USA for analysis. See the **Resources** section for an address.

There is a blood test you can have at your doctor's office for progesterone levels and, if you suspect that your own progesterone levels are tailing off earlier in the cycle than they should, the test can be carried out around days twenty to twenty-four of your cycle. Low progesterone levels late in the cycle can exacerbate oestrogen dominance symptoms and also be responsible for failing to maintain a pregnancy.

There are tests available for the three main oestrogens – E1, E2 and E3. These can be carried out at your doctor's office by taking a blood sample, and the best time to do this is seven to ten days before your period, if you are still menstruating.

At the moment there is no method available for testing environmental xenoestrogen levels. Experiments have taken place examining the chemical residue levels in various body tissues, including breast tissue, but these are invasive and are not available to the general public. This makes the issue of xenoestrogens an invisible problem and it becomes a question of guesswork as to whether, or to what extent, these damaging oestrogens are part of an individual woman's health problems. It is quite possible that any woman who has spent the last thirty years in the West, and who has oestrogen receptor positive breast cancer, is at least partially affected by these xenoestrogens.

It is probably not very useful to have tests done repeatedly, because all that a test will show is what was happening on that particular day. It is more helpful to be aware of the symptoms of oestrogen dominance, and how they respond to treatment – if your symptoms improve, the treatment strategy is working.

How can you obtain natural progesterone?

Because natural progesterone is a hormone, it is only available on prescription and therefore you need to obtain it from your doctor. But here there is a dilemma, because it is not yet widely used by the medical profession. Indeed, because it has had this double life – as a natural product and as a medicine – it is difficult to find doctors who are versed in its use. The **Resources** section tells you how to find a doctor who is familiar with prescribing natural progesterone. The product is available over the counter in other countries. I do not advocate self-prescription as it is a hormone, and therefore open to misuse, and, in the case of breast cancer management, this can be damaging or even dangerous.

Uses of natural progesterone

Natural progesterone can be used by both pre- and post-menopausal women, and the way they use it is governed by their cycle, or absence of cycle – the manufacturer's leaflet describes this.

From the point of view of breast cancer I believe that natural progesterone is one of the most interesting products on the market. It is particularly noteworthy that the presence of progesterone receptors on breast cancer cells is an indication of response to Tamoxifen treatment, and it is possible that we will find, in years to come, that this is a reason for the efficacy of natural progesterone. It is also of interest that soya has been shown to improve progesterone receptor function significantly.[12]

There is no research yet on the use of natural progesterone with

Tamoxifen. In an animal study progesterone is effective at counter-acting oestrogen, as is Tamoxifen.[13] Dr Lee has been using natural progesterone successfully for the management of breast cancer for twenty years, and has elected to do this instead of using Tamoxifen.

I have a personal anecdote about natural progesterone which shows how attitudes may be changing. I have been using natural progester-one, on and off according to need, for six years now. I was not offered Tamoxifen originally, as it was fairly new then, and I would have been considered too young to use it. When I first started using natural progesterone I rather tentatively asked about it when I went for my regular check-ups at the Royal Marsden Hospital in London. At that time the Registrar I talked to did not know anything about it. On subsequent visits I mentioned it occasionally and over time it became clear that the Registrar obviously knew about its existence but would not comment on its usefulness. At my last visit, a year ago, I mentioned it once again and the Registrar said to me without hesitating that as I had not had Tamoxifen, natural progesterone was probably a good thing. Things were really moving along!

Does natural progesterone have any downsides?

Natural progesterone is a hormone and, as such, its effectiveness is subject to being in the correct balance with other hormones. It can certainly be over-used and because a little may be good, it does not mean that a lot is better. It is very important to follow dosage instruc-tions carefully and to monitor your symptoms of oestrogen domin-ance. Natural progesterone should really not be the first option you turn to. It is far more important to deal with diet and lifestyle first and, in so doing, establish which symptoms are relieved and which remain. Once you know this you can decide, with your doctor, if natural progesterone is for you.

One of the downsides of natural progesterone could be that as a precursor to oestrogen it may increase oestrogen levels, which is obviously not desirable when aiming to prevent breast cancer. Dr Lee has expressed the view that as the body has the ability to decide on the pathways for conversion of progesterone into oestrogen, or into a number of other hormones, it will do so in a balanced way – unless you overdo the dosage. A small minority of women do have adverse reactions to natural progesterone and it is possible that some women's biochemistry behaves differently to the majority, and these women may have to seek other solutions.

It is a mistake to view natural progesterone as a panacea, and it is not necessarily appropriate for every woman to take it as a preventive measure – it is a hormone which should be treated with respect. Where there are indications for its use, it is probably a much safer option than some of the drug therapies that are offered – in particular HRT.

The use of natural progesterone has largely been led by the ground-swell of women who have noted the benefits from using it. In some quarters of the medical profession there has been an attempt to ignore it, and there remains a significant degree of dissent about its use. Unfortunately some doctors dismiss it without having read the available literature on the subject. We are at the point now where natural progesterone is being taken seriously, and significant trials are being conducted.

Other benefits of natural progesterone

There are many other benefits to using natural progesterone where necessary, sometimes in conjunction with a small dose of oestriol (E3) cream if you are post-menopausal and have low oestrogen levels (oestriol is non-carcinogenic as it does not go down the metabolic pathway that leads to harmful oestrogens). Using these two in combination is really 'natural HRT', while using natural progesterone alone is aimed at balancing out oestrogen dominance (or progesterone deficiency). Benefits can include easing of menopausal symptoms such as hot flushes and a dry vagina, increased bone density conferring protection against osteoporosis, reducing cardiovascular risk and improved thyroid function.

The thyroid

One factor which is frequently overlooked in the management of breast cancer patients is an investigation of their thyroid function.[14] Recent research is confirming the suspicion that underactive thyroid function is a contributing risk factor to developing breast cancer.[15] Higher than average breast cancer rates have been noted in the goitre

257

belts of several countries, including the Great Lakes region of the USA. The goitre belts are areas with low iodine contents in the soil leading to underfunctioning, bulging, goitrous thyroid in many of the population. Countries with high iodine intakes from seafood and seaweed, such as Japan and Iceland, have low levels of goitres and low levels of deaths from breast cancer. The thyroid hormone, thyroxine, favourably influences the conversion of pro-carcinogenic oestrogens E1 and E2 into the benign E3 in the liver, via a process called hydroxylation. In the exercise of balancing hormones, it is worth spending a few minutes to consider if low thyroid activity may be part of your health picture.

The thyroid gland is a small butterfly-shaped gland in the throat which produces thyroxine, also called T4 because it has four iodine molecules attached to it. T4 is relatively inactive and is converted as needed into the more biologically active T3 hormone (you guessed, it only has three iodine molecules). These hormones regulate metabolism – our internal engine. And because metabolism governs the uptake and expenditure of energy for every cell in the body, the impact of thyroid hormones is far-reaching.

If you think that low thyroid is relevant to you, it is worth asking your doctor for a blood test, which is easy and inexpensive, to determine your thyroid hormone levels. The test should include the TSH levels, to measure how much thyroid-stimulating hormone is being secreted by the pituitary. The less efficiently the thyroid is working, the harder the pituitary has to pump out TSH, and levels are elevated. Normal T4 levels and high TSH levels would mean an under-active thyroid. The test should also look at free-T4 levels to see if T4 is being under-produced. Some people will also be inefficient at making the conversion from T4 to T3, and so free-T3 levels need to be checked as well. If any of these are outside the normal parameters it is a simple thing for your doctor to prescribe some thyroxine, or occasionally tertroxin (T3) – supplementation of these hormones has not been linked to an increased risk of breast cancer.[16] Levels should then be checked regularly because an excess of thyroid hormones can be damaging. Excess can lead to hyperactivity, osteoporosis and atrophy of the thyroid gland and this makes it even more important not to overdo the prescription.

It is not unusual for tests to register in the normal range and for the person to have a sub-clinically under-active thyroid. This was my experience. I insisted on being tested about four times in fifteen years, to be told on each occasion that my thyroid levels were normal. This was despite having a number of symptoms and one of my parents having an under-active thyroid. Some years later I had a test and was informed that I definitely had an under-active thyroid (by then the tests were more sensitive, but presumably I had also been sliding towards this point for a number of years). Addressing the thyroid deficiency subsequently became part of my strategy for preventing a recurrence of breast cancer.

If you do not have a clinically measurable under-active thyroid, but are exhibiting some of the symptoms above and suspect that you may have a sub-clinical condition, there are a number of measures that can be taken to improve thyroid function:

Diet

Because thyroid deficiency also usually leads to blood-sugar imbalance, it is common for low-thyroid sufferers to crave sweet foods, refined carbohydrates and other stimulants. The advice in this book is particularly appropriate for balancing blood-sugar levels and therefore managing low thyroid function. Substitute complex carbohydrates for refined or sugary foods and ensure that a little protein is eaten at each meal – for example nuts, seeds, yoghurt, eggs, fish, tofu, pulses. Dilute juices with water, minimize alcohol, and reduce coffees and teas to a bare minimum, substituting herbal coffees or infusions. The brassica (cabbage) family and soya fibre, which are so useful for the prevention of breast cancer, can have an effect on reducing thyroid function if they are eaten to excess. For this reason it is a good idea to cook cabbage and other brassicas lightly to reduce this effect, and keep to the suggested amount of 50 mg of phytoestrogens daily from soya products and not to exceed it by too much.

Wheat

Some thyroid problems are triggered by a sensitivity to wheat and it is not uncommon for thyroid problems to improve dramatically when wheat products are cut out of the diet – these include bread, pasta, pies, cakes and biscuits. Good substitutes include oatcakes, cornbread, buckwheat noodles, porridge, rye bread and rice.

Iodine

Iodine is the core molecule for the thyroid hormone and is frequently deficient, especially if you are avoiding salt which may be iodized. Iodine can be obtained from seafood and seaweed. It may also be useful to supplement with kelp or other thyroid-specific supplements which include iodine (see the **Resources** section) – a dose of 100 mcg iodine daily is recommended for low thyroid function. Thyroid-specific supplements also usually include the amino acid tyrosine and the mineral zinc, as these are needed for thyroid hormone production. Occasionally an adverse reaction can be experienced by those who are low in iodine suddenly being exposed to high doses, so it may be wise to add iodine into your regime slowly.

Selenium

The conversion of T4 and T3 involves selenium-dependent enzymes. In some studies, supplementing selenium alone has been sufficient to improve thyroid hormone activity. A supplemented dose of 100–200 mcg is advisable. Selenium is also protective against breast cancer.[17] See under **Minerals** (page 167) for sources of selenium – the richest sources are Brazil nuts, seafood, seaweed and brown rice.

Natural progesterone

One of the effects of natural progesterone is to improve thyroid hormone function – this means that if you are a borderline case, natural progesterone may be sufficient to enhance your thyroid function. However, it also means that if you are already taking thyroxine, you need to have your dose checked by your doctor, in case the addition of natural progesterone means that you are now taking too much thyroxine. Natural progesterone should not be taken specifically to boost thyroid activity, but on its own merits.

Managing your menopause naturally

Compared to women in the West the average Japanese woman has a noticeably different experience of 'the change', with very few complaints of menopausal problems.[18] It has been noted that the Japanese have much higher levels of phytoestrogens than their American or European counterparts. 'High levels of isoflavonoid phytoestrogens may partly explain why hot flushes and other menopausal symptoms are so infrequent in Japanese women,' commented the researcher Herman Adlercreutz in a letter published in the *Lancet*.[19]

The interesting thing about soya phytoestrogens is that they seem to have a dual effect. If there is an excess of oestrogens in the body, they have the effect of blocking them, but if there is a deficiency of oestrogens, they have the effect of replenishing them, though at a lower level of intensity without the negative implications of excess oestrogens. In this way they can help to combat osteoporosis and menopausal symptoms. According to research from the Royal Society of Medicine, regular consumption of legumes reduces menopausal symptoms by 60 per cent, risk of breast cancer by 50 per cent, and coronary heart disease by 30 per cent.

The information throughout this book covers many of the measures that can help you to manage your menopause without resorting to HRT. Here are some of the key points:

- Once again the soya bean, linseeds, chick-peas, and other phytoestrogen-rich foods come to the rescue. An Australian study used high doses of phytoestrogens – 160 mg daily – and reported a significant reduction in menopausal symptoms, and in particular in the incidence of hot flushes.[20] Another study reported a 40 per cent decrease in hot flushes after six weeks of adding 45 g/1½ oz of soya flour daily to the participants' diets (wheat flour also had an effect but not as pronounced or as quick).[21]
- Many women find that they can contain the number and intensity of hot flushes by using 1,000 ius of vitamin E daily and/or 1–2 g of evening primrose oil. Use these doses for at least two or three months to see if they work for you. Research which was inconclusive made the mistake of using lower doses for only four weeks.

■ Remedies for menopausal complaints include:

- Herbal complexes which include the Chinese herb Dong Quai (Chinese angelica) and the herb Black Cohosh can dramatically limit hot flushes.
- The herb St John's wort is as effective as anti-depressants at relieving mild to moderate depression (but should not be used alongside other anti-depressant medication).
- The herb Gingko Biloba helps to combat memory loss and confusion. It works best alongside B-complex supplement.
- Weight gain of about 7 lb around the menopause is not unusual, but if it goes much beyond that, make sure you are keeping up exercise levels and eating healthy meals and snacks to keep your blood-sugar levels in check. If bloating is a problem, have a wheat-free trial period of a month to see if this helps to stabilize the situation. Replace wheat with rice, potatoes, rye and corn products.
- Headaches and migraines often start, or get worse, around the menopause. Foods that make these worse contain amines – cheese, wine, alcohol, oranges, chocolate, yeast extract and pickles. Caffeine, wheat and dairy products are other frequent triggers. Ginger can help to reduce headaches and migraines by dilating blood vessels in the head. You may also find that muscular tensions contribute and it may be helpful to have neck massages or to practise relaxation exercises.
- Libido can frequently become an issue around the menopause, and this is not helped by vaginal dryness. An energy-boosting diet, with lots of vegetables, fruits and juices can help to keep the spark alive, and phytoestrogen-rich foods such as soya and linseeds have a positive effect on vaginal tissues.
- Insomnia is an often reported complaint. If hot flushes and night sweats are the cause, upping the intake of soya foods can help as can natural progesterone (see below). The herb valerian is a useful sleep-inducer, without side-effects (but should not be used with other sedating medication). A few drops of aromatherapy oils added to your bath just before bedtime can be useful – lavender, geranium and marjoram are all calming.

- Using natural progesterone[22] can reduce menopausal symptoms for many women. If some symptoms persist, such as a dry vagina, it may be appropriate to use a little topical oestriol (E3) cream directly to the area. E3 is the non-carcinogenic oestrogen and is not contra-indicated for use by women who have had breast cancer. Discuss this with your doctor.
- The main worry for women who do not wish to take HRT relates to developing osteoporosis. Again, the diet recommended in this book offers strong preventive measures against this disease:

  – Eating lots of green leafy vegetables, fruit and seeds to obtain the most usable sources of calcium and magnesium.
  – Avoiding salt, alcohol, sugar, smoking, sodas and coffee, all of which leach calcium out of the bones.
  – Soya phytoestrogens have a significant bone-building effect even post-menopausally.[23]
  – Moderate weight-bearing exercise increases bone density. Fast walking, skipping, tennis or using a mini-trampoline, four times a week, are ideal. Swimming and bike-riding do not have the same positive effects as your weight is supported.
  – Keeping animal protein to a minimum as excess protein encourages the loss of calcium from the bones.
  – Using natural progesterone which helps to remineralize bones. Oestrogens stop bone loss, but do not build new bone significantly, while progesterone has a greater impact on increasing bone mineral density.
  – Reducing stress levels as stress depletes calcium from the bones.
  – The nutrients needed for bone health are calcium, in the correct balance with magnesium and phosphorus (phosphorus does not need to be supplemented as it is widely available), the sunshine vitamin, vitamin D, available from oily fish in the diet, zinc and vitamin C for the building process, and boron which, at 3 mg per day, has been found to decrease calcium loss in urine by 44 per cent. Essential fats from oily fish, linseeds, evening primrose oil and eggs also contribute to bone health. A daily supplement that includes these bone-builders can be much more useful than the calcium that many women take in isolation from the other nutrients.

- A dietary supplement, ipriflavone, which is an organically synthesized derivative of phytoestrogenic isoflavones. Over sixty studies attest to its safety, and it has been shown in double-blind, placebo-controlled studies to have a positive effect on increasing bone density and maintaining vertebral and peripheral bone mass in osteoporotic post-menopausal women, without side-effects.[24] It seems to induce bone formation while inhibiting bone breakdown. 200 mg three times a day (a total daily dose of 600 mg) is the optimal dose.
- Fluoride hardens bones in the same way that it hardens teeth. This is not as good as it sounds, because bone is living tissue and successful bone-building is dependent on mineral turnover. Fluoride encourages brittle bones, which in turn can lead to fractures.[25] Teeth are hardened by adulthood and the need for fluoride beyond childhood is highly questionable. Good oral hygiene, regular dental checks, a low-sugar and high-vegetable diet, using vitamin C and CoQ10 to ensure healthy gums are all measures to maintain healthy teeth. Buy fluoride-free toothpaste today.

Bone Broth

In the 'good old days' the stock pot was a regular feature in the kitchen. One of the best sources of the correct balance of minerals for bone health is – bones. By making a stock or soup out of chicken, fish or meat bones and cartilage, you are automatically benefiting from the calcium, magnesium and phosphorous that make up the bone, and the muco-polysaccharides that make up the cartilage.

Beg, borrow or steal some bones from your butcher or fishmonger, cover with filtered water and add assorted vegetables (carrots, celery, cabbage, onion, garlic). Make sure you also add something acidic to help leach the minerals out of the bones – a couple of tablespoons of lemon juice or vinegar, or some tomatoes. Bring to the boil, then allow the pot to simmer for several hours, making sure it does not boil dry. When the stock is cool you can refrigerate it to set, and skim off any fat. Use the broth as a basis for soups and sauces.

A much-advertised benefit of HRT is a reduction in cardiovascular risk. After the menopause, a woman's risk of cardiovascular disease increases to the same level as a man's as her oestrogen levels drop and possibly also because her blood iron levels increase when she stops menstruating. Contrary to the supposed benefits, the progestogens in HRT have been shown to have a constrictive effect on the arteries leading to the heart (progesterone was shown to have a dilating effect). Cardiovascular disease is largely a dietary problem, and the measures which are important to reduce the risk of cardiovascular problems include:

- Eating at least five fruits and vegetables a day and preferably seven to ten portions.
- Making sure you get 25 g/1 oz of fibre a day as fibre eliminates cholesterol as well as oestrogens.
- Keeping salt below 6 g a day, and preferably less – check all packaged products to determine the level you are getting.
- Keeping sugar to a minimum as it raises fat levels, triglycerides, in the blood.
- Eating a low-saturated fat and low-trans-fat diet.
- Again, soya phytoestrogens come to the rescue. Soya has been shown to have a significant effect on lowering cardiovascular risk[26] and reduces overall cholesterol, reducing damaging LDL cholesterol levels and raising beneficial HDL levels. Genestein in soya may also inhibit platelet aggregation.
- Enjoy one measure of alcohol a day if post-menopausal and not on HRT.
- Again, exercise significantly reduces cardiovascular problems and it is ideal to take exercise at least three times a week at a level that increases your heart rate for thirty minutes, without making you speechless.
- If you feel you are permanently under stress, address this as it contributes to high blood pressure.
- The following nutrients have a marked effect on cardiovascular health:

- Vitamin E, at levels of 400–800 ius, has been shown to have powerful cardiovascular protective effects, probably because of its anti-coagulant and antioxidant effects.
- Magnesium relaxes the smooth muscle of the arteries, bringing blood pressure down. It can also reduce or stop heart palpitations. It improves the use of calcium which is also needed for cardio-vascular health and the two should be supplemented together in a ratio of 2:1 magnesium to calcium – a dose of 500 mg magnesium to 250 mg calcium is sufficient for most people to derive a very real benefit.
- Vitamin C strengthens artery walls, which stops plaque being laid down and repairs damaged arteries – 1–3 g daily is an ideal preventive measure, while more might be needed if cardiovascular problems have been diagnosed.
- Co-enzyme Q10 allows the heart muscle to use oxygen more effectively – 100 mg daily is highly beneficial.
- Chromium reduces LDL cholesterol levels (the 'bad' cholesterol), and 200–500 mcg can be very effective.
- B vitamins lower levels of homocysteine, a toxic metabolite implicated in a large number of cardio-vascular problems.
- Natural progesterone may also protect against cardiovascular disease in women. In women arteries tend not to be clogged, instead they spasm, often induced by stress. The death rate for cardio-vascular surgery for women is twice that of men because of this spasm effect. According to Dr John Lee a leading HRT preparation causes the arteries to become a little more dilated, but does nothing to stop the spasm. Progesterone, on the other hand, widely dilates the arteries and eliminates the spasm.

Healthy Digestion

We eat around 900 g/2 lb of food a day. Every cell, hormone, enzyme and neurochemical in the body is dependent not only upon the quantity and quality of the food we eat, but also on *what we manage to digest, absorb and assimilate from that food.*

A poorly functioning digestive tract can have a negative effect on immune function, increase the absorption of toxins into the body and encourage elevated levels of circulating oestrogens. A properly functioning digestive tract is vital for health.

It is not unusual to view the digestive tract as nothing more than a tube. It is, in fact, a vital, highly complicated and rather large organ. To give an idea of its size, if the small intestine were flattened out, it would be about the size of a tennis court. The numerous vital functions of the digestive tract include:

- Secreting digestive enzymes
- Absorbing nutrients
- Acting as the front line against the outside world in the same way as our outer skin and producing immune antibodies. It is the largest immune organ in the body
- Acting as a home for the colonies of beneficial bacteria in the bowel
- Elimination of waste

Oestrogens are eliminated via the colon

Concerning ourselves with our bowels, when we are principally interested in our breasts, may seem strange. Oestrogens are meant to be eliminated via the bowels, and if they are not, blood levels of oestrogens are raised. Raised oestrogen levels mean that more circulating oestrogens are available to latch on to breast cells, and this is where the trouble can start.

There is a relationship between constipation and breast cancer, and resolving the problem of infrequent and poor-quality bowel movements must be a priority. If you are not emptying your bowels once daily, comfortably, without any straining, then you must consider yourself constipated. It is interesting to note that more money is spent annually in the UK on laxatives (£79 million) than on chemotherapy (£59 million). Just think – with a few simple measures perhaps the budgets for both could be slashed.

The circuit that oestrogens make on their way to elimination begins in the liver. The liver processes spent oestrogens and forms substances called glucuronides (and also some sulphates). These are then sent to be eliminated from the bowel. Insufficient fibre in the diet can lead to an overgrowth of 'bad' bacteria which, in turn, increase levels in the bowel of a bacterial enzyme called beta-glucoronidase. This has the unfortunate effect of re-activating the oestrogens from the glucuronides, resulting in their reabsorption and raising blood oestrogen levels. Maintaining sufficient fibre in the diet helps to reverse this negative spiral.

This is what you can do to improve your bowel movements and increase elimination of oestrogens:

- Eat at least 25 g/1 oz, and preferably 30–35 g/1½ oz, of dietary fibre a day, from a wide variety of plant foods such as fruit, vegetable, pulses, grains and seeds (see the fibre chart (page 215) in **Your Basic Nutrition and Supplement Plan**).
- If you are on a very low-fibre diet, are severely constipated, or have irritable bowel syndrome, increase the amount of fibre in your diet slowly, say by 5 g every couple of weeks, to allow your bowels time to get used to the extra work they now have to do. If you introduce more fibre too fast you may find that your symptoms get worse rather than better.
- Do not be tempted just to add spoonfuls of wheatbran fibre on to your food. Wheat causes a lot of allergy-type problems in sensitive people, and in any event is a very harsh source of fibre.
- If you want to sprinkle fibre on to your food, the best source is linseeds – which I have suggested you use for their phytoestrogenic lignans. Another amazingly useful standby for anyone who is constipated is powdered psyllium husks. These come from the outer

coating of plantain seeds and are also effective in lowering cholesterol and balancing blood-sugar levels. There are also the old
standbys of prunes and figs; eight prunes a day or three or four figs
usually have the required effect.

Why a good diet may not mean good health

Before looking at the whys and hows of improving digestion, it is
important to take a look at what we really are eating. We don't always
get what we imagine we should from our diets. One consideration
is the food we eat in the first place. Is it grown in a nutrient-rich
environment? Is it whole and not stripped of valuable vitamins and
minerals, as are refined foods? Is the food cooked in such a way as to
preserve the nutrients, or are they all boiled away in the cooking
water? Are other things being ingested which might interfere with
the absorption of useful nutrients? These include tea, coffee, alcohol
and drugs, including over-the-counter drugs as well as all the more
familiar prescribed items, such as antibiotics, the contraceptive pill,
steroids and other anti-inflammatory medication.

Even if the diet is perfect – organically grown food from nutrient-rich
soil, lightly cooked to preserve vitamins and minerals, and with no
interfering stimulants or medicines – many people still have a compromised nutrient status. A blood test, or other appropriate test, will show
that the majority of people who complain of health problems have
deficiencies in several nutrients.

So we have to look at the ability of the digestive tract to absorb
these valuable building blocks. And in many people the ability to
absorb nutrients, for one reason or another, is severely compromised.
This becomes even more important if recovering from breast cancer
as, in many instances, the person will be having to overcome surgery,
chemical and radiation assault – and further impairment of nutritional
status.

Properly digested food ensures maximum uptake of nutrients from foods

How much thought do you give to what happens to the food you eat? Many people believe that it just goes in at one end and eventually comes out of the other. In fact, what happens in between is a complex and fascinating process of breaking down the food into individual components, sorting out the good from the bad, selectively absorbing food and nutrients at specific sites along the way, and eliminating the waste products. This takes twelve to twenty-four hours in the healthy digestive tract. It is only when something goes radically wrong – constipation, indigestion or an ulcer – that we give our digestive tract much thought.

Factors to consider are:

Do you chew your food properly?

Chewing food has a number of functions. Breaking down the food to increase the surface area for digestive enzymes to work effectively is critical. If food is being passed along the system not fully digested it could cross the digestive barrier and set up allergy or intolerance reactions. Why should your stomach and small intestines work unnecessarily harder than they do already? Many, if not most, people chew their food four or five times and then swallow. Far better to pulverize it.

Chewing also triggers the digestive enzymes further along the digestive tract. It is a clever process – if you are eating steak and chips, steak and chip-digesting enzymes will be stimulated; if it is bean casserole and salad, bean casserole and salad enzymes will be produced.

Saliva is rich in a substance called epidermal growth factor (EGF) which helps the lining of the digestive tract to repair itself. EGF needs to be properly mixed with food to encourage repair of the digestive tract and to keep it healthy. It takes time to establish new habits, and this is no different. Initially, you will find that you have to remind yourself constantly to chew. It helps to take time over your food, eat in a relaxed environment, and to put your knife and fork down in between mouthfuls.

Are you producing sufficient digestive enzymes?

We should produce around 9 litres/15½ pints of digestive juices every day. In view of this large volume, it seems impossible that anyone would not have enough digestive enzymes to break down their food properly, but lack of digestive enzymes is a major factor for many people with digestive health problems. The stomach produces hydrochloric acid and pepsin for protein digestion, the pancreas produces enzymes for carbohydrate and fat digestion, the gall bladder produces bile for fat emulsification, and the small intestine produces enzymes for fat and carbohydrate digestion. In particular, it is not uncommon for hydrochloric acid levels and pancreatic enzyme levels to be low, and this is often the case when someone has been under medical treatment for a while. This can create a vicious cycle, because a low uptake of nutrients can lead to low production of digestive enzymes, which in turn means that food is not broken down properly. This leads to further impaired release of nutrients from foods – and so it goes on.

Symptoms which may indicate that there is insufficient production of these valuable juices are: burping, bad breath coming up from the stomach, indigestion, bloating around the middle (especially within a couple of hours of eating), diarrhoea, constipation, or any food allergy- or intolerance-related problems (including, possibly, arthritis). Solutions for the problem include:

- Drinking sufficient filtered water overall to stimulate production of digestive enzymes – around 2 litres/3½ pints a day is ideal. Very diluted fruit juices or non-dehydrating herbal or fruit teas or dandelion coffee may replace plain water.
- For some people it is helpful not to drink too much water with meals, or half an hour either side of a meal, to prevent digestive enzymes being diluted at the critical time when they are needed to do their hardest work. Yet for others it is helpful to drink a large glass of water fifteen to twenty minutes before a meal to stimulate digestion.
- Avoiding substances which interfere directly with healthy digestion, including strong tea, coffee, alcohol and over-the-counter medication.

- Increasing your consumption of exotic fruits, especially fresh pine-apple and papaya, which come packed with their own rich source of digestive enzymes which help you digest your food. You can also liquidize them and add them to juices and 'smoothies'.

- Having a trial period to see if food-combining alleviates digestive problems. To food-combine, avoid eating protein foods – meat, fish, eggs, cheese, milk, soya, beans and pulses – with carbohydrate foods – pasta, rice, potatoes, bread, cakes, crackers, pie crusts. Either of these two food groups can happily be eaten with vegetables and salads. So a meal would consist of (for example) either fish and vegetables or salad, or a baked potato with vegetables or salad. But you would not combine the fish and potato at the same meal. The principle behind food-combining in this way is that different foods are digested in different locations along the digestive tract, and this stops foods from 'fighting' with each other, and so improves digestion. Food-combining also conserves energy for healing the body overall and repairing tissues. People with excess weight to lose frequently benefit from such a regime. There are many other rules to food-combining, but keeping protein and carbohydrate foods separate is the most important principle. It is worth food-combining for at least two weeks to see if it works for you. If it does, there are many books on the subject to take you further.

- Taking a three-month course of supplemental digestive enzymes. These are readily available from health food shops. Mail-order suppliers are listed in the **Resources** section. A good-quality, broad-spectrum digestive enzyme will have a variety of digestive enzymes for breaking down a number of different food constituents. It is good fun to break a capsule into a bowl of warm porridge and watch what happens – in about five minutes it turns the porridge into a liquid, demonstrating what it will do inside you, and obviously making the porridge more digestible. The instructions on most bottles of digestive enzymes will suggest taking one or two with a meal, but if your digestion is very badly impaired you may even need as many as three or four with a large meal. How long you carry on depends on your symptoms. Three months is sufficient to tell if they are making a difference to your overall health, and there is no harm in carrying on for quite a bit longer, though you may get fed up with popping pills at each meal.

As a general rule, the worse your overall health, or the older you are, the longer you will need to take digestive enzymes. Our digestive capacity reduces dramatically with age, and taking digestive enzymes can be a very easy way to ensure that we are getting what we ought to from our food. A recent Government study of 1,682 people over the age of sixty-five found that although the average intakes of most nutrients were above the RDAs, as many as one in fourteen people suffered serious vitamin deficiency. Intakes of minerals were even more deficient than vitamins, with low levels of magnesium, zinc, iron, calcium and iodine reported.[1]

■ For many people, their digestive problems relate to low hydrochloric acid (HCl) in the stomach. The pH in the stomach should be around 2.0, but in many people, as they get older, or if they have been unwell, the levels decrease, reducing their ability to break down proteins. Unfortunately, not only are the signs and symptoms of low stomach acidity almost identical to those of high acidity, but this is an almost unrecognized phenomenon. The reason why low acidity is so misdiagnosed is that, confusingly, it is often relieved by acidity-lowering medicines. This is because when the antacids create a more alkaline environment in the stomach – which is already erring on the side of too little acidity – it puts the stomach acid-producing cells into overdrive and they produce more acid to compensate. This, in turn, relieves the symptoms of low acidity.

Buying HCl supplements (Betain Hydrochloride with pepsin) is straightforward and a dose of two capsules with each meal helps many people. If, however, you have digestive problems accompanied by reflux of your meal back up into your throat (which is not caused by a structural imperfection) you can suspect high stomach acidity. Do not take HCl supplements if you have had ulcers or gastritis diagnosed.

If you find that you get a slight burning sensation when taking the supplements, stop them – it probably means that you do have excess acidity – however, this is unlikely to happen for most people. If you are currently on a course of chemotherapy, it could be that there is a problem with over-acidity which is caused by the treatment, which will stop when the chemotherapy stops, and if this is the case, supplementing HCl is not appropriate.

The merits of taking HCl supplements, if appropriate, are the same as for digestive enzymes. If you are not digesting your food properly, you are not getting the full range of nutrients from your food which you should be. Once again, to rephrase an old nutritional saying: you are not what you eat – you are what you digest, absorb and assimilate.

Integrity of the lining of the digestive tract affects absorption

When the cells, or the gaps through the cells, are more permeable to food substances than they should be, absorption of nutrients is reduced. While it sounds as if increased permeability might lead to increased absorption of nutrients, exactly the opposite happens because the incorrectly absorbed, and usually insufficiently broken-down, food molecules interfere with the uptake of nutrients. Many factors can combine to wear out the villi lining the digestive tract or increase permeability, including stress, food intolerance (especially to gluten grains such as wheat, oats, rye and barley), prescribed or over-the-counter drugs, alcohol, stimulants such as tea and coffee, and a diet low in factors which boost repair of the digestive lining. Luckily, the measures to help both reduced absorption and increased gut permeability are similar. The repair of the digestive tract lining needs to be encouraged, and the body will sort out which way to do this if you give it the right building blocks.

The cells lining the digestive tract are different to most other cells in the body in one significant way. To a large degree they feed locally, and not from the blood supply. This means that the contents of the digestive tract intimately affects the health of the lining. A key nutrient for the cells lining the intestines is a group of fats called the butyrates, which are actually manufactured by the bacteria in the gut, as long as the right balance of bacteria is being maintained. Stress also has a major effect on the integrity of the gut lining, as elevated levels of cortisol (a stress hormone) reduce the repair mechanism.

If a disrupted digestive tract lining is suspected, it is most important to avoid foods and substances that are likely to disturb the digestive tract lining for a period of two months, to see if it makes a difference. If it does, continue for at least another four months. Foods and substances which can be a problem include:

- Wheat and possibly other gluten grains
- Dairy products, especially milk and cheese (yoghurt may be tolerated)
- Alcohol, coffee and excess tea
- Aspirin and other non-steroidal anti-inflammatory medication
- Any foods to which you may be sensitive or allergic
- Sugar and refined carbohydrates, which feed unfriendly bowel bacteria, which in turn has a knock-on effect on gut permeability

Nutrients and herbals which help boost repair of the digestive tract (see **Other Useful Supplements** (page 173) for further advice) include:

- Essential fats, needed to bring down inflammation and used in the structure of the cells lining the gut. A lack of these fats is a major contributor to inflammation, and flax oil provides these useful fats.
- The nutrients vitamin A, biotin (a B vitamin) and zinc, which help to maintain the integrity of the lining of the gut wall.
- L-glutamine, which is used as fuel for the cells lining the digestive tract and has been shown to be effective at repairing damaged digestive tract lining.
- Butyric acid (this can be taken supplementally; however, it is best to eat a fibre-rich diet which enhances production of butyrates in the digestive tract).
- Aloe vera (make sure that it is good quality, and that it is diluted).
- The herb slippery elm, which is soothing and restorative to the digestive tract.
- Some specific products which combine a number of different ingredients targeted at repairing damaged digestive linings. These are in the **Resources** section.
- Cabbage juice, which contains cabagin (or vitamin U), effective at helping to heal the gut wall. It may sound

unappealing, but when mixed in with other juices, such as carrot and apple, cabbage juice tastes delicious and has a fresh 'green' taste.

Food allergies and sensitivities can tax the immune system

The digestive tract is the largest immune organ in the body. It acts as a barrier between the outside world (food and micro-organisms such as bacteria, viruses and parasites) and our inside world. Today we are seeing an explosion in reported food allergy and intolerance problems. This may be due in part to increased awareness of this type of health problem, but it is also true that we are constantly exposed to substances which disturb the fine balance of the digestive tract. In addition, we tend to eat a restricted number of food items, with insufficient variety in our diets. This means that we become susceptible to wear and tear associated with repetitious exposure to certain foods.

It is a little like tennis elbow – tennis is a good sport, but overdo it and you get wear and tear of certain joints. In order to reduce further damage you need to rest from tennis and eventually turn to a variety of other activities in order to avoid exacerbating the damage. In Europe we are heavily dependent on wheat and dairy products. We might eat each of these substances five or even six times a day: cereal and milk for breakfast, biscuits and milky coffee as a snack, cheese sandwich at lunch-time, cake and tea at tea-time, and pasta with a cheesy sauce in the evening – this is very common. Also, if you buy packaged products, you will see in the ingredients list that wheat-based starch and milk products are used in the majority of products, and this increases our exposure. Other foods to which people are commonly sensitive or allergic are the gluten grains (oats, rye and barley), eggs, soya products and citrus fruit.

The significance of this from the point of view of breast cancer is that when we are eating foods to which we have become intolerant and which may have compromised the integrity of the digestive lining, the digestive tract is likely to let large molecules through into the bloodstream which are recognized by the immune system as 'foe' rather than 'friend', producing an immune response called an IgG reaction. If this happens on a regular basis, it means that the immune system is burdened with an extra job, which will distract it from its main functions, including dealing with cancer. These foods become more excess cargo which has to be dealt with. Identifying food intolerances is extremely important, not only in reducing overall stress on the immune system, but also in providing relief from symptoms which can drag you down. Avoiding foods to which you may be sensitive also often leads to some loss of excess weight, and is beneficial for maintaining a 'clean' lymph system.

Until quite recently the idea of food intolerances was scoffed at, as it was considered that the only allergy was a 'true' allergy – one that triggered an immune reaction called an IgE reaction. This manifests as an instant allergic reaction such as hives, or, more seriously, anaphylactic shock. However, a reaction has been identified which explains the immune system's response to food intolerances – foods that do not produce an immediate reaction, but result in delayed symptoms. This is an IgG reaction and is measurable, though at present the blood tests for it are not very reliable. The phenomenon of increased gut permeability is also measurable, though these tests need to be conducted via a trained nutritionist (see **Resources** section).

The way to resolve food sensitivities is to avoid the offending foods in the first place, in order to reduce the strain on the digestive and immune systems. Avoid the possible offending foods for at least two weeks, to see if you feel better and if any symptoms you are experiencing abate. If this proves to be successful, you need to continue to avoid the food, or foods, for at least six months before seeing if you can tolerate them on a rotation basis. Rotating foods by only eating them once every four or five days allows many people to remain symptom-free.

Buckwheat Pancakes

Makes about 20 × 10 cm/4 in pancakes

Originating in Russia, these pancakes, or blinis, are ideal if you crave a bread-type base to a meal, but need to avoid gluten grains. Traditionally they are made with all-buckwheat flour, but they are a bit lighter if you substitute part of the flour with rice flour.

Buckwheat and rice flours are available from good health food shops. If you are not gluten-intolerant you could use whole-wheat flour instead of the rice flour.

1 × 6 g sachet easy-blend yeast
225 ml/8 fl oz soya milk or semi-skimmed milk
100 g/4 oz buckwheat flour
125 g/5 oz rice flour or wholewheat flour
200 ml/7 fl oz thick yoghurt or crème fraîche
2 eggs

Put the milk into a small saucepan with the yeast and warm up. Do not heat too much as this will kill off the yeast. Place the milk and yeast mixture together with all the other ingredients in a blender and whizz. Pour the mixture into a bowl, cover with a clean tea-towel, and leave in a warm place for two hours (the bowl could be placed in a larger bowl of warm water). The batter should be spongy and bubbly.

To cook the blinis, brush a pancake pan with a tiny amount of melted butter or olive oil. Heat the pan and place in it a tablespoon or two of the batter, depending on the size you want the pancakes (they should be fairly thick). Cook for 30–40 seconds, then flip the pancake over and cook on the other side.

You can interleave the pancakes, when cool, with greaseproof paper, and freeze them. (I usually make a double or triple batch, which lasts quite a long time in the freezer.) When ready to use, just take out what you need, pop them into a toaster and toast from frozen.

Toppings are limited only by your imagination and can be savoury or sweet. Try: pickled herrings with onion and yoghurt; smoked salmon with dill; smoked mackerel pâté (page 208); falafel with tahini; tomato and avocado; cottage cheese with chives; nut butter with 100 per cent fruit jam, banana slices; apple sauce; or berries and Greek yoghurt.

Imbalanced bowel bacteria can overload the immune system

We have around 2 kg/4 lb of bacteria in our small intestines and bowels and these are being replenished all the time. About half our stool weight is made up of bacteria which we are shedding. We have a mutually advantageous relationship with these bacteria: we give them a home and food and they, in turn, manufacture B vitamins and vitamin K, act on lignans to produce stronger phytoestrogenic compounds, and manufacture butyric acid to help feed the cells which line our intestines. They are to a degree self-supporting and produce their own food from the constituents in our gut.

Around 20 per cent of this bacteria is meant to be 'good' bacteria, while 80 per cent is pathogenic or putrefactive bacteria. Problems can arise when the balance goes out of sync between the two. If we have too much of the putrefactive bacteria, they produce toxins which place a further burden on the immune system. A high-meat diet can lead to more of these putrefactive, or anaerobic, bacteria getting a foot-hold. Toxic by-products of 'bad' bacteria can include ammonia, phenols, nitrites, nitrosamines, ethanol and acetone. The main symptom of imbalanced bacteria in the bowels is an excess of wind. Cystitis can also indicate bacterial imbalance. If it has got really out of control, it is possible that a yeast infection will also set in, and again the by-products of such an infection can overload the immune system. Signs of yeast infections could include thrush, athlete's foot, fungal infections of nails and other areas and skin problems, and is most common when there is a history of antibiotics and consumption of high levels of sugar and stimulants. It is also frequently signalled by fatigue and other non-specific problems. The importance of the good bacteria may be even more specific to women with a risk of breast cancer as usefulness of the phytoestrogens in soya and lignans from flax seeds and other sources depends on the relative ability of the gut bacteria to degrade or convert these compounds.[2] It has been suggested that antibiotics can sufficiently imbalance the bowel bacteria to limit the ability to prevent the development of breast cancer.[3]

There are many problems that can throw out the balance of the bacteria, but the main ones to consider are:

- A high-sugar or refined carbohydrate diet. These are great food for the bad bacteria at the expense of the good bacteria. This can lead to enhanced growth of the pathogenic and putrefactive bacteria over the benign bacteria.
- A low-fibre diet will encourage the bad bacteria. Fibre acts as a food substrate for the good bacteria, from which they manufacture their food. A diet which is consistently high in fibre will encourage the growth of the good bacteria, over time.
- Antibiotics wipe out a major quantity of the colony of bacteria in the bowels, good or bad. Antibiotics are not selective and in targeting the pathogenic bacteria for which you are being medicated, will also destroy the fine balance of bacteria in your bowels. As the bad bacteria are more opportunistic, this means that they grow back at a faster rate than the good bacteria, creating an imbalance.
- Stress hormones have a direct impact on the digestive tract and bowel, changing the climate, and therefore the ecology, of bacteria in the region. Stimulants have a similar effect by producing a stress reaction, and alcohol in particular is a culprit as it both produces a stress reaction and raises sugar levels.
- Yeast-based foods may need to be cut out of the diet, in particular bread, cheese and alcohol.

Addressing these issues will, in due course, improve bowel bacteria balance and reduce the negative effect on the immune system. There are also particular foods and supplements which are helpful:

- Garlic is a powerful natural anti-bacterial agent which selectively targets the bad bacteria. It also attacks yeast infections, and olive oil too has a potent anti-yeast effect. Including as much of these two Mediterranean standbys in your cooking as you are able will help to redress the balance of bacteria. You can also take garlic capsules, but the odourless variety have had the active compound removed, so stick to the ones that make you less kissable.
- Cranberry juice has a selective effect on the bacterial overgrowth in the urinary tract which leads to thrush. Drink liberal amounts if you feel a urinary infection coming on, or take cranberry supplements.
- Live yoghurt is a source of the good bacteria we need to help

replenish our stocks, and a small pot a day can work wonders. If you have thrush, yoghurt can also be applied topically to the affected areas.

- Papaya is useful for restoring the balance between good and bad bacteria. When it is in season, having some slightly unripe papaya daily can be a great boon to bacterial balance.
- Apart from the pro-biotics, such as acidophilus mentioned above, there is also a compound which is pre-biotic. This means that it acts as the fibre substrate from which the good bacteria make their food. It is called FOS (fructo-oligo-saccharides) and is a sweet-tasting powder which is ideal to sprinkle on cereals as a sugar substitute. It is not sugar, even though it tastes like it, but a non-digestible fibrous relative which promotes growth of the good bacteria.

Detox Your System

Over the course of a year, every man, woman and child in the UK takes in about 6 kg/14 lb of chemicals, and since the Second World War 60,000 chemicals have been added to our environment, 3,000 foreign chemicals to our food alone, and more are being added year on year.

Our bodies have mechanisms for dealing with unwanted chemicals that we ingest or absorb. We probably developed these mechanisms since many common foodstuffs have toxic chemicals that have to be eliminated – potatoes, red kidney beans, peanuts, all have some toxic compounds. This does not make these foods bad, as we have devised means of using what is helpful and getting rid of the rest. The problem, as ever, arises when we overload our systems with more chemicals than we can cope with.

Our lymph system acts as a cleansing system for each cell in our body. The liver should turn harmful toxins into harmless by-products. Some toxins are stored in the liver and fat cells, while the majority should be eliminated via our skin, breath, urine and bowels. If any of these channels of elimination are not working to maximum efficiency, or if they are overloaded, we run the risk of excess toxins having an effect on the efficient working of cells and taxing the healing process.

Additionally, many of these chemicals have a negative oestrogenic effect which directly influences the progress of breast cancer. When recovering from breast cancer you certainly want to have all your restorative faculties working.

The simple reason why you should seek to detoxify your body is to reduce the total load that you are carrying, while also reducing your exposure to potentially harmful chemicals.

Your housekeeping system

The lymph system can be regarded as the body's housekeeping system. It collects up fluid which bathes our cells and performs a sort of mopping-up operation by cleaning up debris and germs. The lymph is filtered through lymph glands where this operation takes place. Lymph nodes contain fixed macrophages (white blood cells) which destroy bacteria and clean up debris and are probably instrumental as a first line of defence against the spread of cancer. The spleen, which is part of the lymph system, also acts as a store cupboard with a reservoir of white blood cells, which it programmes and releases when needed. About 4 litres/7 pints of fluid a day are drained into the lymph system. The lymph vessels do not have a pump like the cardiovascular system, which has the heart. So to keep the fluid moving, the lymph vessels are dependent on differences in pressure, surrounding muscles contracting and releasing, the action of breathing, and valves to stop backflow.

If lymph becomes too static and viscous, it is unable to do its job properly – circulating and cleaning up toxins and helping to fight cancer. In extreme circumstances, and especially after an operation on lymph glands in a particular area, such as the axillary glands, lymphoedema can result. This is a build-up of lymph in the tissues in certain areas of the body, for instance the upper arm. It is also common for women to get pooling around the ankles. To keep lymph flowing, there are several easy steps that can really help:

- Keep well hydrated by drinking filtered water, diluted fruit juices and herbal teas, and avoiding dehydrating liquids such as excess tea and coffee. Eating a diet high in water-rich fruits and vegetables is a key contributor to our liquid levels and helps to cleanse the lymph system. Freshly made fruit and vegetable juices also provide effective cleansing for the lymph system.
- You may find it useful to have a detox day once a week, during which you drink only water, herbal teas and freshly made juices, and eat only fresh fruits, raw or lightly steamed vegetables flavoured with lemon juice, and vegetable soups. This is not the same as fasting, which I would not advocate under any circumstances if you have a diagnosis of cancer. Detox days have a marked cleansing

effect, but should not be attempted if you are faced with a very busy day, feel faint or dizzy, or if your doctor advises against. You should not detox for more than one day a week, as you need a steady supply of good-quality proteins and healthy fats. (When children or animals are unwell, they reduce their food intake quite naturally.) The digestive system uses a massive amount of energy digesting food. Freeing it from time to time channels energy into the healing process. Also, by eating high-water foods and avoiding foods which are a burden on your system, you allow your lymph system to do a better job in cleaning up debris and getting rid of toxins.

- Avoid foods which tend to make lymph more viscous, especially excess fats and dairy produce. Fats are circulated in the lymph and can clog it up, making it less effective. Salt increases the tendency to retain water and slows down lymph.

- If you are retaining water, a mild and effective diuretic is to drink about ten cups of camomile tea in one day.

- Take regular exercise to keep your skeletal muscles moving lymph along the channels and to stop it stagnating. Of particular use is the rebounder which I have already mentioned (see page 185). The reason for this is that you are working against gravity and gently applying pressure on the lymph system to move the lymph upwards against gravity. For a second, on the way up, you are weightless, and when you hit the rebounder the G-force is about three times the usual gravitational force, which helps to push lymph towards the heart in a dynamic way. If lymph is not moved upwards, it would pool permanently around the feet. It is just below the shoulder area that the lymph system drains back into the blood system, and obviously it has to get there first. The bouncing motion on a rebounder can be very gentle, but for the more energetic, a really good cardiovascular workout is possible, with even better results.

- A gentle form of massage, called manual lymphatic drainage, is very effective at encouraging lymph flow and maximizing its cleansing ability. See the **Resources** section.

- Dry skin-brushing is a wonderful technique for improving lymph flow. Take a natural bristle bath brush and on your dry skin, before taking a bath or shower, use long sweeping motions up the body in the direction of the heart. This stimulates the lymph to circulate and encourages the skin to eliminate toxins. There is no need to apply undue pressure and you should end up tingling, not red and raw. Avoid brushing over any broken skin.

■ Epsom salt baths help to draw out impurities from the skin. Put a cup of Epsom salts into the bath and lie in it – there couldn't be an easier way to eliminate toxins.

Breakfast Rice*

Getting the brown-rice habit is excellent for speeding up detoxification, balancing blood-sugar levels and avoiding eating an excess of wheat. Breakfast rice also makes use of leftover brown rice from last night's meal. You can make brown rice in bulk and then freeze it in portion sizes, defrost and refresh in a sieve by pouring boiling water over it

Allow one bowl of cooked brown rice per person, and a selection from the following:

Fresh nuts and seeds	Finely diced dried fruit
Desiccated coconut	Stewed dried fruit
Spices, e.g. nutmeg	Chopped fresh fruit
Soya milk or soya yoghurt	Stewed fresh fruit
Fruit juice	Carob powder

It is a good idea to keep nuts, seeds, chopped dried fruit, etc., in clear glass jars in the fridge. Then you can quickly add toppings to a bowl of warm or cold rice. Children love the idea of helping themselves to toppings.

Suggested combinations for one bowl of rice:
– ½ chopped banana, a few raisins, few cashew nuts
– ½ stewed apple, pinch cinnamon, sunflower seeds
– ½ pear, chopped dried apricots, desiccated coconut
– Liquidize ½ peach and ½ banana and pour over the rice
– Stewed prunes and soya yoghurt
– Stewed dried apricots and chopped almonds

* This recipe has come from *Cooking Without*, a gluten-, dairy-, yeast-, salt- and saturated fat-free cookbook (Thorsons, 1996), with kind permission from the author Barbara Cousins.

The liver

The liver is a complex organ, which works a twenty-four-hour shift reorganizing proteins and fats, making cholesterol, manufacturing oxygen-carrying pigments, secreting bile, storing glycogen, processing hormones, manufacturing enzymes *and* detoxifying pollutants and toxins. All chemicals have to be processed via the liver, where they are either neutralized or stored. They are also despatched for elimination, and if elimination channels are not effective, the chemicals are stored in fat cells. One theory as to why women carry more fat around their hips is that this is a storage area for toxins which might otherwise affect a developing foetus. Reducing body fat helps to minimize body stores of toxins.

The process of detoxification of chemicals and carcinogens by the liver works in two phases: Phase I which, depending on what is being modified, can produce an even more toxic product, and Phase II which deals with the by-product from Phase I, neutralizing and getting rid of it. This process involves an enzyme system, the cytochrome P450 system. In some people, the two phases work out of sync, which means that they end up with toxic metabolites after Phase I which Phase II does not deal with effectively. This can lead to symptoms such as headaches, fatigue, skin problems, nausea, inability to handle alcohol, coffee or aspirin, among many. It is very important for the liver to be working optimally if breast cancer is present because it is responsible for dealing with carcinogens as well as converting pro-cancerous oestrogens into benign oestrogens. Liver health can be improved by:

- Avoiding alcohol, coffee, smoking and excess tea, all of which have to be dealt with by the liver.
- Reducing saturated fats and increasing unsaturated fats. The cell structure of a healthy liver is dependent on good-quality unsaturated fats in the membranes to work optimally.
- Eating organic food to minimize the number of chemicals that the liver needs to detoxify and eliminate.
- Carrot juice and lemon juice are potent liver detoxifiers. See **Your Basic Nutrition Plan** for other juice ideas (page 205).
- The cruciferous vegetables, broccoli, cauliflower, Brussels

sprouts and so on, are potent liver protectors and detoxifiers. The sulphur amino acids found in garlic, onions, eggs and cottage cheese promote one of the key liver detoxification enzymes.

– The amino acid L-glutamine is very useful for encouraging the liver to detoxify (see information in **Vitamins** (page 159) and **Minerals** (page 167)).

– The herb milk thistle has liver-specific compounds which many trials have shown to improve liver function (see information in **Vitamins** and **Minerals**).

– The herb dill works on both the Phase I and Phase II stages of detoxification. You can freeze it when it is in season and steep it in boiling water and drink it, and you can also use the dried herb.

– If you are on chemotherapy, or have been in the past, this information becomes doubly important, because the treatment chemicals all pass through, and are sometimes activated by, the liver. Reducing the effects of this burden becomes a priority.

Heavy metals

A number of metals to which we are exposed are toxic and have to be eliminated. These metals also have an antagonistic action against useful nutrients. The heavy metals we commonly encounter include:

Lead: 10 per cent of the population have excess blood levels sufficient to impair nerve function. The main source of contamination is our water supply.

Cadmium: The main source is cigarettes and cigarette smoke.

Copper: An important antioxidant mineral which we need, but which is toxic in excess. Sources which can lead to excess are copper water pipes through which our household water may run (particularly in new houses) and the copper contraceptive coil. The contraceptive pill and HRT also significantly raise copper levels in the blood.

Mercury: There is dispute about whether amalgam fillings lead to raised mercury levels. The school which argues against the use of amalgam points out, quite rightly, that mercury is a highly toxic poison. It is probably wise to have white composite dental fillings when having new fillings, or when old ones are replaced.

Aluminium: Sources include aluminium foil and pans, though they are quite stable unless you use them to cook acidic foods such as tomatoes, lemons, rhubarb or vinegar. Other sources of aluminium include antacid preparations and anti-perspirants. When cooking, you can ensure aluminium foil does not touch the food by creating a hood, or use baking paper instead, and replace aluminium pans with stainless steel or ceramic pans.

There are two ways to reduce heavy metal load. These are avoidance as described above, and competition. Certain nutrients either compete for absorption with the heavy metals, or actually latch on to them and escort them out of the body. Useful measures to include in your regime daily if you think that heavy metals might be a problem for you include:

- Seaweed, which is a potent anti-cancer food anyway, and is high in alginic acid, which is a great heavy metal detoxifier.
- Chlorella is known as the 'unpoisoner' because it is so effective at ridding the body of the heavy metals, especially lead and cadmium.
- Pectin, found in vegetables and fruits, especially apples, bananas, berries, peaches, onions and carrots, detoxifies heavy metals well. You can also buy pectin from good health food shops to sprinkle on your food.
- The sulphur amino acids found in onions, garlic, shallots (plus other members of the onion family), eggs and cottage cheese are all potent detoxifiers.
- The nutrients which are most useful for latching on to, and getting rid of, heavy metals, or competing with them for absorption, are vitamin C, zinc, selenium, calcium and magnesium. Silica found in the herb horsetail is also very useful at getting rid of aluminium. (Horsetail will also make your nails grow long and strong.)

Fluoride

Fluoride is a highly toxic mineral which is recognized as toxic in concentrations of only two parts per million in water. Yet one part per million is the amount recommended for dental health.

Fluoride has a strong affinity with calcium, which is why it is used to harden teeth. The fluoride in toothpaste is sodium fluoride. As fluoride does not have as strong an affinity with sodium, it loosens (disassociates) from the sodium and latches on to the calcium in our teeth. But there is a catch: it does not do this directly. It is absorbed into our body via the mucous membranes in the mouth, with a small amount swallowed in saliva, and so it gets to work from the inside out. But this means that it affects other aspects of our health as well. It hardens calcium in the bones, which means that bone turnover is reduced. You may think that this sounds fine with respect to osteoporosis, but bone is living tissue and is not meant to be hardened. The bone becomes brittle and becomes more liable to fracture. Fluoride interferes with many different enzyme functions in the body, including DNA-repair enzyme systems, and thyroid hormone production.

Natural fluoride comes in the form of calcium fluoride, which can be used more safely and does not interfere with enzyme functions to the same degree as sodium fluoride. Children may need fluoride, but adults, in whom teeth have already hardened, do not need further fluoride. Incidentally children can have a fluoride coating painted on their teeth by the dentist every so often, which obviates the need to take fluoride into the body where it can affect developing bones.

It is very hard to judge if you are within the 'safe' level of fluoride. If you are in a fluoridated water area, you may be getting too much when you use toothpaste and mouthwash. We are also exposed to fluoride from non-stick coatings in kitchen pans. Brown mottling of teeth is an indication of toxicity. I do not believe it is wise to use sodium fluoride if maximizing your fight against breast cancer, and there are a number of fluoride-free toothpastes available from health food shops. Tea is a natural source of fluoride and Rooibos tea (see page 134) contains enough natural fluoride to resist tooth decay.[1]

Reducing Your Stress Load

It is no secret that stress – or dis-stress as I prefer to call it – has an impact upon the immune system, lowering white blood cell counts.[1] It is quite common for women to develop a detectable cancerous lump in their breasts after a bereavement, divorce or other major trauma.[2] Studies at King's College Hospital, London found that of 100 women diagnosed with early-stage breast cancer, 50 per cent had experienced at least one severe adverse event such as a marriage break-up or death of a close family member in the preceding year. It is also the case that those suffering a relapse of breast cancer are more likely to have suffered major stress.[3] It is quite possible that stress has accelerated the growth of an existing breast cancer and brought it more quickly to the point where it is detectable. By the same token, I have lost count of the women who have told me that this disease has enabled them to sort out their priorities and not let minor situations become more stressful than they need to be. Getting life into perspective seems to be one universal benefit of breast cancer!

Stress does not just mean mental stress or, for that matter, taxing life events – such as being diagnosed with breast cancer. 'Total load' stress includes chemical stresses, environmental stresses and dietary stresses as well as mental stress. For many people it is this superfluous baggage that it is most useful to eliminate initially – food chemicals and additives, artificial hormones, excess stimulants, unhelpful fats, unnecessary jobs and obligations, and so on. Simplifying our lives is often the best way forward in reducing an overall stress load.

Mental stress is the domain of this chapter, along with nutritional strategies to create a 'shield' to protect your body against the physical damage of stress.

Whether stress is mental, physical or dietary, the stress reaction, that of producing the hormones adrenaline, noradrenaline and cortisol, profoundly affects the various body systems.

The knock-on effects of these stress hormones are to:

– Impair the actions of the digestive tract by diverting the blood supply away from it and therefore reducing the uptake of nutrients from the diet.
– Increase blood-sugar levels which trigger increased levels of insulin. Controlling insulin release is important for reducing the risk of breast cancer.
– Interfere with the actions of sex hormones, which include the stress hormone cortisol, binding with progesterone receptor sites and therefore competing with progesterone.
– Reduce the number of white blood cells.
– Increase oxidation damage.
– Have a catabolic effect on body tissues. Catabolic is simply the reverse of anabolic. Anabolism builds body tissues, while catabolism breaks them down. If the balance is out, tissue repair is not effective.
– Raise blood pressure, which is a predictor of cardiovascular ill-health.

Any stressor has these effects, whether it is comparatively minor, such as being late for an appointment, or more serious, such as having to deal with ill-health; the difference is just one of degree. But what is not often appreciated is that dietary stresses can have a similar impact. One of the reasons why stimulants have the effect that they do is because they stimulate the stress hormones. In particular adrenaline is triggered by – you guessed it – smoking, alcohol and caffeine. Even more surprising to many people is the revelation that foods to which they tend to be addicted have a similar effect. This is why real wheat addicts, for instance, will feel almost instant relief when they eat bread or pasta. These foods affect other chemical reactions in the body, influencing certain brain chemicals, for example, but the food also triggers adrenaline almost instantly.

More of what you want

Changing habits is about more than just changing the food on your table. It is about making room in your life for more of what you want – more of what makes you feel good, and less of what drains you. We can talk endlessly about diet and exercise, but never forget that laughter also boosts the immune system.

I have often heard women say that breast cancer has completely changed their focus. They have made a shift in perception which has benefited them hugely. You quickly learn to get your priorities into the right order. Suddenly, it doesn't seem so important if the train is late, or if the balance on your bank account is not quite what you expected.

This may be the right time, whether you have been diagnosed with breast cancer or are interested in prevention, to sit down and make a list of all the things that give you pleasure, then start doing more of them. Spending more time with your children or grandchildren, taking more bubble-baths, reading more books, going to the cinema – whatever it is that you enjoy, resolve to do more, now.

There is endless discussion about the 'cancer personality'. Some will say that there is a type of person who is most likely to get cancer, while others will dispute this and say that there is no such thing. It is probably dangerous to categorize people – we are all individuals. When talking about prognosis, it is particularly unhelpful to fix on a particular type of person as more likely to recover than another – whether that person is a 'fighter', or more passive, or the type to 'get involved', or whatever.

We are all individuals and behave differently when under duress. However, I have noticed one trait that is probably worth working on. Women quite often have different nurturing roles – they are mothers; they may support the family emotionally; they contribute to the family income, or are solely responsible for it; they are home-makers; they do charity work; they look after elderly parents. And many will fall into the trap of putting everyone else first, thinking of the needs of others before they think about themselves. I am not advocating total selfishness, after all you cannot suddenly change your nature or instincts, and you need to live in harmony with others. But the ability to say no when you need to, or to ask others to help you out, or to feel that you need to take time out for yourself are all useful skills, and worth honing now. And if you feel that this is the right moment to concentrate wholly on yourself, then do so.

Changing habits takes energy, it means rearranging your priorities, and it means putting yourself first some of the time. There are some good books on this subject; see the **Resources** section. Learning to delegate is not a cop-out, it's real life. There is nothing wrong with that.

The mind matters

Some interesting research by Sam Leinster in the *Journal of the Royal College of Surgery*, Edinburgh, evaluated the effects of surgery on breast cancer patients. The theory was put forward that situations of loss lead to depression while situations of threat lead to anxiety. Their results confirmed their hypothesis. Patients who had undergone mastectomy (loss) had higher scores for depression, and patients who had reconstruction surgery (threat) scored higher for anxiety levels. The good news is that the scores did not reach pathological levels; however, knowing what might be bothering you could be a first step to addressing the issues. The research also found that when a patient had matters taken out of her hands in terms of decision-making and was 'swept along on a tide of events until her treatment is completed . . . had worse scores on a number of psychological parameters compared to those where alternative (choices of hospital) treatments were possible'.[4]

Our theories about what choices we will make if confronted with a diagnosis of breast cancer may not hold up. In another study, women who did not have cancer predominantly chose options which allowed them control, while cancer patients generally preferred to leave all the decisions to their doctors.[5] Leinster's paper concluded that women do want information about the disease, its treatment and prognosis,[6] and that the communication skills of the surgeon are paramount in ensuring the best effect of treatment on prognosis.

Burying the ghosts

Many people who have been through a life-changing experience, which a diagnosis of breast cancer can be, will find that the situation replays itself in their minds, over and over again. Obviously, the reaction is different from individual to individual.[7] Some people don't have time to 'be ill', and just get on with their lives as if nothing had happened – one book that sees the situation from this point of view is, amusingly, called *Breast Cancer? Let Me Check My Schedule . . .* However, I have often been told by women that they lie awake at night worrying that they are going to die, that they will never see their children again, that the cancer will come back at a later date, and other terrible scenarios. For some, these are very real issues and they are traumatized. If you find that this is the case it is important to seek out someone to talk to, and preferably professional help. Sometimes the slightest headache or bad back can mean imagining that the cancer has returned. It can take a long time to realize that you can feel ill, just as any other person can, without it indicating something more sinister.

Anna Stopford's story

Sometimes you can also feel that there is a conspiracy against keeping a positive frame of mind and that you are being thwarted at every turn. When Anna Stopford was in hospital after her mastectomy she declared to a house doctor, 'I'm going to be positive', and his reply was, 'Well, I hope you're not going to be disappointed' – a totally thoughtless reply. To really put the dampers on her determination to be positive, the charity she contacted for support and information sent her a newsletter that absolutely terrified her with lots of statistics about life expectancy (she was only aged twenty-nine at the time).

Things have changed dramatically since Anna's experience nearly nine years ago and the medical profession and support charities are far more aware of the impact of their communication skills. But there are still echoes of it – one current book by an expert on the subject of breast cancer lists eight books in the reading list, and the first five have the words death and dying in their titles. The best advice is to ignore it all. Careless talk hurts. Unfortunately, it is likely that you will encounter at least one or two experiences similar to Anna's – people don't mean to be tactless, but they can be. Keep to the forefront of your mind that you are an individual and not a statistic.

Time is a great healer and for most people these concerns begin to fade as they get on with their lives. The worry at the back of your mind may never leave you completely, but your reaction to it gets more into proportion: 'After all, I could get run over by a bus anyway.' The fearful vision fades in its intensity and frequency, and is seen almost through a haze. I liken my own experience to feeling almost as if it had happened to someone else. At the time it was living hell, but the memory has faded. There are so many other more positive things to focus on, especially if you take my advice above – to do more of what makes you feel good.

Helping others to help you

You may not realize it, but when you have to start telling people that you have a diagnosis of breast cancer, you may need to support them through it. Just when you need other people to lean on, you may find that they do not know how to cope with your illness. Husbands may be scared, children uncomprehending, friends embarrassed or nervous. You may find yourself telling people that actually you feel fine, mainly to save them from worry, rather than telling them the truth, that you feel frightened, or tired, or depressed.

Chris Kerrigan's story

Discussing your thoughts and emotions is often the best policy, and trying to guess what others are thinking can lead to uncertainty and unhappiness. When Chris Kerrigan came back from hospital after having a mastectomy (see page 308), she worried that her husband would think her less of a woman. She was saddened on her first night back from hospital when he suggested that he should sleep in the guest bedroom, and Chris spent the whole night feeling tearful and low. This continued for a few nights, when eventually she was able to express her sense of

295

rejection. Her husband was completely shocked that this had been her interpretation, as he had been worried that he would hurt her if he rolled over in the night. His support of her had not wavered for a moment and his actions were based on concern and love, not on revulsion as she had feared.

It becomes quite important to be honest about your feelings. This may not be easy for some people, who are not used to being open about their emotions, but it can be a relief to family and friends to know what you are thinking. If you express yourself gently and without recrimination, it is usually fine to tell people what you want of them, and what you need from them. You may be reticent about asking them to change their behaviour, but once you do so, you may find it a huge relief. One woman I know found that her husband's reaction to her diagnosis of breast cancer was to start frantically doing up the house, and making everything perfect, always being on hand to do everything and anticipating her every wish. While she appreciated his endeavours, she found this quite wearing, and gently, very gently, explained that a more normal pace would be welcome.

When children are old enough to understand what is going on, it can be worse than when they don't understand. Often they may have their own ideas about what breast cancer means, and find it hard to express their worries; they may even be teased at school about their mother. These are all problems which add to the burden of dealing with your health in a positive framework. If any of them get too much, don't try to struggle through – find some help by talking about it with someone who can really help you.

Support groups

A diagnosis of breast cancer is uncharted territory for each of us. With no one to talk to who has had the same experience, it can seem very lonely out there. Fortunately there are an increasing number of support groups and facilities available to those who feel the need for some outside help. They are not for everyone – some women prefer to keep themselves to themselves – but before dismissing the possibility of attending one of these groups, try talking to someone with personal or professional experience of them, or going along to one or two sessions.

The focus is different from group to group. Some will spend time discussing issues to do with the disease, some will offer one-to-one matching with a woman of similar background to you (for example matching for age, age of children, professional status), and others will spend little time talking about the problems of breast cancer but meet for exercise sessions, or for tea and biscuits with people who just happen to have this one common problem. A four-year study at Stanford Medical School in the USA has shown that breast cancer patients who participated in long-term therapy groups live longer and that the women seemed less worried, more able to cope and ultimately to do better. Dr Maggie Watson, principal psychologist at the Royal Marsden Hospital, London, is taking a lead from this study and instigating a similar programme. A number of such groups already exist – see the **Resources** section.

Nutrition to limit damage by stress

Dealing with the mental and physical manifestations of stress is of great importance in seeking optimum health, and following the advice in this book will help cast off some of the chemical and dietary stresses that build up and reduce the effectiveness of the healing mechanism. Here is a check-list of the nutritional strategies that can help to reduce the impact of stress on the body:

- Vitamin C is the supreme anti-stress nutrient. The adrenal glands, which produce the stress hormone adrenaline, are the only storehouses for vitamin C in the body. We are one of only about seven species on this earth that have lost the ability to manufacture vitamin C from glucose in our blood, and we are totally dependent on our diet for this essential nutrient. When animals are under stress (injury, illness or capture), the rate at which they manufacture vitamin C goes up from around 1 g a day to 5 g a day (in human terms, and dependent on species). We are unable to do this. Our predecessors had a more heavily plant-based diet which provided more vitamin C than we have today, and it is useful to supplement around 3 g or more of vitamin C daily, in divided doses throughout the day, if you are under stress.

■ The other nutrients which the production of adrenaline uses up in vast quantities are magnesium and the B vitamins. Magnesium is used for 300 different biochemical processes, and if it is being used up when we are under repeated stress, this means that many functions will not be working properly. B vitamins, magnesium and vitamin C are all used for energy production, so it is no surprise that when we are stressed our energy levels plummet. Supplementing with a 50–100 mg B-complex and 500 mg of magnesium during periods of stress can help to alleviate some of the impact.

■ When we are under stress the first thing we turn to is our favourite prop. However, this is one time when it is best to resist the temptation of the double espresso, gin and tonic, or the family-sized bar of chocolate. The effect of all these pick-me-ups is to start off the blood-sugar roller-coaster, and a key mechanism of reducing the impact of stress is to balance blood-sugar levels (see page 246). And of course elevated blood-sugar levels in turn depress the immune system – it is a vicious cycle that needs to be broken. Adrenaline triggers the hormone glucagon, which raises blood-sugar levels, and in turn can lead to a blood-sugar dip soon after. Regulating this mechanism has a positive feed-back on the production of stress hormones. You will be much better served by turning to a snack which is high in fibre and includes a little protein, such as an oatcake with chopped egg, rye cracker with salsa dip, yoghurt and fruit; all these have little effect on blood-sugar levels, provide you with nutrients (rather than depleting you) and give you an energy boost.

■ As anyone in whom anxiety and stress trigger irritable bowel syndrome will know, stress affects the functioning of the digestive tract. When we are producing a lot of adrenaline and its sister hormone cortisol, blood is shunted away from the digestive tract and repair of its lining is arrested. This leads to a lowering of digestive efficiency and can reduce the amount of 'goodness' or nutrients which we get from our food. If you feel your stress in your digestive system at all, turn to the advice in the chapter **Healthy Digestion** (page 267).

- The aromatherapy oil ylang-ylang is noted for its relaxing properties. A few drops in a bath during times of stress can help to alleviate some of the symptoms and aid restfulness before retiring to bed.
- If stress-induced sleeplessness is a problem, the herb valerian is a side-effect-free solution for many people and has been shown in trials to be as effective as sleeping pills in some cases. The suggested dose is between 150 and 300 mg daily.
- Depression is a common side-effect, or in many cases cause of, stress. The herb St John's wort has been shown in trials to be extremely effective in mild to moderate cases of depression. The daily dose is 340 mg (divided into two lots of 170 mg), giving a total of 1000 mcg of the active compound hypericin.
- Kava is a well-known herbal remedy for anxiety and has some pain-suppressing qualities as well as being a muscle relaxant. 150–200 mg of Kava daily, or 1–3 ml of liquid Kava tincture are the suggested doses. Higher intakes of Kava can produce side-effects such as stomach upset or rashes, so it is not advisable to exceed the dose.

Herbs should not be taken if you are planning a pregnancy, or are pregnant.

Part 5 **Supporting your Medical Treatment Choices with Nutrition**

Your Medical Treatment Choices

I have used the words 'treatment choices' because it is increasingly the case that women are given the option of different treatments – when what they are expecting is to be told what their treatment plan is. This informed choice can be wonderful for some women who want to be involved with, and understand, what is happening, but for others it can create difficulties. To be faced with the choice of a lumpectomy or a mastectomy, or whether to have chemotherapy or not if their case is borderline, can be very difficult, and to make a rational decision means going through a steep learning curve – fast!

Other women will not be given the full set of choices and will not find out until later that there were other options which might have been available to them. They could find themselves in a health district that has a limited budget for some treatment protocols, which might have been offered if they lived just one mile away. A patient who is not being treated at a specialist unit may find out later that the full range of choices had not been offered. It does happen.

It is extremely important to have a rapport with your surgeon or oncologist. Most doctors are kind and considerate – despite being under huge time pressures – however, switch doctors if you are unhappy. Professor Gordon McVie, Director General of the Cancer Research Campaign, has commented that much of the suffering and anxiety that a patient experiences can be induced by a doctor who may have poor communication skills.[1] If you are not happy about the way you are being treated, or feel you are being patronized, then you are entitled to seek another specialist.

The principal criterion for choosing a treatment plan is to maximize the therapeutic effect while minimizing the side-effects, which your specialist will discuss with you.

Insist on the best

In 1997, Professor Karol Sikora, Director of Cancer Services at Hammersmith Hospital in West London, was quoted as estimating that 15,000 people a year in the UK died unnecessarily as a result of never seeing a cancer specialist.[2] And the treatment received in different parts of the country can be dramatically different with, for example, 60 per cent of women at one treatment centre receiving radiotherapy versus 20 per cent in another district.[3] The Department of Health has now created a national standard for cancer care and has directed health authorities to provide a cancer centre which provides specialist treatment for every type of cancer. The National Cancer Alliance publishes a directory detailing the individual interests of almost every cancer specialist in the country. See the **Resources** section for information. You have the right to decide at which centre you would like to be treated, and it is worth doing some investigative work, asking current and former patients about their experiences, and checking out league tables comparing success rates.

Diana Miller's story

In 1991, at the age of forty-seven, Diana was on holiday on a Greek island when she noticed a bruise on her breast. On her return she was referred to a major teaching hospital as a lump was detected beneath the bruise. Unfortunately Diana was seen by a general surgeon, rather than a specialist breast surgeon. After the biopsy she was told that the lump looked like fatty tissue, but a week later she was told that it was in fact malignant. Diana's lymph glands began to swell, and she went in for further investigation. To her horror, during the first operation the surgeon had sliced through the tumour and it had bled heavily into the surrounding tissue. She was told diplomatically that 'We need to get more margin.' The next surgery was conducted by a registrar who was more focused and a wider excision was made along with removal of the infected lymph glands. Diana was only seen by the Oncology Department at the point when she embarked on chemotherapy and radiotherapy, and they were excellent. Eight years on Diana is thriving and has started up her business again.

Diana became very focused on her own needs during her treatment and she knows that she behaved quite selfishly, but has no regrets – she feels that it helped her to get through the experience. Her husband and children were supportive throughout. Diana's commitment to buying organic food and drinking bottled water is total and she makes sure that she eats a diet that is heavily dependent on fruits and vegetables. Her initial strong supplement regime saw her through the treatment programme, and if there is a hint of illness the vitamin C comes out of the cupboard, as she knows that it works for her.

How quickly do I need treatment?

I have already mentioned that early diagnosis vastly improves survival rates and it follows that early treatment is important. It is certainly the case that treatment should be started within three or four weeks. However, that does not mean that you do not have the time to reflect on your best options. One of the key considerations is psychological – many women feel that if they are doing something proactive they can be more at ease with themselves. But rushing into an instant decision is usually not necessary:

- If the surgeon you want is not available for two weeks this probably will not change the outcome. Indeed, it can be positively advantageous if the surgeon has superior technical skills and judgement relative to another who is more immediately available.
- If you want to arrange surgery for a particular time in your menstrual cycle that is probably fine.
- If you want to make time to consider the options of lumpectomy versus mastectomy, which your surgeon may be offering you, do so – within reason – as it is a major decision.
- If you want to discuss the impact of treatment on your home and working life with your family and work colleagues, do so.
- You can use this time positively to prepare yourself for surgery or chemotherapy using the nutritional tools in this book.

305

■ For some women the waiting period can become a time of increasing stress and confusion as they may be bombarded with conflicting advice and grow more uncertain about the right course of action. This is something to be wary of.

Women diagnosed with breast cancer can be made to feel like invalids as a result of the treatment rather than the disease. At this stage the cancer has caused no untoward symptoms and it is the physical trauma of treatment, together with the psychological strain of feeling a victim, or of facing the prospect of mortality, which can cause damage. One day you are fine, the next you are having an operation or nausea-inducing chemotherapy. This is a shock for many women, yet others take it in their stride. There is no right or wrong, but being aware of your reactions helps you to deal with them. I recall sitting in the hospital brimming with tears, while all the women around me seemed to be perfectly normal, taking the treatment in their stride. I was struck with the thought that I was the only person who seemed to be a 'wimp'. It did not occur to me at the time that everyone was different – some would be coping well, some would be hiding their emotions, and others, like me, would have their feelings very near the surface.

The following are the major investigative and treatment options which you may be offered, along with ways to help yourself through the process.

Investigative Scans

Mammography

There are no immediate side-effects from mammography, other than boredom while waiting in the queue! However, there is criticism of the mammography technique within the natural health movement, and this can be alarming for a woman with a lump or other irregularity in her breast, who may feel caught between a rock and a hard place – forgive the pun. On the one hand, she may be told to have a mammography by her doctor, and on the other, she may hear that there are risks associated with mammography. The anti- lobby is particularly opposed to regular mammography screening of older women. In working out the risk to benefit ratio, what are the facts as we know them at the moment?

- Taking one set of X-rays for the purposes of assessing the nature of a breast abnormality probably gives no significant radiation risk.
- Mammography techniques have improved over the years and use lower doses than previously.
- Mammography is the best, if not the only, tool for detecting very early cancers before they can be detected by touch.
- The risk of exposure to mammography X-rays has to be weighed against the risk of undetected breast cancer.
- Unless there are particularly suspicious circumstances, women under thirty-five are not advised to have mammography. The technique is not as sensitive for younger women with more active breast tissue. The breast tissue of young women, in their teens and twenties, is also more sensitive to low-level radiation than in older women.
- A study of 62,000 women aged over thirty years by the Health Insurance Plan of Greater New York has reported that the use of mammography to screen for early, otherwise undetectable,

307

breast cancer results in a reduction in mortality of almost a third.[1]

– If repeat mammograms are likely to be given over time, the radiographer can be asked to calculate the specific likelihood of increased risks from cumulative exposures for individuals, depending on dosage used and their particular details, such as age when mammograms started. I have calculated that if I continue to have mammograms every two years until I am eighty years old, I will have had twenty-eight X-rays, twice over, to each breast – a total of 112 X-rays. I am not sure that this is wise.

Chris Kerrigan's story

In 1989 Chris found out, by accident, that she had breast cancer: 'I saw the practice nurse for a routine smear test and I asked if there was any point in also having a mammogram – even though, in every way, I felt healthy and had no outward symptoms. At the age of fifty I was only just within the range for the screening programme. To my horror I was recalled for further investigation and six weeks later I had a mastectomy. I suspect that nowadays I would have been offered a lumpectomy, but it was the only option given to me at that time. I was so terrified of the operation that if I had had access to my clothes that evening in hospital, I think I would have walked out. I gained a lot of strength from my family, who really pulled together, and my husband was a tower of strength. I was scared that he would be repelled by my appearance, but he didn't flinch for one minute. The experience has made me a much stronger person, and I live more for the moment – I never put off for tomorrow any fun that I can have today. I'm just so grateful that the cancer was detected early and believe I am a monument to early investigation by mammography.'

Assessment of secondary spread

Some simple tests are used to assess the possibility of the cancer having spread to other sites, even if there is no outward indication that this is the case. They include:

- Chest X-ray, to see if any secondaries show up on the lungs, or in the surrounding membranes.
- Blood tests, to look for anaemia or other abnormalities that could suggest bone marrow involvement. Blood tests may also show blood chemistry indication of secondaries in the bone or the liver. Of particular interest for breast cancer are elevated levels of alkaline phosphatase, which could indicate bone or liver involvement, though there are other possible reasons, unconnected to breast cancer, for raised levels.
- Bone scans and X-rays, to look at possible sites for bone spread (most often skull, spine, pelvis and hips). A bone scan involves the injection of radioactive isotopes, or markers, which concentrate in the bone and show up on a 'skeletal survey'. The scan will show up areas of increased circulation, called 'hot spots'. These hot spots could also be arthritis or bone fractures as well as cancer spread. Bone scans are not always offered, and opinion is divided as to how often they should be used. However, if any persistent back, joint or bone pain is experienced, a bone scan should be insisted upon. I have seen several cases where women reported such problems and were told not to worry, only to go back a year later for treatment following a bone fracture resulting from bone weakened by tumours.
- Ultrasound, of the type used on pregnant women to look at the developing foetus, may be used to assess the condition of the liver.
- CAT scanning is a type of X-ray which produces cross-section pictures and may be used if there is a suspicion of spread to the brain.

Surgery

Lumpectomy

Lumpectomy is also called excisional biopsy or breast-sparing surgery. This is the most conservative surgical approach, involving removal of the lump and the tissue surrounding it. It usually leaves a minimal scar and conserves as much of the breast tissue as possible, including the nipple, often necessitating no change in bra size and no reconstructive surgery. Six or seven out of ten cases of breast cancer are dealt with by lumpectomy rather than mastectomy and, according to the leading breast surgeon, Professor Michael Baum, 'It can now be said with confidence that attempts to preserve a woman's breast do not pose a hazard to her life.'[1]

Axillary gland removal

The axillary glands lie in the armpit and are the glands that are most likely to become infected if the cancer has started to spread. For this reason it is usual for the axillary glands to be removed if necessary, or at least to be sampled. Axillary gland removal is unlikely to be carried out if the primary tumour in the breast is 'in-situ' (i.e. shows no sign of spreading). If it is uncertain whether the glands have been infected, sampling may be suggested, and the glands nearest the breast removed for laboratory investigation. If they are shown to be clear, further removal may be unnecessary.

It is of concern to some people that removal of the lymph glands will impair the immune system as these glands are an integral part of it. There are many areas of nodes throughout the body and, generally speaking, the body adapts well and compensates for the loss of a group of axillary glands. However, there is a chance of local infection as the drainage is impaired in that particular area, consequently it is a good idea to support your immune system, and your lymph system, to the full in the future (see the chapters **Building Powerful Immunity** (page 239) and **Detox Your System** (page 282). You will find that any future blood samples will be taken from the other arm in order to reduce the risk of infection of the area.

Mastectomy

This is surgical removal of the breast and every woman's reaction is different. Some really dread it, while others are relieved to have the cancerous tissue removed, and no doubt many women feel a mixture of both. There are several different types of mastectomy and your surgeon will discuss the merits of each as they relate to your particular case. Mastectomy is usually suggested where the tumour is of a significant size, if several tumours are diffuse throughout the breast, or if aggressive malignancy is detected. Mastectomies can be:

Partial	Somewhere between a lumpectomy and a mastectomy, also called wide-excision, segmentectomy (wedge) or quadrectomy.
Complete	Or total, removes all soft breast tissue.
Modified	Removes tissue and lymph nodes.
Subcutaneous	Removes breast tissue leaving skin intact.
Radical	Removes all muscles of chest wall as well as the breast. Radical surgery is hardly ever performed these days and has almost been consigned to the history books.

Reconstructive surgery, to return you to your former glory, is possible after a mastectomy.

Delaying surgery

It is sometimes suggested by the cancer specialist that surgery should be delayed. It may be that it is more appropriate to have chemotherapy and radiotherapy first to shrink any cancer masses, and to consider surgery later. In these circumstances the eventual surgery may be more conservative as the tumour mass is smaller. This is a fairly new and successful approach and is aimed first and foremost at dealing with any cancer spread, before addressing the primary tumour. It can speed up systemic (whole body) treatment by four to six weeks, which in some cases may be an advantage. It is even possible that chemotherapy and/or radiotherapy offered first may remove the need for surgery later.

Timing of surgery

Interesting research[2] has shown that there are better survival rates for pre-menopausal women who are operated on in the second half of their menstrual cycle (i.e. days 14–30). The probable explanation for this is hormonal.[3] In the second half of the cycle levels of progesterone, which antagonizes oestrogen, are high, whereas in the first half of the cycle oestrogens are unopposed.[4] The overall figures quoted are:

Surgery on day 1–12	54 per cent chance of survival for ten years
Surgery on day 13–28	84 per cent chance of survival for ten years

The difference was most impressive when axillary nodes were involved:

Surgery on day 1–12	33 per cent chance of survival for ten years
Surgery on day 13–28	78 per cent chance of survival for ten years

The figures quoted are for ten years as this was the length of the study – survival was no doubt longer for many women.

Not all studies which have tried to confirm this finding have been as positive, and consequently most doctors will view this effect as interesting but unproven. Nevertheless, if surgery can be timed accordingly – why not?

Breast reconstruction

While most women have lumpectomies instead of mastectomies, for some women conservative surgery is not appropriate. Many women will be happy to have a well-fitting prosthesis (false breast). I have even heard one woman with a double mastectomy cheerfully talk about changing her bosom size depending on her activity – small for every day and more buxom for evening pursuits. Other women will opt for reconstruction.

Reconstructive surgery is now available to most women. Some women will be quite happy with a prosthesis instead of undergoing further surgery, but for many women this ability to 'return to normal' is a wonderful boost to their confidence and self-esteem. Reconstructive techniques have improved dramatically and it is no longer a question of 'filling the bra'. The aim now is to build a breast which is cosmetically attractive and matches the other breast.

While reconstruction is available, it is not automatically offered in all cases, and you may need to initiate the discussion. Availability is usually a question of the treatment centre you are attending and you may need to move to another centre to have access to a plastic surgeon specializing in breast reconstruction. The operation is becoming increasingly popular and is available on the National Health Service. If your surgeon is not willing to offer reconstruction, you have the right to ask your GP for a referral to a different surgeon.

If reconstruction is available it may take place at the same time as the mastectomy though some surgeons prefer not to do this. It is best discussed prior to an operation because, if reconstruction is delayed, many women will simply not be able to face a second operation at a later date. However, a simultaneous operation is not always possible because it usually requires a breast cancer surgeon and a plastic surgeon to be available at the same time.

Overall, 5 per cent of women who have had mastectomies have reconstructive surgery, but in treatment centres where it is available about half choose to have it done, which indicates that if reconstruction were more widely available, more women would opt for it. The outlook is improving for the breast cancer 'graduates' of the early twenty-first century as the breast cancer surgeons now coming off the production line are automatically being trained in reconstruction techniques.

Reconstruction does not affect any other aspects of treatment (chemotherapy, radiotherapy or hormone therapy). Nor does it create difficulties at follow-up sessions or in detecting recurrence. What it does do, for many women, is offer increased self-esteem and optimism and cuts out the need for prostheses and special or restrictive clothing.

Several different methods of reconstruction are possible and your surgeon will discuss the best option for you. They fall into three categories:

Tissue expanders: More suitable for women with larger breasts. A type of balloon is inserted and is gradually inflated with salt water (saline).

Silicone gel implants: A soft bag filled with silicone gel, the same as that used for breast enlargement surgery, is inserted. The body reacts to silicone by forming a capsule around it, and sometimes this can contract causing a hard feeling in the breast. There is concern that silicone leakage can lead to auto-immune diseases such as arthritis, allergies and rashes – or even, possibly, cancer. In response to these concerns in the UK, the Department of Health has taken the situation seriously enough to set up a register of women with breast implants, to monitor possible side-effects.

Musculocutaneous flaps: Skin and muscle are taken from somewhere else on the body to create a breast shape. If they are taken from the abdomen you can have a tummy tuck at the same time! More frequently it is taken from an adjacent area to the breast and swivelled round into place. The main disadvantage is the need to inflict surgery on another part of the body.

Nipple reconstruction: Many women do not feel the need to have this extra procedure which is best done separately, allowing the breast to settle and the nipples to end up at the same height. Tissue may be taken from the opposite nipple, if large enough, or the inner thigh. Coloration can be darkened by tattooing and in some cases cartilage from an earlobe might be used. Another option is to have stick-on nipples made. My local hospital uses the services of the local denture maker to take casts of the opposite nipple to get an exact match – I'm sure this is welcomed extra business as the demand for dentures is decreasing these days.

> ### Katrina Davison's story
>
> You do need to keep a sense of humour to see you through the whole breast cancer experience. Katrina found herself, at the age of forty-one, facing a mastectomy, but she managed to have the surgery combined with a reconstruction. On the big day she found herself in a plastic surgery ward, rather than a cancer ward, surrounded by women in the other beds who were due to have cosmetic breast reductions. A young registrar, touring the ward, peered over his glasses and said in a loud voice, 'And what are we in here for? . . .' His tone became slightly more hushed when he realized Katrina's procedure was more than cosmetic. In the end her reconstruction was superb and a massage therapist, who was treating her at a later date, asked her how she had lost her nipple – the rest of the breast looked so natural that this was the only obvious difference between her new breast and the opposite breast. With a smile she told the therapist that she had lost it in the supermarket while shopping one day!

Side-effects of surgery

Post-operative pain can be well managed by giving a costal nerve block, meaning that the patient can wake up without pain, and is able to get up and move around quite soon after surgery. Apart from the obvious effects of surgery, including some discomfort, bruising and possible complications around the scar tissue, there are other specific problems which a breast cancer patient may encounter.

There is often some degree of weakness around the shoulder inhibiting movement immediately after surgery. A physiotherapist will examine the extent of the problem and give remedial post-operative exercises to free movement. Sometimes there is a tightness in the ligaments which lasts for quite a long time, though this does not cause pain and can be remedied by movement.

Swelling of the arm, especially the upper arm, called lymphoedema can be caused when lymph nodes are removed or damaged. This problem has been reduced considerably by the drop in the number of radical mastectomies carried out. The combination of removing axillary nodes and following up with axillary radiotherapy is usually avoided as it worsens this problem. For information on managing lymph circulation problems see the chapter **Detox Your System** (page 282).

Sometimes the nerves to the muscles at the base of the armpit are damaged during radical surgery and this can lead to instability of the shoulder blade, but this is now extremely rare.

There may be psychological changes that need to be dealt with. For example, some women are distressed by the change in their physical appearance, while others are not in the least troubled by this. The availability of reconstructive surgery has gone a long way towards overcoming such problems – however, if you are greatly upset by the change in your body, or the reactions of others, talk to a counsellor instead of bottling up your feelings.

If a tumour is encapsulated in a collagen envelope (meaning it has been naturally isolated from surrounding tissue), it is best to remove it without piercing the capsule. One problem that is not often spoken about is the possibility of spreading cancer by surgery. This is a rare occurrence in the hands of an experienced breast cancer surgeon, and is yet another reason to go to a specialist. Many people do not realize that when they have an operation, the surgeon may be a generalist and not a specialist. The survival rates of women operated on at specialist centres tend to be considerably better than at non-specialist centres.

Tips to help you through surgery

You will usually have a few days to prepare for surgery and there are a number of positive things you can do to minimize the impact. The first thing is to be as informed as you think you need to be. Studies consistently show that patients who were given good pre-operative information had a lower need for pain-killers, faster post-operative recovery and shorter post-operative hospital stays than those who did not receive the same information.[5]

Prepare yourself nutritionally by cleansing your system as much as possible. Drink a lot of water, at least 2 litres/3½ pints a day, to hydrate yourself, and avoid dehydrating drinks such as alcohol, coffee and caffeinated drinks. Your liver is going to have to deal with the anaesthetic and giving it a break for a few days beforehand is probably wise. Eat lots of organic fresh fruit, make fresh juices and eat salads and vegetable soups to encourage vitality. Aim to keep in mind that you are nurturing yourself and stocking up on dietary sources of vital nutrients.

Tomatoes, aubergines, peppers and potatoes, members of the deadly nightshade family group of plants, contain compounds called solanaceous glycoalkaloids, which may inhibit the way the body disposes of anaesthetic, so it may be a good idea to avoid eating large amounts of these foods the week before, and a few days after, surgery.

Drinking plenty of water can also help to ward off the constipation which often results from having an anaesthetic. You will probably find that you have little appetite after the operation as your body conserves energy to speed up healing, and avoids wasting it on digestion. You may want to take a supply of fresh organic fruit into hospital with you to nibble on, as the average hospital menu is a sad affair.

The most valuable nutrients for repairing tissues following an operation are vitamin C and zinc. Vitamin C is used to manufacture collagen, the glue that sticks our cells together and is a tremendous boost for wound healing. Zinc is necessary for repair of tissues as it is used for all protein synthesis. Taking at least 3 g of vitamin C and 15 mg of zinc, along with a multi-vitamin and mineral supplement daily, can really boost healing. Conversely, it is best to avoid vitamin E in excess of 100 ius a day for around seven to ten days prior to an operation as it is a blood-thinning agent. Vitamin E and aspirin need to be avoided before an operation to avoid excessive bleeding. You should, however, start to take vitamin E again just after your operation as it can significantly reduce scarring.

The homeopathic remedy Arnica is fabulous for reducing bruising and alleviating shock after surgery or any other trauma. Starting a couple of days before surgery take five drops four times daily, or one tablet four times daily, until you are better. Arnica cream is particularly good for clearing bruising, but do not use it on broken skin. If you are very nervous about the operation you may find that the Bach flower homeopathic remedy, rescue remedy, helps to calm you down – place a few drops under your tongue every couple of hours for as long as is necessary.

The herb comfrey's popular name is 'Knitbone' because it has such remarkable healing properties on bone and other tissues including muscle, ligaments and skin. It is currently 'voluntarily' restricted by herbalists as it is difficult to maintain consistent levels of alkaloids in preparations, so it is not advised to take it internally. You can however buy comfrey tea from health food shops, and use it to make a poultice to apply topically to a wound. It is soothing and can help to speed up repair. To make a poultice make a thick damp mixture with the tea and then spread it on to the wound. Apply damp cotton gauze on top, then lightly bind with some bandage to keep it in place for an hour or so, while resting. Juice taken from the aloe vera plant can also be used topically to speed up healing of wounds, and can be spread on the area and allowed to dry. Do not apply this poultice until any surgical drains have been removed.

You will probably find that the hospital you are in does not like you taking any supplements while under their care, or at any rate not without their consent. They usually have rules about all medication being dispensed by the nurses. You may want to discuss this with them before admission.

Your length of stay in hospital is likely to be between three days and a week. You can use the time to good effect and relax and sleep as much as possible. You may enjoy having visitors, but some people may be almost too kind and overwhelm you with visits when you feel the need to rest. If this is the case don't worry about asking people not to visit until you get home – that is usually when you will need the extra support and help that visitors can give.

Lymphoedema, swelling of the arm after surgery to the axillary glands, used to be much more common, but now less than one in ten women develop this problem. The left side is most likely to be affected because the lymph system is unilateral and there is more pressure on the left. MLD, manual lymphatic drainage, a gentle form of massage that specifically targets the lymph channels, has been available as a medical treatment on the National Health Service at a few centres

318

since 1995. The lymphoedema clinic in your hospital may have a list of MLD practitioners, otherwise see the **Resources** section. MLD can reduce the swelling significantly – the massage should always go in the direction away from the tumour site. You should check that the therapist is qualified to use MLD for cancer treatment as there are different levels of qualifications. It has been used in Europe and the USA for many years but is only now being taken seriously as a treatment option in the UK.

Surgery also suppresses the immune system and you may want to review the information in the chapter **Building Powerful Immunity** (page 239) to see what measures you want to take to reduce the impact of surgery on your immune system.

Movement after surgery

Movement can be uncomfortable after any surgery, however it does seem that the earlier someone begins to move around, the earlier their recovery (though you should move at your own pace – it was the last thing I wanted to do on day one). You may be worried about stitches pulling apart, but this is highly unlikely to be a problem. Obviously you have to be sensible about the types of movement that you attempt as you build up strength in the area. Initially, a physiotherapist will visit you and give you some suitable exercises to stretch and regain use of the muscles. You can take a shower once any surgical drains or staples have been removed, and you can take a bath when the wound has healed. In the long run swimming is ideal exercise for the arm area and you can resume other normal activities once the wound has healed, but serving overarm at tennis or lifting weights may not be a good idea in the first few days after surgery!

Radiotherapy

Radiation (X-ray) is used for local treatment of cancer cells and is given to women with the highest risk of local recurrence – about 30 per cent of those with breast cancer. Where this risk is evident, the rate of recurrence can be reduced by three- to four-fold.[1] Radiation works best on small areas, hence the need, usually, for surgery first. Radiotherapy is not normally given after mastectomy, to avoid problems with lymphoedema.

Radiotherapy is usually given after surgery and is targeted at the affected area – the breast, the chest wall and, occasionally, the armpit and the collar-bone. A course of treatment is usually scheduled for five days a week for about six weeks. Apart from having to lie very still for several minutes during treatment, it is not an uncomfortable procedure. The requirement not to wash the area for six weeks causes much more discomfort than anything else.

Radiotherapy to the breast area is carefully targeted these days so that the radiation burns experienced by women in earlier decades rarely occur. Occasionally, the top part of the lung may be affected, becoming stiff and fibrous, which can cause a dry cough or breathlessness. Radiation to the breast does not cause infertility, nor does it trigger hair loss. Some people do find radiotherapy tiring and it may cause nausea. However, in most cases there are no adverse reactions.

The most likely short-term side-effect is a dark patch which develops at the site of the radiotherapy, akin to sunburn, which may be itchy or sore. Much can be done to reduce this sunburn effect, as we shall see later. People with fair or red hair, and fair skin, are most at risk of this. As the tissues absorb radiation they can tend to retain water so there may be some local swelling. Sunbathing should be avoided for a year or two after radiation treatment.

The radiographer will decide on a total overall dose to be given over a number of weeks and then divide that dose by the number of treatments to be given. There will either be lower individual doses with more frequent treatments or higher individual doses with fewer treatments. The number of treatments will be governed, as much as anything else, by pressure on resources. So if there is a heavy work load the hospital may run three visits per week (with a stronger dose), versus five visits per week (with a lower dose) if less busy. If there is an option, it is probably better, in terms of ensuring fewer side-effects, to go for the more frequent visits with lower individual doses.

Side-effects of radiotherapy

A key worry for women undergoing radiation therapy is the possibility of it leading to an increased chance of cancer later on. In the past there was certainly a risk of an increased incidence of sarcoma (a cancer of connective tissue, bones and blood vessels) from the use of low-energy X-rays.

The high-energy X-rays used today do not seem to produce this effect. Radiation doses are in excess of 4,500 rads, and at this level the risk of radiation-induced malignancies is minute. The risk occurs at lower doses, especially in the 300–1,000 rad range, after which the risk begins to decrease. The reason why lower doses have this effect is that healthy cells can mutate into malignant cells in this range, while at higher doses the cells are simply killed off. In Hiroshima, where a large increase of breast cancer was noted as a result of the nuclear fall-out, women were exposed to about 300–400 rads – the dangerous zone. Historically, there was an 80 per cent higher incidence of breast cancer in women who had fluoroscopic investigations for TB than in the general population. This was because each examination delivered up to twenty rads and fluoroscopies were administered to the same women many times.

Here are some of the side-effects and facts about radiotherapy:

- Any swelling of the breast usually settles down after a few weeks, though if the nipple and areola area are affected, it may take a little longer as the skin in this area is much thinner and therefore harder to repair.
- The ovaries receive about thirty to forty rads which is due to scattered radiation throughout the body (this cannot be reduced with protective lead coverings). Fertility and menstrual periods are not affected

by this level and there does not appear to be evidence of foetal problems later on.

■ A woman is unlikely to be able to breast-feed a baby from a breast that has had radiation treatment but should be able to produce sufficient milk from her other breast. I had no trouble nursing my baby with only one breast – the only problem was cosmetic, with one breast much larger than the other during the months of feeding, though this settled down afterwards.

■ If the tumour is in the middle of the breast, there is an increased risk of damage to the lymphatics in the area from radiation treatment.

■ There are immunological changes, including a lowering of white blood cell count, after a course of radiation therapy – however there is no statistical difference on the course of cancer.[2] It must also be remembered that the thymus, an important immune organ which programmes white blood cells, lies uncomfortably close to the breast and may be susceptible to damage from radiotherapy.

■ Younger women are at greater risk of radiation-induced cancer, although after the age of thirty-five the risk is negligible.

■ The incidence of new cancers in the opposite breast is identical for women treated with radiation therapy versus those who received chemotherapy alone, and radiation does not increase the incidence.

■ Once a breast has been treated with a course of radiotherapy, it is seldom used for treatment again.

Reducing the side-effects of radiotherapy

The most important first step is to make sure that you are taking your antioxidant supplements on top of a diet which is rich in natural sources of antioxidants from fruits, vegetables and legumes. Radio-therapy creates free radicals and the antioxidants can help to protect tissues against damage.[3] Another supplemented nutrient which may help to reduce the side effects of radiotherapy is vitamin B6.[4]

You can also contact a homeopathic doctor (see the **Resources** section) to find out about remedies, such as X-ray or Radium, which can reduce the side-effects of radiotherapy.

Protease inhibitors, found in pulses, beans and soya, are thought to protect cells from ionizing radiation, which includes the X-rays used in radiotherapy, so including these in your diet as often as possible before, during and after radiotherapy treatment may be a bonus. French scientists have shown that alfalfa can reduce tissue damage caused by radiotherapy[5] and you may want to include a daily sprinkling of alfalfa sprouts on your salads.

Along with other medical treatments, radiotherapy can interfere with the immune system. This means that supporting your immune system nutritionally becomes more important. Follow the advice in the section Building Powerful Immunity (page 239).

As the tissues in the breast area may tend to retain water when absorbing radiation, as they do after sunburn, you may be more comfortable wearing a soft cotton T-shirt instead of, or under your bra to prevent abrasion.

Generally radiation is fairly symptom free though occasionally women complain of fatigue. This seems to build up as the treatment goes on, so it may be wise, especially towards the end of the treatment period to allow more time to rest, as and when you need to.

You will be asked not to wash the treated area and not to use cosmetic creams. Aloe vera is extremely soothing and encourages the tissues to heal quickly. Aloe vera juice, squeezed directly from the leaf of the plant itself and applied topically to the site, is superb at reducing the superficial irritation and sunburn effect often experienced as a result of the radiation. It does not reduce the effectiveness of the radiotherapy on the target tumour site. Failing this, use a brand of aloe vera gel which has no other potentially irritating substances (see the **Resources** section). Apply it just before you go to have your radiation treatment and allow it to dry. You can also apply it afterwards.

Hormone Treatment

Tamoxifen

Tamoxifen (Novaldex) is a drug which has been the subject of great excitement in the medical community in recent years as it seems to offer increased protection from recurrence of breast cancer. Tamoxifen is now prescribed to about 80 per cent of women with breast cancer. There are undoubtedly considerably fewer side-effects to Tamoxifen when compared to the treatment options that have been available historically. While incidence of breast cancer is on the increase, mortality has finally taken a downswing of 15 per cent since 1990. The reported view of Professor Trevor Powles, director of the breast unit at the Royal Marsden Hospital, London, is that this reduction in mortality has come too soon for it to be attributable to improved screening or chemotherapy, but is likely to be due to the increased use of Tamoxifen.

Tamoxifen seems to be protective as it acts as an oestrogen regulator. This means that it stops the negative effects of oestrogens at receptor sites in the breast. It is most useful for post-menopausal women, though it is also given pre-menopausally. Tamoxifen also acts as a prolactin blocker; prolactin is the hormone responsible for initiating breast milk production. Levels are high in breast cancer patients and prolactin may be an even more potent stimulator of tumour growth than oestrogen. Additionally Tamoxifen reduces circulating blood levels of IGF-1 (insulin-Pike growth factor-1). IGF-1 encourages cell division in breast cancer tumours. It is even possible that it acts to suppress blood vessel formation by breast tumours.

The drug is given in tablet form and treatment is usually continued for two to five years – more usually five years. Post-menopausal women will quite often be given Tamoxifen irrespective of oestrogen receptor status or lymph node involvement. As it may trigger menopause or threaten fertility, pre-menopausal women are not given it routinely, especially as it has less clear benefits for this group of women.

There is a move towards giving Tamoxifen as a preventive measure to women who have a high risk, in particular women with a significant family history of breast cancer. There are major trials under way at the moment to assess its relevance for this scenario, but serious concerns are being expressed as, if taken for prevention, longer courses of the drug are required, which may well exacerbate the risk factors associated with Tamoxifen. As with any drug, it is a case of weighing up the risk-to-benefit ratio – what may be acceptable to a woman with diagnosed breast cancer may not be appropriate to a woman who is so far disease free.

Side-effects of Tamoxifen

The immediate side-effects of Tamoxifen are likely to be those associated with the onset of menopause, including cessation of menstruation – often permanently. Others include weight gain (sometimes significant), sweats and hot flushes. Less common, but possible, are problems of vaginal dryness or discharge. Other short-term effects that have been reported are the triggering of asthma, and depression. If the last two are suspected, the way to find out if they are being caused by Tamoxifen is to discuss with your specialist the possibility of a trial period during which the medication is avoided.

More serious is the continuing debate about the long-term safety of Tamoxifen. This is not surprising as the drug has only been in large-scale use for around fifteen years. It is only after a considerable period and many trials that we are truly able to evaluate any drug. Although there seems to be no doubt that Tamoxifen is effective at reducing recurrence of breast cancer, the anti- lobby cite side-effects such as increased risk of endometrial cancer, liver cancer and eye damage. The pro- lobby argue that Tamoxifen not only protects against breast cancer, including a reduction in the development of breast cancer in the other breast, but also seems to reduce cardiovascular risk by lowering serum LDL cholesterol. It also has the effect of increasing bone density and helping to prevent osteoporosis.

There is considerable debate among researchers about the best way forward. A recent joint US–UK study into the use of Tamoxifen as a breast cancer-preventive measure for healthy women who might be at risk was halted in the USA. The results were found to be so remarkably protective that it was deemed that it would be unethical not to give women at risk this drug. In the UK, however, the researchers distanced themselves very quickly from this decision, pointing out that the trial had only been going for two years, and that the data relating to very long-term use of Tamoxifen in healthy women is simply not there. It appears that after two years the number of women developing endometrial cancer (of the lining of the womb) doubles, while after five years it quadruples. Incidence of endometrial cancer amongst the general population is three in 10,000 each year. So this means that the incidence increases to six in 10,000 with two years' use, and twelve in 10,000 after five years' use. This may be a risk worth taking for women who have had breast cancer and enjoy a markedly reduced risk of recurrence, but may not be such a great idea for women who have never had breast cancer but are considered at greater risk. Instigating protective nutritional and lifestyle changes may be the best way forward for this group of – usually young – women. One group of researchers raised 'the question of whether dietary intervention with soy protein should be considered as an alternative approach to drug therapy or breast cancer prevention' (they were referring directly to Tamoxifen).[1] Another unanswered question is whether an optimally nourished woman is less likely to develop endometrial cancer if on Tamoxifen – it will be a long time before this question is answered, but if you elect to use Tamoxifen it may be good insurance to improve all other dietary and environmental risk factors.

There is much to be learnt about Tamoxifen. For instance, it has been assumed that it works as a hormone-blocker – stopping the action of oestrogens on breast tissue. Yet if this simple explanation is correct, we would probably see a reduction, instead of an increase, in the risk of endometrial cancer, which is also an oestrogen-related cancer. In fact, Tamoxifen seems to have a dual effect, both anti- and pro-oestrogenic, depending on the site in the body. Additionally, if the theory of oestrogen-blocking was correct we would expect to see a greater effectiveness in younger women, who are more hormonally active, than in post-menopausal women who have lower oestrogen levels. This is not the case, indeed the opposite is true, with post-menopausal women benefiting more. It is probably correct to say that

Tamoxifen is better understood in terms of its clinical effect than its biochemical action.

A round-up of the effectiveness of Tamoxifen on treatment of breast cancer looks like this:[2]

- The drug is of most benefit to post-menopausal women with oestrogen receptor positive breast cancer.
- Post-menopausal women with oestrogen receptor negative breast cancer also benefit, and the benefits probably outweigh the risks.
- It is in the balance whether pre-menopausal women with oestrogen receptor positive breast cancer benefit significantly, and statistically the potential benefits are small.
- A woman who is pre-menopausal with oestrogen receptor negative breast cancer will probably enjoy no benefit.
- Breast cancers that are progesterone receptor positive are more likely to respond well to Tamoxifen, and these receptors may even be a better indicator of a good outcome than oestrogen receptor status.
- There is more benefit for women where the cancer has spread to the lymph nodes than for women where it is contained in the breast tissue.

Tamoxifen seems to have benefits for many women without the toxic side-effects of chemotherapy, which may well make it a treatment of choice. Whilst it seems that Tamoxifen is a step forward in the treatment of breast cancer, it is important not to gloss over potential problems. The considerations to weigh up are:

- Little is known of the effect of Tamoxifen on a developing foetus, so it is advisable to take contraceptive precautions while on the drug. The contraceptive pill and the 'morning-after' pill are not advised for women with breast cancer.
- About 1 per cent of women on Tamoxifen experience blood-clotting problems, which can be very serious. Women with a history of thrombotic disease are advised not to take the drug.
- Trials have reported damage to the eyes of women taking Tamoxifen, and even a trial using low doses has reported 6 per cent of women experiencing ocular toxicity, the symptoms of which are 'floaters' – black spots clouding vision. Most of the damage seems

to be reversible after the drug is stopped, but the decreased vision may be accompanied by actual damage to the eye. Regular eye checks are obviously a good idea.

- As already discussed, the risk of developing uterine or endometrial cancer seems to be about twice that of women not using Tamoxifen after two years, and four-fold after five years on the drug. Research at Yale University concluded that the uterine cancers were of a high grade with a poor prognosis. The researchers did however use 40 mg of Tamoxifen in their study, when the more usual dose is 20 mg.[3] The risk-to-benefit that has to be worked out here is whether the risk of uterine cancer is worse than the risk of breast cancer. It would appear, statistically, that for women for whom Tamoxifen is most useful (see above) the benefits of a reduction in breast cancer risk may outweigh the risk of uterine cancer – but the individual is not a statistic and this is a personal decision to make.

- Women on Tamoxifen are more likely to grow polyps and show hormonal changes on cervical smears, both of which are risk factors for cervical cancer.

- Liver cancer is another concern. Tamoxifen is a potent liver carcinogen in laboratory rats, and humans are usually affected by the same carcinogens as these rodents. Though very few cases of liver cancer have actually been reported in Tamoxifen-treated women, there is still concern. In women with breast cancer it is possible that subsequent liver cancer could be missed or mistaken as secondaries from the original breast cancer (the liver is a common place for breast cancer secondaries). Also, most Tamoxifen trials are for five or seven years and liver cancer usually takes longer to develop than this. If the small and theoretical risk of liver cancer is real, it will probably take years to show up. This is an important consideration as liver cancer is much more serious than breast cancer – but then you may have gained many intervening years, possibly as many as twenty to thirty. As with uterine cancer, the risk has to be weighed against the possible benefits.

- A rare but serious reaction may occur between Tamoxifen and the drug Warfarin (a blood-thinning, anti-coagulant medication) and Tamoxifen may increase blood levels of Warfarin. If you take Warfarin, regular blood tests to check on its effectiveness during the use of Tamoxifen is prudent, and you should make sure that you notify your doctor of any signs of bleeding, including excessive menstrual bleeding or severe bruising.[4]

Ovarian ablation

This means removing, switching off or blocking the ovaries or the ovarian hormone, oestrogen.

Surgical removal of the ovaries is called oophorectomy. Radiotherapy may also be used to destroy the ovaries. These treatments are aimed at reducing the output of oestrogen in pre-menopausal women and have been shown to increase survival rate of such women by about 30 per cent. Indeed, for women under fifty, a recent trial showed that ovarian ablation was slightly more effective than chemotherapy for survival rates, especially in women with oestrogen receptor positive breast cancer rated over 100.[5] It is a treatment that is usually not suggested as it causes infertility and brings on early menopause, but it is a good example of how hormone management improves survival rates – the critical issue is to work out how to manage hormones without such drastic measures.

Another option is a drug called Goserelin (Zoladex), administered by injection, which turns off oestrogen production. It works by interfering with hormone triggers from the pituitary gland which would normally encourage the ovaries to make oestrogen. Menopausal symptoms may be brought on by this drug, but when the drug is stopped, the symptoms may cease.

Chemotherapy

Drug therapy, or chemotherapy, is a systemic treatment – in other words, one that affects the whole body. The primary, or original, tumour may have been cut away, but chemotherapy is given when spread may be suspected. This is most frequently indicated by cancer being detected in the lymph glands. As previously mentioned, it is becoming increasingly common to use chemotherapy before surgery, to shrink the tumour and deal with any rogue cancer as a priority, operating on the – hopefully shrunken – tumour later. Overall, if chemotherapy is used as adjuvant treatment, fairly quickly after surgery and radiation, risk of recurrence is reduced by one-third.[1] It is now also being advocated that chemotherapy should be used for breast cancer without apparent lymphatic involvement, as this improves survival rates by 5 per cent. It is presumed that this is the case because cancer is not always detectable and may be missed at the moment when the decision is taken whether to use chemotherapy or not. The proximity of the tumour to the underarm area will have a bearing on this decision. Of course this decision is not to be taken lightly as chemotherapy drugs are very powerful. Breast-feeding should not take place while on chemotherapy.

Drugs that are used to combat cancer are called cytotoxic. 'Cyto' means cell, so they are toxic to cells. They are administered by injection or drip, and sometimes in tablet form as well. The doses are very carefully controlled in order to do maximum damage to cancer cells, but minimum damage to normal healthy cells. They are designed to have more effect on fast dividing cells, which is exactly what cancer cells are. However this means that they have an effect on other fast-dividing cells – in particular those in the lining of the digestive tract, and in the bone marrow where immune cells are produced. A blood test is carried out before each chemotherapy treatment to check that white blood cell levels, important for defence against infection, have not been overly affected by the drug treatment. Chemotherapy is becoming more finely tuned, and it is no longer the case that patients will necessarily be completely debilitated by their treatment, or automatically lose their hair. The type of reaction that you have largely depends on the type of drugs that you receive and your resilience. The most commonly prescribed course of chemotherapy for breast cancer, CMF, is well tolerated by most people.

Chemotherapy is most likely to be offered to pre-menopausal women, while hormone treatment is most likely to be offered to post-menopausal women, but this varies depending on the individual case. The goal-posts on the issue of whether to give chemotherapy or not are being moved so quickly, that it is now becoming increasingly common to prescribe it alongside Tamoxifen. No doubt the criteria for whether or not to give chemotherapy will continue to change in the next ten years.

Side-effects of chemotherapy

Being on the receiving end of chemotherapy is certainly not a picnic, but for the majority of people it is not as bad as they probably imagine and the chemotherapy regimes for breast cancer are nowhere near as dramatic in their effect as regimes for other cancers. They have been fine-tuned in recent years and many women find that they sail through the chemotherapy treatment with little more than a bit of tiredness. In fact, the imagination can work overtime and be your worst enemy. I found that, when I was having treatment, I would be instantly nauseous and by my third treatment was vomiting before I got into the treatment room. When questioned by a hospital psychotherapist about how I viewed the chemo, I realized for the first time that I was imagining it as a toxic, greenish-yellow liquid (I never actually saw it, as I looked away during the whole treatment – a hangover from a phobia of injections as a child). He asked me to visualize the liquid as a clear, sparkling, health-giving fluid, and lo and behold, I experienced no nausea for the remaining treatments. I may be more suggestible than most, but this is a small illustration of the power of the mind.

The following list may serve to increase your anxiety about chemotherapy, but it is worth remembering that it is unusual to experience all these side-effects and that many of them can be managed or contained. The main possible side-effects of chemotherapy that may concern you are:

Discomfort

Receiving the chemotherapy injection is not at all painful once the needle is inserted, and only one needle is required for any combination of drugs. Chemotherapy nurses are very experienced at finding veins, so inserting the needle is not usually a problem even if, like me, your veins disappear at the mere thought of an injection. Occasionally the drugs may feel cold as they pass into the vein, but this only lasts a few seconds. An anti-sickness (anti-emetic) drug is usually given at the same time and this may be felt briefly – a few seconds only – as a buzzing sensation in the vaginal area.

Nausea

This is usually the most feared side-effect, along with hair loss. It is rarely as bad as people anticipate it to be. The queasiness is caused by excessive acidity in the stomach triggered by some of the drugs. Nausea is not usually felt immediately unless the drugs are being administered too fast, in which case you can ask the nurse to give them more slowly. If feeling sick is going to be a problem, it is more usual for the sensation to arrive in the twenty-four hours following the chemotherapy session. It is probably a good idea to take this possibility into account, and ensure a restful period following chemotherapy.

While it is unusual during treatment for breast cancer, nausea combined with a change in taste sensations or mouth ulcers can severely limit appetite. It is best to maintain a good nutritional status during treatment by eating a varied diet, but if this is being made difficult by how you feel, you may need to resort to easier meals that 'slip down the throat' without too much chewing. These could take the form of soups, pâtés and spreads, minced chicken or fish patties, porridge, purées, fools, mashed soft fruits, yoghurt or breakfast-in-a-glass (see page 118).

Ginger or peppermint tea, either on their own or in combination, are very helpful for reducing nausea induced by chemotherapy. The tea can be drunk as often as needed – you can even take a flask of the tea with you to sip while you are having your chemotherapy treatment – or ginger capsules can be taken every three or four hours.

Cooked oatmeal can be very effective at reducing the nausea associated with chemotherapy, perhaps because it is effective at 'mopping up' excess gastric acid.

The homeopathic remedy Nux Vomica is helpful for lessening chemotherapy-induced nausea. Take one dose of 6 C as needed.

Ginger and Mint Infusions

These herbs are wonderful at settling feelings of nausea. In trials ginger has been shown to be as effective as anti-nausea pills for travel sickness and morning sickness and it is a great boon for chemotherapy-induced nausea.

Peel a ginger root and put it into the freezer for use at any time. When you want to make the tea, just grate some of the frozen root into a cup and return the unused portion back to the freezer. Pour boiling water over the grated ginger and let it steep for a couple of minutes. Ginger and lemon or honey are other delicious combinations to try. For peppermint tea just steep some washed, fresh leaves in boiling water for a couple of minutes. Peppermint grows really well in the garden or in pots and needs almost no attention. Dried leaves can be kept in jars to use as needed. (Strong aromatic teas may interfere with the action of homeopathic remedies, so allow an hour in between the teas and any remedies you may be taking.)

Hair loss

Many women seem to worry about this more than any other side-effect. They may be feeling particularly vulnerable, and now, on top of everything else, they must worry about potential hair loss. The most popular chemotherapy regime, CMF, is the least likely to cause hair loss (there may be slight thinning). For those who are on other regimes where hair loss is more likely, it may help to remember that all their hair will grow back, sometimes stronger than ever. The drug Adriamycin will definitely cause hair loss. With some of the other protocols hair loss can be avoided for many women by using a cuff type of tourniquet during treatment. This physically stops the majority of the drugs reaching the scalp. For those who are likely to lose their hair the hospital should automatically offer a wig-fitting before treatment starts. It may also be an idea to invest in some stylish scarves and hats to use for the few months of treatment.

Vitamin E in daily doses of 1,000 ius can dramatically reduce hair loss from chemotherapy. Take it for at least two weeks prior to starting chemotherapy treatment and continue for the duration. Do not take vitamin E for a week before surgery, as it can thin the blood sufficiently to cause excess bleeding. High doses of vitamin C – 10 g daily – can also be protective against hair loss.

Fatigue

This is most likely to be a problem on the first two or three days after the injection. After this, as long as you pace yourself, there is no reason to expect undue tiredness over and above tiredness later in the day. It is sensible to rest whenever you feel this way. If you feel particularly tired, especially if you feel flat out, it could be that your drug dose is too high, and you should report this to your specialist.

Metallic taste

It is possible to find that taste perceptions change with chemotherapy. You could experience a metallic taste, or the flavours of foods may seem bland. You may need to eat stronger-tasting dishes flavoured with herbs and spices to conceal the strange taste.

Fertility

About 40 per cent of women on chemotherapy will become infertile so if a woman wants to have children at a future date this is something to think about. It is more likely that fertility will be affected if the woman is getting close to her menopause, or in the case of more severe drug regimes. It may be that you will want to discuss the possibility of preserving eggs in case of infertility. If periods continue throughout chemotherapy, it is unlikely that fertility has been affected, and if they cease then it is possible that they will restart once treatment has finished, especially in younger women. There is no evidence that a single course of chemotherapy causes mutations to a woman's eggs, or causes birth defects, though workers in laboratories that produce these drugs and who have repeated exposure have a higher incidence of birth abnormalities. I felt lucky to conceive about five years after my treatment, and have a healthy and boisterous son running around as I write.

Infection

Because chemotherapy affects bone marrow, the immune system is suppressed. This is why a white blood cell count is taken prior to each treatment session to evaluate immune status. If a fever develops, or there are other signs of infection, this should be reported to your specialist at once.

All the points covered in the chapter **Building Powerful Immunity** (page 239) are appropriate to ensure that your immune system is kept in top shape during chemotherapy, and if you look after yourself you can successfully keep your white blood cell count in the healthy range. Of particular use are high doses of vitamin C, and I would recommend up to 10 g taken at intervals during the day (for example five doses of 2 g each). Vitamin C is a key component for manufacturing white blood cells.

The herb astragalus (*Astragalus membranaceous*) helps to support the immune system while undergoing chemotherapy and to reduce some of the side-effects, including poor appetite, hair loss and depression. Take one capsule two to three times a day.

Phlebitis

This is inflammation of the vein and very occasionally can occur in the legs as a side-effect of chemotherapy. It needs prompt treatment with anti-inflammatory drugs and, in some cases, antibiotics.

Weight

Weight gain is common during chemotherapy – around 3–5.5 kg/7–12 lb, but this usually reverses after the treatment phase. The weight gain often seems to occur without any increased food intake, though some women find they eat more, to settle their stomachs when feeling nauseous – the excess stomach acid caused by the drugs can be mistaken for hunger signals.

Hot flushes

Women near to their menopause may be tipped into menopausal symptoms by chemotherapy. Symptoms such as sweating and hot flushes are not uncommon.

Oral ulceration

Occasionally some chemotherapy regimes will cause ulceration of the mouth. These can be healed quickly by piercing a capsule of 400 ius vitamin E and rubbing the contents on the ulcers twice daily.

Preparing for chemotherapy

You will usually have at least a couple of weeks' warning that you are going to have chemotherapy treatment. And that is a lot of time to get yourself ready.

It is generally a good idea to downtune your activities during the chemotherapy course, which usually lasts six months. You may need to take time off work, or at least to reduce your work load. You may be able to keep your work ticking over by doing some at home, if appropriate, and many people find that this helps to keep them occupied. While you may feel a little tired in the couple of days immediately after chemotherapy, you may well find that your energy levels are not too bad in the couple of weeks between treatments. But do not be tempted to do too much, even if you feel fine. Chemotherapy is an onslaught on the body and it is as well to rest as much as you can in order to give your healing mechanisms the best possible chance to maintain your health. This may be a time to find a quiet pastime that allows you to feel as if you are doing something, but not stretching yourself too much. Perhaps it is the ideal opportunity to read the *Complete Works of Shakespeare*, or write that book you have had in mind for a while. I found that I became a crossword fiend – a great time-waster that needs no more effort than crossing the room to check the dictionary from time to time.

You may find that there are changes to your appetite, moods and sleep patterns. These usually right themselves after treatment has stopped, but in the meantime do not worry if you feel less or more hungry than usual, just aim to eat as healthily as possible, following the guidelines in this book. You may find that you sleep more than usual, or if you find that sleep is interrupted, the herb valerian is a useful, non-addictive, natural sleep aid.

Moods can be affected and some women may get depressed or anxious during this time. It is probably a combination of the diagnosis of breast cancer really sinking in, along with a distaste for the treatment, and the chemotherapy itself affecting moods by upsetting body chemistry. This is the ideal time to learn some visualization, relaxation or meditation techniques which some people find revolutionize their ability to deal with the disease. Alternatively, you may want to join a local support group or to seek out someone to talk to who has been through the same experience, via one of the support charities. Read the chapter **Reducing Your Stress Load** (page 290) for suggestions of how to support yourself at this time.

Protecting your body tissues

Taking supplements during chemotherapy is a controversial area. Some oncologists will quite happily go along with supplements and agree that if they make you feel better then it is a good thing, while others will be more conservative and ask you to avoid supplements during chemotherapy. There is no hard-and-fast advice that can be given in this instance and it is a matter for personal decision-making. Having read the information available on the subject, I have decided quite firmly that if I were to have chemotherapy again (and I expect not to have my bluff called on this one!) I would use all the supplements I could to bolster myself physically. Supplements that may be of particular use during chemotherapy are discussed below – read on before making any decisions about this with your oncologist.

There are three main criteria for using supplementation in preparation for and during chemotherapy:

■ The first is effectively to create a shield around healthy cells, and reduce their susceptibility to the chemotherapy, by using

337

antioxidants, which protect the heart and liver against direct damage from specific chemotherapy drugs. Cancer cells do not take up antioxidants as well as healthy cells do, meaning that, come the start of treatment, the drugs can work more selectively on cancerous cells. The other reason to use antioxidants during and after chemotherapy and radiation treatment is that both these treatments produce free radicals in abundance and the antioxidants can help to offset some of the cellular damage this can lead to.

- The second criterion is to help repair damage to healthy cells that may have been done by the drug therapy. For instance, healing the lining of the digestive tract, which is frequently damaged by chemotherapy, will allow it to return speedily to correct functioning and therefore allow good uptake of the fifty or so essential nutrients that we need to get from our diet, reducing the possibility of malnourishment in cancer patients.

- The third important action of nutrients and herbs is to detoxify the chemotherapy at the end of the course of treatment. Once they have done their job it is of no advantage to patients to have these potent drugs persisting in their livers. The object is to accelerate the removal of toxic metabolites that remain after the liver's enzymatic breakdown of the drugs. Helping to eliminate these drugs allows a speedier return to full health and may avoid the possible long-term damage attributed to many chemotherapy drugs.

What does the research tell us so far about using supplements to reduce the side-effects of chemotherapy?

Most of these methods of reducing the side-effects of chemotherapy drugs have not been rigorously tested in randomized clinical trials, as they should be. However, the use of supplements does not have the serious side-effects associated with chemotherapy.

The twice Nobel Laureate Linus Pauling observed: 'Vitamin C . . . controls to a considerable extent the disagreeable side-effects of the cytotoxic chemotherapeutic agents, such as nausea and loss of hair, and that benefit seems to add its value to that of the chemotherapeutic agent.'[2] Dr Charles Simone has summarized dozens of studies which suggest the possibility that vitamin and mineral supplements, and especially antioxidants, enhance the potential of chemotherapy drugs to kill cancer cells.[3] 'Vitamins and minerals do not interfere with the anti-tumour effects of chemotherapy and radiation . . . on the contrary some vitamins and minerals used in conjunction with chemotherapy . . . protect normal tissue and potentiate the destruction of cancer cells.[4]

Twenty years from now perhaps we will see nutrition and supplements being used alongside other hospital treatments as a matter of course, with the current debates consigned to the history books.

This is what the picture looks like at the moment:

- Vitamin E, in doses of 1,000 ius daily, is important to consider to help prevent cardiac toxicity with the chemotherapy drug Adriamycin whilst not affecting its anti-tumour activity.[5] It has also been shown in animal and test-tube experiments to reduce the toxicity of 5-Fluorouracil, Methotrexate, Cyclophosphamide and Vincristine, while enhancing their action.[6] Vitamin E at 1,600 ius per day can reduce hair loss.[7]
- Vitamin C increases the cytotoxicity of chemotherapy as well as blocking heart damage from Adriamycin.[8] It also potentiates chemotherapy drugs without inducing toxicity.[9] (Some of these studies used vitamin C alongside vitamin K3, which is not available as it can have toxic side-effects.)
- Co-enzyme Q10 can help to reduce cardiac toxicity from the chemotherapy drug Adriamycin.[10]
- The fish oil EPA seems to improve the response of tumour cells to chemotherapy agents by altering properties of the tumour cell membranes.[11]
- Nicotinamide (vitamin B3) partially reversed the toxicity of the drug cis-platin in mice,[12] while selenium enhanced its actions at the same time as reducing its toxicity.[13]
- Vitamin A, in combination with chemotherapy in post-menopausal women with metastasized breast cancer, significantly increased the numbers of complete responses,[14] and experiments have been shown to increase the effects of Adriamycin while protecting against cardiotoxicity and protecting cells against oxidative stress.[15] It has also been

shown to protect the small intestine, in animal studies, against damage from Methotrexate administration, while not interfering with the other activities of the drug and it was concluded that '[vitamin A] will be of great use in Methotrexate cancer chemotherapy'.[16]

■ The amino-acid L-glutamine has been shown to be protective of the digestive tract against the effects of chemotherapy (see **Other Useful Supplements**, page 173). Studies show that L-glutamine significantly enhances the effectiveness of chemotherapy against tumours,[17] while protecting normal body tissues.[18] One review concluded: 'These studies suggest that oral glutamine supplementation is safe in its administration to the tumour-bearing host receiving Methotrexate.'[19]

■ The herb astragalus (Chinese Huang Qi) has protected the liver in animal studies against damage from chemotherapy,[20] in addition to improving immune function in cancer patients.[21] A Texan trial concluded that 'reversal of cyclophosphamide-induced immunosuppression [by astragalus] was complete'.[22] No toxicity has been reported for this herb.

■ *Lactobacillus* bacteria, commonly found in cultured milk products (*L. casei*) inhibits the growth of tumours in mice, in combination with the drugs Dyclophosphamide, Mitomycin, 5-Fluorouracil and Bleomycin.[23]

■ Aloe vera has been shown to increase the anti-tumour effects of 5-Fluorouracil and Cyclophosphamide. Purified aloe vera has no known toxicity and is protective of the digestive tract.

Chemotherapy is disruptive to the lining of the gut wall, which reduces its efficiency

Chemotherapy was developed from mustard gas. It was noticed in the early days that mustard gas affected fast-dividing cells. This is the whole premise behind chemotherapy's effectiveness against cancer cells since, compared to normal cells, they are very fast-dividing. But other fast-dividing cells in the body include bone marrow, which compromises immunity, and also the cells of the digestive tract. Astoundingly, the lining of the digestive tract takes only four days to replace itself. This means that it is susceptible to disruption during and just after chemotherapy, and this can manifest in a number of symptoms, including nausea, vomiting, diarrhoea and constipation. Repairing, and preferably reducing, this damage is a high priority.

Research has shown that L-glutamine, an amino acid, can make a significant difference to chemotherapy damage to the digestive tract if taken in high doses three days before starting chemotherapy and all the way through treatment. It can also help to repair the gut wall, if taken after treatment. Despite the fact that the lining of the digestive tract replaces itself every four days, it still can take several months to repair any damage as the replacement will improve in small increments, as long as the conditions are right to do so. For more information about L-glutamine including dosages, see under **Other Useful Supplements** (page 173).

Chemotherapy might destroy the enzyme-producing cilia of the small intestine. Taking supplemental digestive enzymes to enhance digestion during chemotherapy may be helpful if you feel that your digestive capability has been affected. The cilia should grow back after chemotherapy has been stopped.

Other support for the lining of the digestive tract includes drinking aloe vera juice which should be taken diluted as it is too strong in its undiluted form. Ensure that you buy a good-quality brand with sufficient active compounds (see the **Resources** section). The herb slippery elm is also supportive of the digestive tract.

Protect your liver from damage

The cells of the liver are susceptible to lipid peroxidation as chemotherapy has to pass through the liver for activation and detoxification. Keeping the liver healthy during this time is a priority for returning to full health. A number of compounds are helpful for ensuring this:

- Milk thistle is the king of liver protectors and there are no contra-indications to taking this supplement during chemotherapy.
- Siberian ginseng has long been known to help protect the liver from chemotherapy-induced damage.
- Detoxifying the liver is enhanced by carrot juice and lemon juice. Taking these two juices at regular intervals helps the liver to regulate itself.

- Substitute dandelion coffee for your usual brew as dandelion root has a cleansing action on the liver.
- As well as its other reported actions, the amino acid L-glutamine also helps the liver to detoxify.
- Drinking at least 2 litres/3½ pints of water daily helps to keep the liver 'flushed out'.
- A high-fat diet puts an extra strain on the liver. Keeping to below 30 per cent calories from fat in the diet, and ensuring that the fats you eat are mainly unsaturated – especially from omega-3 rich sources – will lessen the burden on your liver.
- 60 g/2 oz of dried seaweed daily during treatment can help to protect the liver. It also provides a concentrated source of nutrients, including trace nutrients, which can be useful if you have elected not to take supplements.

There are three main categories of chemotherapy drug:

Alkylating agents

These damage the genetic programmes which control tumour growth. Cytoxan (Cyclophosphamide) is the most widely used and is given by mouth or intravenously. It is not activated until it is processed by the liver. Other alkylating agents are Thiotepa, which has to be carefully monitored as it is highly toxic to bone marrow, and Adriamycin (Doxorubicin) which also needs to be carefully monitored as it can induce cardiac toxicity.

Antimetabolites

These interfere with the manufacture of DNA in the cells. The most frequently used for breast cancer treatment are Methotrexate and 5-Fluorouracil, and are usually given intravenously, though Methotrexate may also be given by tablet where appropriate. Methotrexate interferes with the metabolism of folic acid, a vitamin which is needed for cell division. Sometimes Leucovorin, which is a derivative of folic acid, is given in combination with Methotrexate to modulate its activity.

Extracts of natural products

Not to be confused with the term 'natural' applied to vitamin, mineral or herbal supplements. These extracts are indeed natural in that they are plant extracts and have not been synthesized. However, they are very toxic and interrupt cell division and interfere with cell structure. Taxol, extracted from the Pacific yew tree, is one such drug, which is very powerful and rarely given for first-time breast cancer. It is usually kept in reserve for a second line of treatment if there is recurrence and where cancers show a resistance to other chemotherapy treatments.

A variety of soups

Different standard protocols are used, which have been tried and tested over several years. The two most common regimes are CMF (Cytoxan, Methotrexate and 5-Fluorouracil) and CAF (Cytoxan, Adriamycin and 5-Fluorouracil). Most regimes are administered in two injections during a four-week period. This is then repeated each month for six months. The regime that your specialist advises may be different to these.

Drug/drug and drug/nutrient interactions

Pain-killers: Methotrexate is the 'M' in the CMF chemotherapy regime used for breast cancer. Methotrexate is also used to treat severe cases of psoriasis and rheumatoid arthritis. Aspirin and other NSAIDs (non-steroidal anti-inflammatory drugs), such as ibuprofen, may have the effect of potentiating Methotrexate, and high blood levels of Methotrexate can be reached when the two are combined. As well as making the Methotrexate more powerful, the combination can also increase its toxicity. Check with your doctor before taking aspirin or any other NSAID while on Methotrexate.

Folic acid: Methotrexate acts on the intestinal wall and interferes with the absorption of folic acid, vitamin B12 and beta-carotene. Because of this it is possible for deficiencies to arise. It is important to replace these nutrients to reduce the overall toxicity of the drug on healthy body tissues. Methotrexate is believed to work precisely because it interferes with the action of folic acid, a lack of which slows down, or stops, cell division. It is unclear whether the low doses in multi-vitamin supplements (400 mcg) are sufficient to interfere with the action of Methotrexate.[24] The standard text states that 'folic acid itself provides poor protection against the toxicity of such drugs as Methotrexate',[25] implying that it may not interfere with the actions of the drug. It is best to discuss the situation with your oncologist before taking any folic acid or folate. Some folic acid-free B-complexes are available (see **Appendix**).

Vitamin C: There is some concern that vitamin C may possibly increase the risk of toxicity of the chemotherapy drug Methotrexate as vitamin C in the short term is an organic acid which may inhibit secretion from the kidneys at high doses.[26] It is advisable to avoid vitamin C within twelve hours either side of taking Methotrexate.

Echinacea: One paper has suggested that echinacea should not be used for longer than eight weeks at the same time as chemotherapy drugs as it may have negative effects on the liver.[27]

Alcohol: Chemotherapy drugs need to be closely monitored as they can cause liver toxicity. Since alcohol is also a liver toxin it is advisable to avoid alcoholic drinks while on chemotherapy drugs. You may also want to avoid coffee which is difficult for the liver to handle.[28]

Grapefruit juice: Can potentiate Cyclosporin and should be avoided during chemotherapy treatment. Other citrus juices do not have the same effect. Of course it may be possible in years to come to take grapefruit juice alongside Cyclosporin meaning that the drug levels might be reduced.

Every little helps

Even the most positive and go-ahead person usually feels a little daunted about the idea of hospital treatment for cancer – it is something to be 'got through'. When you read some of the case histories in this book it becomes clear that everyone has a different experience, but many people feel richer for it – lessons are learnt, life is viewed in a different way, and lasting friendships are made.

Not everyone has the stamina to do everything that may make them feel better during treatment, but anything you do can help – taking more rest, reorganizing your priorities, adjusting your diet or taking some antioxidants and vitamin C. Being involved with your healing process can alter the whole experience: easing physical symptoms, maximizing the opportunity for recovery and boosting morale.

To reiterate the point I made at the beginning of the book – cancer is not a disease against which we are helpless. By restoring balance in all areas of our lives – dietary, biological, emotional, environmental – we can adjust the circumstances in which the disease was able to proliferate. This is a powerful statement, with powerful implications for those of us who are confronted with managing and recovering from breast cancer.

A Very Important Message

The most important focus for the next ten years must be to reduce the incidence rate of breast cancer.

Waiting for Government policy to lead the way would take an unacceptable length of time. A groundswell of action is already taking place: women are seeking more information, better facilities and improved options; support organizations and charities are providing what the National Health Service cannot; the complementary fields are filling the gaps in health care and creating a more holistic healing environment.

As a society we must question whether our speedy lifestyle is really driving us towards a glittering future, or is simply accelerating us away from Nature's intentions. In order to halt the incidence of breast cancer and then shift gear to prevent it occurring, there are some very accessible measures that we can take. The inexorable march of statistics can be reversed by creating for ourselves lifestyles which do not act as a breeding ground for breast cancer, or other cancers. We can minimize our exposure to chemical pollutants in our water and our food. We can eat more fruit and vegetables. We can mimic the diets of societies where the risk of breast cancer is far less than in ours. We can be more physically active. And we can avoid our excessive use of over-the-counter and hormonal pharmaceutical preparations.

Every woman, whether touched by cancer or not, has the amazing gift of intuition. She can listen to what her body needs, treat her body with respect and take control of her life. If we take individual responsibility for our health we *can* reverse this heartbreaking trend.

Appendix

Folic acid- and iron-free supplements for use during chemotherapy with Methotrexate (if advised by oncologist)

Biocare
B-plex: B-complex supplement which avoids folic acid and vitamin B12.

Health plus
HH pack: A multi-vitamin and mineral supplement with several supplements in a once-a-day sachet. Avoids folic acid and vitamin B12, and includes a fish oil capsule.

Note: After taking a folic acid- and B12-free supplement during your chemotherapy course, you will probably need to add in these two nutrients as soon as possible after your treatment at levels of at least 400 mcg folic acid and 100 mcg vitamin B12 daily to redress any deficiency.

Multiple-formula supplements with no, or low, iron levels

All.1
No iron. A rice-based powder formula, to mix with water or fruit juice, with good doses of all the main vitamins, minerals and proteins. Also includes lecithin and some other ancillary nutrients such as lemon bioflavonoids. Includes folic acid (400 mcg), so possibly avoid if currently on Methotrexate chemotherapy.

Biocare
Adult multi-vitamins and minerals: No iron, 400 mcg folic acid.

Vita-myns: No iron, 800 mcg folic acid (so may be useful to make up for deficiency if avoided during Methotrexate chemotherapy). Also contains many bioflavonoids.

Mineral complex: A multi-mineral formula which avoids iron. It also contains no calcium, so you may want to supplement as well. However, if you do so, magnesium is frequently needed in higher amounts to metabolize calcium correctly.

Femforte I (tablet): No iron. A 'female formula' multi-vitamin and mineral to balance. Suitable for use before, during and after the menopause and for menstrual problems. Also contains no calcium. Has a low dose of only 75 mcg folic acid.

Femforte II (capsule): No iron. Similar to above, but generally lower doses as it is in capsule form.

Solgar
Solovite tablets: No iron. Good carotene mixture and 100 mcg folic acid.

VM75: 1.3 mg iron in one tablet. A good multi-vitamin and mineral formula with 400 mcg folic acid.

Multi II vegicaps: 1 mg iron in 1 capsule. 400 mcg folic acid and soya protein.

Lamberts
Multi-max: 1 mg iron. A good multi-vitamin formula with, generally, low-dose minerals and 400 mcg folic acid. You may want to take an iron-free mineral supplement alongside it such as the Biocare Multi-mineral formula above.

Thorne
Basic nutrients III (citrate formula): No iron, no copper, 800 mcg folic acid.

Meta-fem: No iron, 800 mcg folic acid, contains Dong Quai and wild yam. Dosage is two to four capsules per day.

IDN

Lifepack European formula: 3 mg iron. Good multi-formula. Slightly low on B vitamins so you may want to take multi-B formula alongside it if you think you are deficient. 500 mcg folic acid. Contains chemopreventive nutrients including broccoli and cabbage concentrate, quercitin, lycopene and lipoic acid.

Resources

If you wish to be kept informed of Suzannah Olivier's books, workshops and other activities visit her website: www.healthandnutrition.co.uk or E-mail: eattobefit@aol.com

Counselling and patient care

BACUP
(British Association of Cancer United Patients)
National charity offering free information and emotional support to people with cancer.
Patient care support: 0808 800 1234
Information booklet: 0171 696 9003

Breast Cancer Care
Aims to match up patients with people who have had a similar experience. Also has experienced prosthesis counsellors, offers support and advice and produces information publications.
Helpline: 0808 800 6000
Administration: 0171 384 2984
Glasgow helpline: 0141 221 2244
-mail bcc@breastcancercare.org.UK

Cancer Care Society
Provides social and emotional support for people with cancer and their families and friends via a national network of branches. Links people with others who have had cancer. Telephone and personal counselling.
Tel: 0117 942 7419

Cancerkin
Provides advice, support and care for breast cancer patients and their families. Also provides information and education for carers.
Tel: 0171 830 2323

Cancerlink
Provides emotional support, on the telephone, for all types of cancer and has links to self-help groups in the UK. Publications in seven languages available.
Information line: 0800 132 905
For publications and written information: 0171 833 2818
Asian language helpline: 0800 590 415
Scotland: 0131 228 5557

The Haven Trust
Offers counselling and support for breast cancer patients and their families. Also provides access to information about complementary therapies. Some complementary treatments will also be available.
Tel: 0171 384 0000

Appendix

Lavender Trust
In association with Breast Cancer Care, aims to raise money to fund services for younger women with breast cancer in the UK.
Breast cancer care helpline: 0808 800 6000
Administration: 0171 384 2984

Macmillan Cancer Relief
Provides support in the form of information and specialist care for patients at every stage of their illness.
Information line: 0845 601 6161

Marie Curie Cancer Care
Provides free practical nursing at home, and specialist care at eleven centres across the UK (a medical referral from a Marie Curie nurse is required). Also conducts research into the causes and treatment of cancer.
Tel: 0171 235 3325

Complementary and alternative cancer information

Bristol Cancer Centre
Seeks to combine the benefits of a holistic approach with an appreciation of the effectiveness of orthodox treatment.
Tel: 0117 980 9500

The Cancer Resource Centre
Offers a holistic approach and offers information, support and a range of complementary therapies. Usually used to support the patient through conventional treatment.
Helpline: 0171 924 3924

The Gerson Support Group
Takes a completely alternative approach using dietary manipulation for people who have elected not to pursue conventional treatment. Send an A5 SAE for information to: 108 Birmingham Road, Litchfield, Staffs WS14 9BW.
Tel: 01372 817 652

The Homeopathic Trust/The Faculty of Homeopaths
Will help you find a qualified local homeopathic doctor.
Tel: 0171 566 7800

Institute of Complementary Medicine
Will supply names of both support groups and reliable holistic therapists. Send a SAE with two first-class stamps and a letter stating area of interest to: PO Box 194, London SE16
Tel: 0171 237 5165

National Institute of Medical Herbalists

Herbs can be a very useful adjunct to treatment for cancer, but as herbs can be quite potent and have medicinal effects such use is best supervised by a qualified herbalist, medical herbalist or Chinese herbalist. To obtain a list of practising herbalists, send an A5 SAE with two second-class stamps to: 56 Longbrook Street, Exeter, Devon BX4 6AH

Royal London Homeopathic Hospital

NHS funded cancer clinic with qualified doctors and homeopaths. Will include dietary advice as well as other therapies which include acupuncture, aromatherapy and relaxation techniques. Usually need a referral from a medical practitioner.
Tel: 0171 837 8833

Society for Complementary Medicine

Practitioners from a number of different disciplines see clients by appointment at the practice in London.
Tel: 0171 436 0821

Society of Homeopaths

Will send you a register of qualified homeopaths on request.
Tel: 01604 621 400

To find a nutritional therapist

Institute for Optimum Nutrition

Publishes the *National Directory of Nutritionists*. Check to find if the nutritionist has experience with breast cancer.
Tel: 0181 877 9993

Society for the Promotion of Nutritional Therapy

Provide a list of nutritional therapists around the country. Check to find if the nutritionist has experience with breast cancer. Send a SAE and £1 to: BCM Box SPNT, WC1N 3XX.
Tel: 01825 872 921

Appendix

University of Westminster Poly-Clinic

Offers concessionary rates for nutrition and other consultations. Consultations are with a qualified practitioner, but they are observed by students. The Poly-clinic also offers acupuncture, herbal medicine, homeopathy, chiropractic and massage.
Tel: 0171 911 5041

Women's Nutrition Advisory Service

Information, advice and self-help books on all aspects of women's hormonal health, including dealing with menopausal symptoms without HRT, or coming off HRT safely. The WNAS offers 'scientifically based tailor-made programmes'. Clinics in London and East Sussex, and postal and telephone consultations available.
Tel: 01273 487 366
Website: www.wnas.org.uk

Pressure Groups and Information

National Cancer Alliance

A voluntary organization of patients and health care professionals to voice concerns and opinions about the service, care and treatment for cancer patients. Supplies *The Directory of Cancer Specialists* which details the individual interests of almost every cancer specialist in the country.
PO Box 579, Oxford OX4 1LP
Tel: 01865 793 566

Rage (Radiotherapy Action Group)

A support group for women who have suffered severe damage from radiotherapy.
Tel: 0181 460 7476

UK Breast Cancer Coalition (UKBCC)

Dedicated to making the voice of women heard by the Government, health authorities, hospitals, etc.
Tel: 0171 720 0945

Women's Environmental Network Trust

Deals with environmental issues that specifically affect women.
Tel: 0171 247 3327
www.gn.apc.orgwen

Useful Websites

Cancernet
From the US Government's
National Institute of Health.
Website: cancernet.nci.nih.gov

Cancerhelp
An academic site from Birmingham
University with professional and
voluntary sector contributors.
Website: medweb.bham.ac.uk/
cancerhelp/indexg.html

Institute of Food Research
Website: www.ifrn.bbsrc.ac.uk

Oncolink
A vast and detailed resource from
Pennsylvania University.
Website: oncolink.upenn.edu

UK Breast Cancer Internet Site
Information, contact numbers,
campaigns and list of other related
sites.
Website: www.easynet.co.uk/aware

Cancer Research

Action Against Breast Cancer (ABC)
Research into the impact of diet,
lifestyle and immunology on breast
cancer.
Tel: 01865 407 384

Breakthrough Breast Cancer
A charity committed to fighting
breast cancer through research.
Tel: 0171 430 2086
Website: www.breakthrough.org.uk

Cancer Research Campaign
A charity which investigates the
cause, distribution and treatment of
cancer, in all its forms, in order to
defeat the disease and promote its
prevention.
Tel: 0171 224 1333
Website: www.crc.org.uk

**Imperial Cancer Research Fund
(ICRF)**
For a range of free leaflets and
brochures send a large SAE to: PO
Box 123, Lincoln's Inn Fields,
London WC2A 3PX
Tel: 0171 242 0200

Supplement Companies

Arovite, Warick
Manufacturer of All-1 powdered
vitamin and mineral supplement
mentioned in the **Appendix** as a
no-iron supplement. Also makes
other nutritional supplements. Mail
order.
Tel: 0800 731 0732

Biocare
Mail order service available.
Supplies a full range of supplements
including iron and folic acid-free
supplements (see **Appendix**). Range
of products include: Replete – an
invaluable intensive bacterial
recolonization programme for use
after a course of antibiotics. Thyroid
support supplement TH207.
Digestive support includes a range
of digestive enzymes and HCl with
pepsin. Enteroguard is Biocare's
product designed for restoring
intestinal health if there is a gut
permeability problem along with
other useful products such as
permatrol and FOS.
Tel: 0121 433 3727

Higher Nature, Sussex
Mail order service available.
Supplies a full range of supplements
including organic flaxseed oil,
organic linseeds, Cat's Claw tea,
digestive enzymes, L–glutamine,
aloe vera.
Tel: 01435 882 880

IDN
An American company which
produces the Lifepack product with
low-iron levels and added nutrients
including indole-3-carbinol,
sulphorophane, quercitin, lycopene
and lipoic acid. Although IDN is a
network marketing company, which
means it 'signs up' distributors and
sells to the public via a network or
salespeople, it does have a good
range of supplements.
Tel: 0800 413 672

Lamberts, Sussex
Has an excellent broad range of
supplements, including digestive
products, herbals and alfalfa, found
in good retail outlets. Also has a
sister mail order company, Nature's
Best.
Nature's Best: 01892 552 117
Technical Dept: 01892 552 121

Malcolm Simmonds Herbal Supplies, West Sussex
A superb range of herbal products
available by mail order.
Tel: 0800 298 6698

Nutri Centre, London W1

The Nutri Centre has an excellent shop, but also provides a 24-hour postal service. It sells a huge range of products including Essiac, Flor-Essence and Cat's Claw teas and combination Essiac/Cat's Claw (from Peruvian Imports Unlimited Inc.). Nutri is the sole importer for products designed by leading US nutrition expert Jeffrey Bland for restoring intestinal and metabolic health – Ultraclear and Ultraclear Sustain.

Tel: 0171 436 5122

Solgar, Buckinghamshire

Stocked at most good-quality health outlets. Mail order not available. Ipriflavone, Milk Thistle, Dong Quai Root, Echinacea, Valerian, Horsetail. Solgar's Greens and More green food powder supplement is an excellent product with alfalfa, spirulina, shlorella, dulse seaweed, maitake, reishi and shiitake mushrooms, licorice, astragalus, milk thistle, ginseng, broccoli, lecithin and other ingredients.

Tel: 01442 890 355 (for information on your nearest stockist)

Thorne

Products only available on prescription from doctors or from qualified nutritionists. Health Interlink can supply Thorne products to health professionals. Contact Health Interlink on 01582 794 4094.

Xynergy Health Products, West Sussex

A range of superb green products including spirulina (tablet, powder and flakes), aloe vera juice, and alfalfa/chlorella/barley juice concentrates.

Tel: 01730 813 642

Appendix

Soya and Linseed Bars

Wallaby Bars, Australia
Wallaby bars are distributed widely in health food shops throughout England, Scotland and Ireland. Planet Organic (Tel: 0171 221 7171) and Wild Oats (Tel: 0171 229 1063) in London are main suppliers. The soya/linseed/calcium bar gives around 60 mg of soya isoflavones. This means that one bar a day will give sufficient isoflavones to confer the benefits indicated in research for hormone modulation. The company is also considering producing a breakfast muesli with linseeds and soya isoflavones – not available yet, but keep a look-out.

Other bars are now coming on to the market, but they contain fairly high levels of sugar and give only around 20 mg of isoflavones. I mention this because it is best to check labels of any new products coming to the market in this expanding area of the health food industry, to establish if the bars give sufficient isoflavones without too many, or any, additives.

Natural Progesterone Information

Higher Nature
Supplies natural progesterone to doctors and arranges hormone saliva tests via Aeron Laboratories in the USA.
Tel: 01435 882 880

Mistletoe, Oxford
Workshops 'Balancing Hormones Naturally' with Sue Pembrey. Sue is a retired nurse, a fellow of the Royal College of Nursing, and has recovered from breast cancer herself. Call for details of the courses she runs.
Tel: 01865 514 988

Natural Progesterone Information Service (NPIS)
For a list of doctors who are familiar with the use of natural progesterone send a SAE to: NPIS, PO Box 24, Buxton, Derbyshire, SK17 9FB.

The Well Woman's International Network
Tel: 07000 437 225 (answerphone service for information and membership – details are mailed out).

Testing Facilities

Aeron Lifecycle Laboratories (USA)
Saliva tests, by post, for female and male levels (also available via Higher Nature in the UK – see above)
Tel: 001 510 729 375

Natural Family Planning

The Billings Method
Write to: Family Life Centre (Billings), North Main Street, Cork, Eire.

Organic Foods

The Soil Association, Bristol
Researches and promotes the use of organic food. Produces a directory *Where To Buy Organic Food*. Before sending a SAE requesting the directory, telephone to check its cost: 86 Colston Street, Bristol BS1 5BB
Tel: 0117 929 0061

Chemical-Free Cosmetics

The Green People, Sussex
A range of natural cosmetic products. Mail order and also available from health shops.
Tel: 01444 401 444

Lymphatic Massage Therapists

ASK (Association of Systematic Kinesiology), Surrey
For a therapist qualified in the 'breast congestion technique' described in the section **Benign breast lump solutions** in the chapter **Lifestyle Choices** (page 193). A recent trial at Guy's Hospital, London, under the direction of Ian Fentiman, has been completed after two years with 200 women participants. There was a general reduction in mastalgia (breast pain), and the paper is currently being submitted to a peer review journal for publication.
Tel: 0181 399 3215

MLD UK (manual lymphatic drainage)
Send a SAE for a list of therapists to: PO Box 149, Wallingford, Oxon OX10 7LD

Water Treatment Suppliers

Suppliers of water distillers
Aquapure Distillation
Tel: 0181 892 9010

Freshwater Filter Company
Tel: 0181 558 7495

Higher Nature
Tel: 01435 882 880

Wholistic Research Company
Tel: 01954 781 074

Other suppliers

Aquathin UK
Suppliers of reverse osmosis with de-ionizer (RODI) filter systems.
Tel: 01252 860 111

The Freshwater Company
Offers delivery service of pre-distilled water in South-East of England.
Tel: 0345 023 998

Juicing machines

Wholistic Research Company
Suppliers of the Champion Juicing Machine.
Tel: 01954 781 074

Self-Help/Stress Management Books

Feel the Fear and Do it Anyway
by Susan Jeffers

The Road Less Travelled
by M. Scott Peck

Women Who Run with the Wolves
by Clarissa Pinkola Estes

Emotional Clearing
by John Ruskan

Out of Pain into Power
by Bill Longridge

You Can Heal Your Life
by Louise Hay

Breast Reconstruction

The British Association of Plastic Surgeons
Tel: 0171 831 5161

Prosthesis and Special Bra Manufacturers

Breast Cancer Care
 Charity with trained prosthesis fitters.
Helpline: 0171 384 2344

Mail Order Companies

Amoena (UK) Ltd, Hampshire
Tel: 0800 378 668

Eloise Lingerie, West Sussex
Tel: 01284 828 787

Medimac, West Sussex
Tel: 01273 441 436

Rigby and Peller, London SW1
Tel: 0171 589 9293

Tru-Life Ltd, Liverpool
Tel: 0151 207 5690

Medical Glossary

This book has been written using the minimum of jargon as not everyone has a penchant for medical terms. You will not find the majority of the words listed below in the book; however, in discussions with your doctor, or when reading other literature, you may well come across unfamiliar terms that need explanation.

Adenocarcinoma   Cancer whose origin is in glandular tissue such as breast tissue.

Adjuvant   Treatment to enhance effectiveness of another, i.e. radiotherapy and chemotherapy are adjuvants to surgery.

Allopathic   Conventional or orthodox medical treatment.

Andi   'Abnormalities of Normal Development and Involution'. A range of non-cancerous breast disorders.

Angiogenesis   New blood vessel growth (to supply the tumour in the case of cancer).

Anovulatory   Menstrual periods when no egg is produced.

Anti-angiogenesis   Inhibits new blood vessel growth to reduce risk of cancer growth.

Antibody   Immune system component in blood and lymph system to fight against specific threats (e.g. virus or cancer).

Anti-emetic   Reduces need to vomit. Often administered with chemotherapy drugs.

Anti-inflammatory   Reduces inflammation.

Anti-mutagenic   Prevents or repairs mutation of DNA.

Anti-tumour   Prevents or shrinks tumours.

Apoptosis   Natural pre-programmed cell death. A cell that does not die is a cancerous cell.

Aspiration   Procedure using hollow needle to draw fluid or cells from a lump for diagnosis.

Atypical cells   Slightly abnormal cells, present in all people.

Atypical hyperplasia	Many abnormal cells, called pre-cancerous. Often can be reversed without invasive treatment.
Axilla	Armpit area.
Axillary node dissection	Surgical removal of lymph nodes in armpit.
Axillary node sampling	Removal and laboratory testing of a few nodes in armpit.
Benign	Non-cancerous tissue mass.
Bilateral	Both sides or both breasts.
Biopsy	Removal of tissue sample for laboratory testing, usually by aspiration or surgery.
Bone marrow	Inner, soft tissue at core of bones. Blood cells and immune system cells are made here.
Bone scan	A radiation test looking for shadows or 'hot spots' that might indicate spread of cancer.
BRCA1	Gene that is abnormal in 5 per cent of patients with breast cancer.
BRCA2	Second breast cancer gene identified in 1995.
Calcification	Small calcium deposits sometimes, but usually not, indicative of cancer. Visible on a mammogram.
Cancer	Unchecked and abnormal cell growth which grows at the expense of surrounding tissue.
Carcinogen	A substance which initiates or promotes cancer growth.
Carcinoma	The most common type of cancer. Originates in epithelial tissue such as skin, glands and lining of organs (i.e. breast, uterine or ovarian cancers).
Chemotherapy	Drug treatment, pills or intravenous injection, aimed at killing cancer cells throughout body. May be used to shrink a tumour prior to surgery.
Chromosomes	Cellular structures that contain genetic coding made of DNA.
Clinical trial or study	Experiments using people (rather than laboratory tests), or overview of records of people/patients. Usually compares with unaffected or untreated people who act as 'controls'. A prospective study looks for differences between those who develop a disease and those who do not.
Cohort study	A type of prospective study that looks at similar groups of people distinguished by one factor only (e.g. contraceptive pill users versus non-pill users).

Medical Glossary

Contra-indicated	Advised against in certain circumstances (e.g. the contraceptive pill should not be used by women with breast cancer).
Contra-lateral	On the other side (e.g. the other breast).
Cyst	Fluid-filled sac or benign growth.
Cytology	Microscopic examination of cells using special staining techniques.
Cytostatic	Inhibits or stops the growth of cells.
Cytotoxic	Poisonous to cells.
Dissemination	Cancer cells that are spreading via the blood or lymph systems.
Double-blind randomized, cross-over controlled trial	Considered the 'gold standard' of trials. More relevant for drug assessment than for nutrition intervention. With drugs, one aspect is measured whereas the complex interplay between food, nutrients and health, in particular their synergistic nature, makes it difficult to apply this type of trial meaningfully for nutrition.
Doubling time	Time taken for a group of cells to double in number.
Duct	Tube for conducting secretions. Breast ducts connect milk lobules to the nipples.
Ductal carcinoma in situ (DCIS)	Mass of cells, with clear boundaries, confined to a duct – non-invasive.
Duct extasia	Common and harmless condition in older women causing nipple discharge, usually from one breast.
Encapsulated	Tumour that is isolated from surrounding tissue by a capsule or collagen envelope.
Endogenous	Arising within the body.
Eosinophils	White blood cells which eat up foreign organisms.
Epidemiology	Studies of populations and relationships to environment, social and hereditary factors. An epidemiological study may look for differences between different populations (e.g. East versus West).
ER status	A measure of the receptiveness of breast tissue to circulating oestrogens. May be positive to different degrees, or negative.
Excision biopsy	Removal of breast lump to examine under the microscope.
Exogenous	From external causes.

364

Fibroadenoma	Non-malignant fibrous breast tumour.
Fibroblasts	Cells in the breast producing chemical messengers, called growth factors, which may communicate with cancer cells, possibly encouraging growth and spread.
Fibrocystic disease	Benign, harmless, breast lumps. May indicate hormone imbalance.
Free radicals	Unstable oxygen molecules which can disrupt and damage cells. Stabilized by enzymes and antioxidants.
Hematoma	Pooled blood in soft tissue which can be a side-effect of surgery.
Heterogeneous	Several types of abnormal cell.
Histology	The study of the minute structure of tissues.
Hyperplasia	Excessive growth of cells which is not cancerous.
Immunoglobulins	Antibodies, which are the body's 'defence army'.
Incidence	Number of new cases which arise in a specified period of time.
Infiltrating or invasive	Cancer which has developed out of its original tissue into immediately neighbouring tissue.
Initiation	Beginning of the cancer process when DNA is damaged and not repaired.
In-situ	Contained within the original site. Not yet invasive.
Interferon	Substance produced by immune system to inhibit viruses and activate T-cells.
Intervention study	A study where an alteration is made in a factor thought to influence a disease outcome (e.g. vegetarianism versus meat-eating).
Intraductal	In between the ducts.
Intraductal papilloma	Non-invasive lump in the lining of the breast duct.
Laboratory study	Experiment conducted in the laboratory either using cell cultures in dishes, or using animals such as mice or rats.
Lipoma	A harmless lump which is a collection of fat cells in the breast. Can be removed if troublesome.
Local recurrence	Cancer of same type recurring in the same site after surgery.
Lumpectomy	Also termed excisional biopsy or breast-sparing surgery. Removal of cancerous or benign lump while leaving whole, or most, of breast intact.
Lymph fluid	Clear fluid that circulates among cells and through

	lymph vessels. Acts as part of the immune system by transporting lymphocytes.
Lymph glands or nodes	Glands that circulate and filter lymph fluid located throughout the body but particularly in the neck, armpits, abdomen and groin. Breast cancer cells may be collected in the glands in the armpits (axilla) and the neck.
Lymph node dissection	Removal of some or all of the lymph glands, usually accompanying surgery to the breast tissue.
Lymph system	A continuous network of organs, nodes, ducts, vessels and capillaries, twice as long as the cardiovascular system, which maintains the fluid balance of cells and is a key component of the immune system.
Lymphocytes	White blood cells with specific immune targets including viruses and tumour cells.
Lymphoedema	Swelling caused by lymph fluid build-up in tissues, possibly after surgery.
Macrophages	Large immune cells that surround and eat up foreign substances to the body.
Malignant	Cancerous.
Mammogram	X-ray picture of breast tissue. May be used for screening or diagnosis.
Mastalgia	Breast pain. Cyclical mastalgia is breast pain that is worse before periods.
Mastectomy	Surgical removal of the breast. May be partial, complete or total, modified (removes tissue and lymph nodes), radical (removes all muscles of chest wall as well as breast), or subcutaneous (removes breast tissue leaving skin intact).
Mastitis	Infection of the breast tissue.
Menarche	First menstrual period.
Menopause	Final cessation of menstruation.
Metastasis/ses, metastasize	Spread of cancer to site elsewhere in the body. Of same type as original cancer. Breast cancer most frequently metastasizes to the liver, lungs or bones.
Mitotic lesion	Disease process arising from rapidly dividing cells. May be a euphemism for cancer when doctors are talking among themselves in front of a patient.
Monocytes	White blood cells that eat up dead cells and debris.

Morbidity	Sickness or handicap caused by a disease or its treatment (e.g. lymphoedema after surgery).
Mortality	Number of deaths attributable to a specific period of time (e.g. one year).
Natural killer cells	A type of lymphocyte which can be cancer specific. NK cells are decreased in cancer patients and the decrease is related to the severity of the disease.
Necrosis	Death of body tissues.
Neoplasm, neoplastic, neoplasia	Cell abnormality including cancer cells. More severe abnormality than hyperplasia. Often a euphemism used doctor to doctor when discussing cancer in front of a patient.
Neutrophils	White blood cells for dealing with infection and the main constituents of pus.
Node status	Whether or not breast cancer has spread to lymph nodes or glands. Either positive or negative. If positive then number of infected nodes is counted.
Oedema	See lymphoedema.
Oestrogen	Female hormone made in ovaries, adrenal glands, fat cells and placenta. Several types (oestradiol, oestrone and oestriol). Also plant oestrogens (phytoestrogens) and oestrogen-mimicking chemicals (xenoestrogens).
Oestrogen metabolism	Body processes by which oestrogens are used or converted into other substances as needed.
Oestrogen receptor sites	All cells have hormone receptor sites that make them sensitive to particular relevant hormones. Breast tissue has sites that make it sensitive to oestrogens.
Oestradiol (E2)	One of the oestrogen hormones, generally thought to encourage breast cancer.
Oestriol (E3)	One of the oestrogen hormones, generally thought to be protective against breast cancer. Produced in larger amounts during pregnancy.
Oestrone (E1)	One of the oestrogen hormones, generally thought to encourage breast cancer.
Oncogene	A normal component of genetic material which helps regulate cell growth. When damaged or 'switched on' starts the cancer process.
Oncologist	Doctor specializing in treatment of cancer.
Oophorectomy	Removal of one or both ovaries.

Ovarian suppression	Treatment for breast cancer to stop the ovaries producing oestrogen. This is carried out by low-dose radiation to the ovaries or by interruptive hormones.
Oxidation	The effect of oxygen on materials (e.g. when iron rusts or apple flesh goes brown on exposure to the air). A destructive cellular process involving free radicals which damages body tissues and is involved in cancer initiation.
Paget's disease	An eczema-like condition of the nipples, which can indicate underlying cancer.
Palliative care	Relief of symptoms and soothing treatment (i.e. pain reduction) but not aiming to cure.
Palpate	Feel with the fingertips, as in breast examination.
Pathology	Branch of medicine looking at cause, origin and nature of a disease. A pathologist will interpret the results of a biopsy.
Pet (positron emission tomography)	A technique of labelling chemicals with radioactive isotopes in order to follow them in the body. Used to see tumours and to follow distribution of drugs.
Phagocytes	Cells that surround and eat up cell wastes and minute organisms; some are fixed and some move around.
Plasma	The fluid of the blood which carries circulating red and white blood cells.
Platelets	Components of blood which repair blood vessels and stop bleeding. Thrombocytes.
Prevalence	Number of cases in a particular population at a particular time.
Primary cancer	First site of cancer, as opposed to recurrence or metastasis.
Progesterone	Hormone produced in second half of menstrual cycle, named for ensuring a pregnancy is maintained (pro-gestation). Balances or opposes oestrogen. Significantly reduced post-menopausally.
Progestogens	Synthetic, pharmaceutical forms of progesterone with slightly different chemical structure to the natural hormone.
Prognosis	Prediction of possible outcome of a disease.
Promotion	The stage following initiation of cancer. Involves substances and events which favour early stage cancer cells evading the immune system.

Prophylactic Treatment given as a preventive measure where no evidence of disease exists (e.g. prophylactic mastectomy or Tamoxifen usage).

Prospective study Study to find the difference between those who develop a disease and those who do not.

Prostaglandins 'Local' hormones which encourage or discourage inflammation. Prostaglandin 2 (PGE2) is often high in breast cancer patients.

Prosthesis An artificial body part (e.g. breast form used to fill out bra after mastectomy).

Protocol Particular programme, for example a particular chemotherapy regime.

Rad Abbreviation for Radiation Absorbed Dose, used to describe a dosage of radiation.

Radiotherapy Radiation treatment to target and kill cancer cells.

Reconstruction As it relates to breast surgery, this is a procedure to return the breast, as closely as possible, to its original state, or to match the other breast.

Recurrence The return of cancer after a period of remission.

Red blood cells Blood cells which use haemoglobin to carry oxygen around the body.

Remission Shrinking of tumour or disappearance of detectable cancer.

Sarcoma Cancer of connective tissues – muscle, bone and cartilage.

Secondaries Cancers which have spread to other parts of the body from the original (primary) site.

Serum The fluid which separates from blood, lymph and other body fluids, a clear, yellowish fluid.

S-phase fraction Number of cancer cells reproducing at any one time.

Staging Cancer classification system that takes into account factors such as tumour size, lymph node involvement and metastasis.

Stem cells The source of all red blood cells, platelets and white blood cells. Found in the bone marrow.

Subcutaneous Underneath the skin.

Systemic Having an effect on the whole body (system) despite the fact that a specific target is sought (e.g. chemotherapy affects the whole body though it is the cancer that is being treated).

Medical Glossary

Tumour   A mass of cells. Can be benign (non-cancerous) or
malignant (cancerous).

Virginal   Breast development around the time of puberty may
 hypertrophy not be symmetrical and may be abnormally large for
the age of the girl – this can cause embarrassment or
discomfort, but no increased risk of breast cancer.

Virus   A minute organism that survives by growing in the
cells of a host. Viruses are responsible for colds,
influenza and AIDS. There are also oncoviruses that
can initiate cancer.

White blood cells Leucocytes. A collective term for immune system cells
which includes: lymphocytes, eosinophils, monocytes
and neutrophils.

Notes

Does Diet Really Influence Breast Cancer?

1. Howe, G. R. et al. Dietary factors and risk of breast cancer: combined analysis of 12 case-control studies, *J Natl Cancer Inst* 1990; 82(7): 561–9.
2. Pierce, J. P. et al. Feasibility of a randomized trial of high-vegetable diet to prevent breast cancer recurrence, *Nutrition and Cancer* 1997; 28(3): 282–8.
   Holm, L. E. et al. Treatment failure and dietary habits in women with breast cancer, *J Natl Cancer Inst* 1993; 85(1): 32–6.
   Stoll, B. A. Diet and exercise regimens to improve breast carcinoma prognosis, *Cancer* 1996; 78(12): 2465–70.
3. Normura, A. M. Y. et al. The effects of dietary fat in breast cancer survival among Caucasian and Japanese women in Hawaii, *Breast Cancer Res Treat* 1991; 18: S135–41.
4. Kohlmeier, L. Future of dietary exposure assessment, *Am J Clin Nutr* 1995; 61 (suppl.); 702S–9S.
5. Riboli, E. et al. Identifiability of food components for cancer chemoprevention, *IARC Sci Publ* 1996; 139: 23–31.

Your Breasts

1. Baum, M. et al., *Breast Cancer*, Oxford, 1994.

Those Fateful Words

1. von Fournier, D. et al. Natural growth rate of primary breast cancer and its metastases. In: Kubli, F. et al. (eds), *Breast Diseases*, Springer-Verlag, Berlin, 1990: 79–96.
2. Baum, M. et al., *Breast Cancer*, Oxford, 1994.
3. Office of National Statistics, National Cancer Registration Database.
4. Hirshaut, Y. and Pressman, Peter I. *Breast Cancer*, Bantam (USA), 1992.
5. Mabuchi, K. et al. Risk factors for male breast cancer, *JNCI* 1985; 74: 371–5.
   Lin, R. S. et al. Epidemiological findings in male breast cancer, *Proc Am Assoc Cancer Res* 1980; 21: 72.
6. Wood, A. J. J. Tamoxifen in the treatment of breast cancer, *Drug Therapy* 1998; 339 (22): 1609–18.
   Kinne, D. Management of male breast cancer, *Oncology* March 1991: 45–8.

Notes

Seeking Medical Help

1. British Breast Group and British Association of Surgical Oncology.

The Impact of Oestrogen on Breast Cancer

1. Cavalieri, E. L. et al. Molecular origin of cancer: Catechol estrogen-3, 4-quinones as endogenous tumour initiators, *Proc Natl Acad Sci* 1997; 94: 10937–42.

Minimizing Risks

1. Eisen, A. and Weber, B. L. Prophylactic mastectomy – the price of fear, *N Engl J Med* 1999; 340(2): 137–8 (editorial).
2. Malins, D. C. et al. Tumour progression to the metastatic state involves structural modification in DNA markedly different from those associated with primary tumour formation, *Proceedings of the National Academy of Sciences of the USA* 1996: 93: 14047–52.

    Challem, J. *Nutrition Science News* August 1997; 2(8). www.nutrition-sciencenews.com
3. Saitoh, S. et al. p53 gene mutations in breast cancers in midwestern US women: null as well as missense-type mutations are associated with poor prognosis, *Oncogene* 1994; 9: 2869–75.
4. Kagawa, Y. Impact of Westernization on the nutrition of Japan: Changes in physique, *Cancer* 1978; 7: 205.
5. Wang, D. Y. et al. Serum hormone levels in British and rural Chinese females, *Breast Cancer Res Treat* 1991; 18: S41–5.

Keep It Complex

1. Kazer, R. R. Insulin resistance, insulin-like growth factor I and breast cancer: a hypothesis, *Int J Cancer* 1995; 62: 403–6.

    Talamini, R. et al. Selected medical conditions and risk of breast cancer, *J Cancer* 1997; 75(11): 1699–1703.
2. Hankin, J. H. et al. Diet and breast cancer: a review, *Am J Clin Nutr* 1978; 31: 2005.

    Horrobin, D. F. and Seely, S. Diet and breast cancer: the possible connection with sugar consumption, *Med Hypotheses* 1983; 11(3): 319–27.
3. Quillin, Patrick. *Beating cancer with nutrition*, Nutrition Times Press, 1994: 53.
4. Franceschi, S. et al. Intake of macronutrients and risk of breast cancer. *Lancet* 1996; 347: 1351–6.
5. Rothkopf, M. Fuel utilization in neoplastic disease: implications for the use of nutritional support in cancer patients, *Nutrition* 1990; 6(4): 14S–6S (suppl).

Santisteban, G. A. et al. Glycemic modulation of tumor tolerance in a mouse model of breast cancer, *Biochem Biophys Res Commun* 1985; 132: 1174–9.

6. Hems, G. and Stuart, A. Breast cancer rates in populations of single women, *Br J Cancer* 1975; 31(1): 118–23.

Seely, S. and Horrobin, D. F. Diet and breast cancer: the possible connection with sugar consumption, *Med Hypotheses* 1993; 11(3): 319–27.

The Fibre 'Movement'

1. Goldin, B. R. et al. Estrogen excretion patterns and plasma levels in vegetarian and omnivorous women, *N Engl J Med* 1982; 307: 1542.
2. Woods, M. N. et al. Low fat, high fibre diet and serum estrone sulphate in premenopausal women, *Am J Clin Nutr* 1989; 49: 1179–93.
3. Stoll, B. A. Nutrition and breast cancer risk: can an effect via insulin resistance be demonstrated?, *Breast Cancer Res Treat* 1996; 38: 239–46.
4. Bruning, P. F. et al. Body measurements, estrogen availability and the risk of human breast cancer: a case control study, *Int J Cancer* 1992; 51: 14–19.

Yam, D. Insulin cancer relationships: possible dietary implication, *Med Hypotheses* 1992; 38(2): 111–17.

Kazer, R. R. Insulin resistance, insulin-like growth factor I and breast cancer: a hypothesis, *Int J Cancer* 1995; 62(4): 403–6.

5. *Food Nutrition and the Prevention of Cancer: A Global Perspective*, World Cancer Research Fund and American Cancer Institute 1997.

Fats – Friends or Foes?

1. Crawford, M. and Marsh, D. *Nutrition and Evolution*, Keats (USA), 1995.
2. Erasmus, Udo. *Fats that Heal, Fats that Kill*, Alive Books (Canada), reprinted 1994.
3. Welsch, C. W. Dietary fat, calories and mammary gland tumourgenesis, *Adv Exp Med Biol* 1992; 322: 203–22.
4. Wynder, E. L. et al. Diet and breast cancer in causation and therapy, *Cancer* 1986; 58: 1804–13.
5. Cameron, E., Director, Cancer Nutriprevention Project, Linus Pauling Institute of Science and Medicine (10 June, 1987) (a study).
6. Willett, W. C. et al. Dietary fat and fibre in relation to risk of breast cancer, *JAMA* 1992; 268: 2037–44.
7. *Food, Nutrition and the Prevention of Cancer: A Global Perspective*, World Cancer Research Fund and American Institute for Cancer Research 1998: 252.
8. Boyd, N. F. et al. Effects of a low-fat, high carbohydrate diet on plasma sex hormones in premenopausal women: results from a randomized trial, *Breast Cancer Res Treat* 1997; 76(1): 127–35.

9. Furst, C. J. et al. DNA pattern and dietary habits in patients with breast cancer, *Eur J Cancer* 1993; 29A(9): 1285–8.

10. Fritsche, K. L. and Johnston, P. V. Effects of dietary alpha-linolenic acid on growth, metastasis, fatty acid profile and prostaglandin production of two murine adenocarcinomas, *J Nutr* December 1990; 120(12): 1601–9.

    Takata, T. et al. Specific inhibitory effect of dietary eicosapentaenoic acid on N-nitroso-N-methylurea-induced mammary carcinogenesis in female Sprague-Dawley rats, *Carcinogenesis* November 1990; 11(1): 2012–19.

    Pritchard, G. A. et al. Lipids in breast carcinogenesis, *Br J Surg* 1989; 76: 1069–73.

    Welsch, C. W. et al. Suppression of growth by dietary fish oil of human breast carcinomas maintained in three different strains of immune-deficient mice, *Nutr Cancer* 1993; 20: 119–27.

    Gonzalez, M. J. et al. Dietary fish oil inhibits breast carcinoma growth: a function of increased lipid peroxidation, *Lipids* 1993; 28(9): 827–32.

11. Borgeson, D. E. et al. Effects of dietary fish oil on human mammary carcinoma and on lipid-metabolizing enzymes, *Lipids* 1989; 24: 290–5.

    Kaizer, L. et al. Fish consumption and breast cancer risk: an ecological study, *Nutr Cancer* 1989; 12: 61–8.

12. Baxevanis, C. N. et al. Elevated prostaglandin E2 production by monocytes is responsible for the depressed levels of natural killer and lymphokine-activated killer cell function in patients with breast cancer, *Cancer* 1993; 72: 491–501.

13. Bougnoux, P. et al. Alpha-linolenic acid content of adipose breast tissue: a host determinant of the risk of early metastasis in breast cancer, *Br J Cancer* August 1994; 70(2): 330–4.

14. Cohen, L. A. et al. Dietary fat and mammary cancer. 1. Promoting effects of different dietary fats on n-nitrosomethylurea-induced rat mammary tumourgenesis, *J Natl Cancer Inst* 1986; 77: 33–42.

    Tinsley, I. J. et al. Influence of dietary fatty acids on the incidence of mammary tumours in the C3H mouse, *Cancer Res* 1981; 41: 1460–5.

15. Keys, A. et al. The diet and 15-year death rate in the seven countries study, *Am J Epidemiol* 1986; 124: 903–15.

    Raloff, J. This fat may fight cancer in several ways. *Science News*, 19 March 1994.

16. Wynder, E. L. et al. Diet and breast cancer in causation and therapy, *Cancer* 1984; 58: 1804–14 (review).

17. Shun-Zhang, Y. et al. A case-controlled study of dietary and non-dietary risk factors for breast cancer in Shanghai, *Cancer Res* 1990; 50: 5017–21.

18. Low-fat diet lengthens menstrual cycle, *J Am Diet Assoc* 1993: 1501 (editorial).

19. Boyd, N. F., Ontario Cancer Treatment and Research Foundation in Toronto. Canadian Diet and Breast Cancer Prevention Study Group.

Nordevang, E. et al. Dietary habits and mammographic patterns in patients with breast cancer, *Breast Cancer Res Treat* 1993; 26(3): 207–15.

Pick Your Proteins

1. Toniolo, P. et al. Consumption of meat, animal products, protein and fat and risk of breast cancer – a prospective cohort study in New York, *Epidemiology* 1994; 5: 391–7.
2. Toniolo, P. et al. Calorie-providing nutrients and risk of breast cancer, *JNCI* 1989; 81: 278–86.
   Goodman, M. T. et al. The association of diet, obesity and breast cancer in Hawaii, *Cancer Epidem Bio Prev* 1992; 1: 269–75.
   Lee, H. P. et al. Dietary effects on breast cancer risk in Singapore, *Lancet*, 1991; 337: 1197–200.
3. Hawrylewicz, E. J. Fat–protein interaction defined 2-generation studies. In Ip, C. et al, (eds), *Dietary Fat and Cancer, Progress in Clinical and Biological Research*, Alan R. Liss Inc, NY, 1986; 222: 4033–4.
   Huang, H. H. et al. Effects of protein diet on release of prolactin and ovarian steroids in female rats, *Nutr Rpts Int* 1982; 26: 807–20.
4. Daniels, R. *Healing Foods*, Thorsons, 1996: 117.
5. Lowry, S. F. et al. Effects of protein malnutrition on host-tumor composition and growth, *Surgical Forum* 1977; 28: 143–5.
6. Drasar, B. S. and Irving, D. Environmental factors and cancer of the colon and breast, *Br J Cancer* 1973; 27: 167–72 (review).
   Lee, H. P. et al. Dietary effects on breast-cancer risk in Singapore. *Lancet* 1991; 337: 1197–2000.
   Lubin, F. et al. Role of fat, animal protein and dietary fibre in breast cancer etiology: a case-control study, *J Natl Cancer Inst* 1986; 77: 605–12.
7. Mills, P. K. et al. Dietary habits and breast cancer incidence among Seventh-day Adventists, *Cancer* 1989; 64: 582–90.
   Mills, P. K. et al. Animal products consumption and subsequent fatal breast cancer risk among Seventh-day Adventists, *Am J Epidemiol* 1988; 127: 440–53.
8. Barbosa, J. C. et al. The relationship among adiposity, diet and hormone concentrations in vegetarian and non-vegetarian postmenopausal women, *Am J Clin Nutr* 1990; 51(5): 798–803.
   Goldwin et al. Estrogen excretion patterns and plasma levels in vegetarian and omnivorous women, *N Engl J Med* 1982; 307: 1542–7.
   Dwyer, J. T. et al. Health aspects of vegetarian diets, *Am J Clin Nutr* 1988: 48 (3 suppl): 712–38 (review).
9. Zheng, W. et al. Well-done meat intake and the risk of breast cancer, *J Natl Cancer Inst* 1998; 90(22): 1724–9.

10. Stoll, B. A. Breast cancer: further metabolic-endocrine risk markers?, *Br J Cancer* 1997; 76(12): 1652–4.

Antioxidant Armoury

1. Chen, J. et al. Antioxidant status and cancer mortality in China, *Int J Epidem* 1992; 21: 625–34.
2. Malins, D. C. et al. The aetiology of breast cancer: characteristic alterations in hydroxyl radical-induced DNA base lesions during oncogenesis with potential for evaluating incidence risk, *Cancer* 1993; 71: 3036–43.
3. Dwivedy I., et al. Synthesis and characterization of estrogen 2,3- and 3,4-quinones. Comparisons of DNA aducts formed by the quinones versus horseradish peroxidase-activated catechol estrogens, *Chem Res Toxicol* 1992; 5: 828–33.
4. Passwater, R. A., *Cancer Prevention and Nutritional Therapies*, Keats (USA), 1993.
5. Katsouyanni, K. et al. Diet and breast cancer: a case-control study in Greece, *Int J Cancer* 1986; 38: 815–20.

    Zarid, D. et al. Diet, alcohol consumption and reproductive factors in a case-control study of breast cancer in Moscow, *Int J Cancer* 1991; 48: 493–501.

    Lee, H. P. et al. Dietary effects on breast cancer risk in Singapore, *Lancet* 1991; 337: 1197–200.
6. *Food, Nutrition and the Prevention of Cancer: A Global Perspective*. 1998, World Cancer Research Fund and American Institute for Cancer Research: 444.
7. Cao, G. et al. Serum antioxidant capacity is increased by consumption of strawberries, spinach, red wine in elderly women, *J Nutr* 1998; 128(12): 2383–90.
8. Graham, S. et al. Diet in the epidemiology of breast cancer, *Am J Epidemiol* 1982; 116: 68–75.

    Brisson, J. et al. Diet, mammographic features of breast tissue, and breast cancer risk, *Am J Epidemiol* 1989; 130: 14–24.

    Garland, M. et al. Antioxidant micronutrients and breast cancer, *J Am Coll Nutr* 1993; 12: 400–11 (review).

    La Vacchia, C. et al. Dietary factors and the risk of breast cancer, *Nutr Cancer* 1987; 10: 205–14.

    Jumaan, A. O. et al. Beta-carotene intake and risk of postmenopausal breast cancer, *Epidemiology* 1999; 10: 49–53.
9. Block, G. Epidemiologic evidence regarding vitamin C and cancer, *Am J Clin Nutr* 1991; 54 (6 Suppl): 1310S–1314S.
10. Howe, G. R. et al. Dietary factors in risk of breast cancer: combined analysis of 12 case-controlled studies, *J Natl Cancer Inst* 1990; 82: 561–9.

11. Wald, N. J. et al. Plasma retinol, beta-carotene and vitamin E levels in relation to the future risk of breast cancer, *Br J Cancer* 1984; 49: 321–4.
12. Foster, H. D. Selenium and cancer prevention, *J Nutr* 1988; 118: 237 (letter).
13. Austin, Steve and Hitchcock, Cathy. *Breast Cancer*, Prima (USA), 1994.
14. Ip, C. and Lisk, D. J. Bioactive selenium from Brazil nut for cancer prevention and selenoenzyme maintenance, *Nutr Cancer* 1994; 21: 203–12.
15. Fürst, C. J. et al. DNA pattern and dietary habits in patients with breast cancer, *Eur J Cancer* 1993; 29A(9): 1285–8.
16. Cao, G. et al. Increases in human plasma antioxidant capacity after consumption of controlled diets high in fruit and vegetables, *Am J Clin Nutr* 1998; 68: 1081–7.
17. Drewnowski, A. and Rock, C. L. The influence of genetic taste markers on food acceptance, *Am J Clin Nutr* 1995; 62: 506–11.

Organic Food

1. Arnold, S. F. et al. Synergistic activation of estrogen receptor with combinations of environmental chemicals, *Science* 1996; 272: 1489–92. (This report was withdrawn 1997 as the information was not later substantiated, but the researchers intend to carry on investigating these issues. My impression of the tone of the withdrawal is that it was erring on the side of caution rather than indicating that the original report was definitely defective.)

     Howard, V. Synergistic effects of chemical mixtures – can we rely on traditional toxicity?, *The Ecologist* 1997; 27(5): 192–5.
2. Colborn, T. et al. Developmental effects on endocrine disrupting chemicals in wildlife and humans, *Environ Health Perspect* 1993; 101: 378–84.
3. *Norwegian Polar Institute*, June 1998.
4. Sharpe, R. and Skakkebaek, N. Are oestrogens involved in the falling sperm counts and disorders of the male reproductive tract? *Lancet* 1993; 341: 1392–5.

     Kunstmann, J. M. et al. Decline in semen quality among fertile men in Paris during the past 20 years, *N Engl J Med* 1995; 332: 281–5.
5. Wolff, M. S. et al. Blood levels of organochlorine residues and risk of breast cancer, *J Natl Cancer Inst* 1993: 85: 648–52.

     Safe, S. H. Xenoestrogens and breast cancer, *N Engl J Med* 1997; 337(18): 1303-4 (editorial).
6. Hoyer, A. P. et al. Organochlorine exposure and risk of breast cancer, *Lancet* 1998; 352: 1816–20.
7. Shekhar, P. V., et al. Environmental estrogen stimulation of growth and estrogen receptor function in preneoplastic and cancerous human breast cell lines, *J Natl Cancer Inst* 1997; 89(23): 1774–82.
8. Residues in food and water, *Pesticides News* December 1995; 30.
9. Westin, J. et al. The Israel breast cancer anomaly, *Acad Sci* 1990; 609: 269–79.
10. Colborn, Theo, et al. *Our Stolen Future*. Little, Brown & Co (USA), 1996: 184–5.

Notes

11. Verma, S. P. et al. Effects of soy-derived isoflavanoids on the induced growth of MCF-7 cells by estrogenic environmental chemicals, *Nutr Cancer* 1998; 30: 232–9.

Phytofacts

1. Ingrams, D. et al. Case-control study of phyto-oestrogens and breast cancer, *Lancet* 1997; 350: 990–4.

   Messina, M. et al. Phyto-ostrogens and breast cancer, *Lancet* 1997; 350: 971–2.

   Adlercreutz, T. et al. Soybean phytoestrogen intake and cancer risk, *J Nutr* 1995; 125: 757S–70S.

   Wang, T. T. Y. et al. Molecular effects of genistein on estrogen receptor mediated pathways, *Carcinogenesis* 1996; 17(2): 271–5.

   Peterson, T. G. et al. The role of metabolism in mammary epithelial cell growth inhibition by the isoflavones genistein and biochanin A, *Carcinogenesis* 1996; 17(9): 1861–9.

   Zava, D. T. and Duwe, G. Estrogenic and antiproliferative properties of genistein and other flavonoids in human breast cancer cells in vitro, *Nutr Cancer* 1997; 27(1): 31–40.
2. Martin, M. E. et al. Interactions between phytoestrogens and human sex steroid binding protein, *Life Sciences* 1996; 58(5): 429–36.
3. Kurzer, M. S. et al. Dietary phytoestrogens, *Annu Rev Nutr* 1997; 17: 353–81.

   Peterson, T. G. et al. Metabolism of the isoflavones genistein and biochanin A in human breast cancer cell lines, *Am J Clin Nutr* 1998; 68: 1505S–11S (suppl).
4. Hughes, C. Phytochemical mimicry of reproductive hormones and modulation of herbivore fertility by phytoestrogens, *Environm Health Persp* 1988; 78: 171–5.
5. Lamartiniere, C. A. et al. Genistein studies in rats: potential for breast cancer prevention and reproductive and developmental toxicity, *Am J Clin Nutr* 1998; 68: 1400S–5S (suppl).
6. Messina, M. J. et al. Soy intake and cancer risk: A review of the in-vitro and in-vivo data, *Nutrition and Cancer* 1994; 21(2): 112–31.
7. Hawrylewicz, E. J. et al. Dietary soybean isolate and methionine supplementation affect mammary tumour progression in rats, *J Nutr*, October 1991; 121(10): 1693–8.

   Hawrylewicz, E. J. et al. Soy and experimental cancer: animal studies, *J Nutr*, March 1995; 125 (suppl 3): 698–708.

   Barnes, S. et al. Soybeans inhibit mammary tumours in models of breast cancer, *Prog Clin Biol Res* 1990; 347: 239–53.
8. Kennedy, A. R. The evidence for soybean products as cancer preventive agents, *J Nutr* 1995; 125: 733S–43S.

9. Hin-Peng, L. Diet and breast cancer: an epidemiologist's perspective, *Crit Rev Oncol Hematol* 1998; 28: 115–19.

10. Knight, D. C. et al. A review of the clinical effects of phytoestrogens, *Obstet Gynecol* 1996; 87: 897–904.

11. Bingham, S. A. et al. Phyto-oestrogens: where are we now?. *Br J Nutr* 1998; 79: 393–406.

12. Adlercreutz, H. et al. Determination of urinary lignan and phytoestrogen metabolites, potential antioestrogens and anticarcinogens in urine of women on various habitual diets. *J Steroid Biochem* 1986; 25: 791–7.

Serraino, M. et al. The effects of flaxseed supplementation on early risk markers for mammary carcinogenesis, *Cancer Lett* 1991; 60: 135–42.

Thompson, L. U. et al. Antitumourigenic effect of mammalian lignan precursor from flaxseed, *Nutr Cancer* 1996; 26: 159–65.

13. Serraino, M. and Thompson, L. The effects of flaxseed supplementation on the initiation and promotional stages of mammary tumourgenesis, *Nutr Cancer* 1992e; 17: 153–9.

14. Wang, C. et al. Lignans and flavonoids inhibit aromatase enzyme in human preadiposites, *J Steroid Biochem Mol Biol* 1994; 50: 205–12.

15. Barnes, S. et al. Chemical modification of isoflavones in soyafoods during cooking and processing, *Am J Clin Nutr* 1998; 68: 1486S–91S (suppl).

Block, G. and Reinli, K. Phytoestrogen content of foods – a compendium of literature values, *Nutrition and Cancer* 1996; 26(2): 123–48.

16. Zava, D. T. et al. Estrogen and progestin bioactivity of foods, herbs and spices. *Proceedings of the Society for Experimental Biology and Medicine* 1998; 217: 369–78.

A little of What You Fancy?

1. Longnecker, M. P. et al. Alcoholic beverage consumption in relation to risk of breast cancer: meta-analysis and review, *Cancer Causes Controls* 1994; 5: 73–82.

2. Quillin, Patrick. *Beating Cancer with Nutrition*, NTP (USA), 1994.

3. Welsch, C. W. Caffeine and the development of the normal and neoplastic mammary gland, *Proc Soc Exp Biol Med* 1994; 207(1): 1–12.

Wet Your Whistle

1. Kaegi, E. Unconventional therapies for cancer: 1. Essiac. The task force on alternative therapies of breast cancer research initiative, *CMAJ* 1998: 158(7): 897–902.

2. Sheng, Y. et al. Induction of apoptosis and inhibition of proliferation in human tumour cells treated with extracts of Uncaria tomentosa, *Anticancer Res* 1998; 18(5A): 3363–8.

Rizzi, R. et al. Mutagenic and antimutagenic activities of Uncaria tomentosa and its extracts, *J Ethnopharmacol* 1993; 38(1): 63–77.

Notes

Anti-Breast Cancer Superfoods

1. Stavric, B. Antimutagens and anticarcinogens in food, *Food Chem Toxicol* 1994; 32: 79–90.

   Stavric, B. Role of chemopreventers in human diet, *Can Biochem* 1899; 27: 319–32.
2. Tyihak, E. et al. Basic plant proteins with antitumor activity, *Hungarian Patent* 1970: 798.
3. De Froment, P. Unsaponifiable substance from alfalfa for pharmaceuticals and cosmetic use, *French Patent* 1974(2); 187: 328.
4. Smith-Barbaro, P. et al. Carcinogen binding to various types of dietary fibre, *J Natl Cancer Inst* 1981; 67(2): 495–7.
5. Kennedy, A. and Little, J. B. Effects of protease inhibitors on radiation transformation in vitro. *Cancer Res* 1981; 41(6): 2103–8.
6. Verhagen, H. et al. Reduction of oxidative DNA-damage in humans by Brussels sprouts, *Carcinogenesis* 1995; 16(4): 969–70.

   Verhoeven, D. T. et al. A review of mechanisms underlying anticarcinogenicity by brassica vegetables, *Chem Biol Interact* 1997; 103(2): 79–129.
7. Michnovicz, J. J. et al. Altered estrogen metabolism and excretion in humans following consumption of indole-3-carbinol, *Nutr Cancer* 1991; 16: 59–66.
8. Wattenberg, L. W. et al. Inhibition of polycyclic aromatic hydrocarbon-induced neoplasia by naturally occurring indoles, *Cancer Res* 1978; 38: 1410–13.
9. Sepkovic, D. W. et al. Catechol estrogen production in rat microsomes after treatment with indole-3-carbinol, ascorbigen, or B-naphthaflavone, *Steroids* 1994; 59: 318–23.
10. Grubbs, C. J. et al. Chemoprevention of chemically-induced mammary carcinogenesis by indole-3-carbinol, *Anticancer Research* 1995; 15: 709–16.
11. Nihoff, W. A. et al. Effects of consumption of Brussels sprouts on intestinal and lymphocytic glutathione-S-transferase in humans, *Carcinogenesis* 1995; 16(9): 2125–8.
12. Helzisouer, K. J. et al. Association between glutathione S-transferase M1, P1, and T1 genetic polymorphisms and breast cancer, *J Natl Cancer Inst* 1998; 90(7): 512–18.

    Kelsey, K. T. and Wiencke, J. K. Growing pains for the environmental genetics of breast cancer: observations on a study of the glutathione-S-transferases, *J Natl Cancer Inst* 1998; 90(7): 484–5 (editorial).
13. Institute of Food Research, Norwich, press release 12 June 1998. www.ifrn.bbsr.ac.uk.
14. Fahey, J. W. et al. Broccoli sprouts: an exceptionally rich source of inducers of enzymes that protect against chemical carcinogens, *Proceedings of the National Academy of Sciences* 1997; 94: 10367–72.
15. Weed, Susan S. *Breast Cancer? Breast Health!*, Ash Tree Publishing (USA), 1996.

16. Homberger, F. et al. Inhibition of murine subcutaneous and intravenous benzo(rst)pentaphene carcinogenesis by sweet orange oils and d-limonene, *Oncology* 1971; 25: 1–20.

17. Guthrie, N. et al. Inhibition of mammary cancer by citrus flavonoids, *Adv Exp Med Biol* 1998; 439: 227–36.

   So, F. V. et al. Inhibition of human breast cancer cell proliferation and delay of mammary tumourgenesis by citrus juices, *Nutr Cancer* 1996; 26(2): 167–81.

18. Thompson, L. U. et al. Flaxseed and its lignan and oil components reduce mammary tumour growth at a late stage of carcinogenesis, *Carcinogenesis* 1996; 17: 1373–6.

19. Ip, C. and Lisk, D. J. Efficacy of cancer prevention by high-selenium garlic is primarily dependent on the actions of selenium. *Carcinogenesis* 1995; 16: 2649–52.

   Ip, C. et al. Mammary cancer prevention by regular garlic and selenium-enriched garlic, *Nutr Cancer* 1992; 17: 279–86.

20. Agarwal, K. C. Therapeutic actions of garlic constituents, *Med Res Rev* 1996; 16: 111–24.

   Sigounas, G. et al. S-allylmercaptocysteine inhibits cell proliferation and reduces the viability of erythroleukemia, breast and prostate cancer cell lines, *Nutr Cancer* 1997; 27: 186–91.

21. Fenwick, G. R. and Hanley, A. B. The genus allium – part 1/2/3, *Crit Rev Food Sci Nutr* 1985; 22: 199–271, 273–377; 23: 1–73.

   Lau, B. H. et al. Garlic compounds modulate macrophage and T-lymphocyte functions, *Mol Biother* 1991; 3: 103–7.

22. Surh, Y. J. et al. Chemoprotective properties of some pungent ingredients present in red pepper and ginger, *Mutat Res* 1998; 402. 259–67.

   Banerjee, S. et al. Influence of certain essential oils on carcinogen-metabolizing enzymes and acid-soluble sulfhydryls in mouse livers, *Nutr Cancer* 1994: 21: 263–9.

   Unnikrishnan, M. C. et al. Cytotoxicity of extracts of spices to cultured cells, *Nutr Cancer* 1988; 11: 251–7.

23. Thompson, L. U. et al. Antitumorigenic effect of a mammalian lignan precursor from flaxseed, *Nutr Cancer* 1996; 26: 159–65.

24. Thompson, L. U. et al. Flaxseed and its lignan and oil components reduce tumour growth at a late stage of carcinogenesis, *Carcinogenesis* 1996; 17(6): 1373–6.

25. Chihara, G. et al. Antitumor and metastasis inhibitory activities of lentinan as an immunomodulator: an overview, *Cancer Detect Prev* 1987; 1 (suppl): 423–43.

26. Nanba, H. Maitake mushroom: immune therapy to prevent cancer growth and metastasis, *Explore* 1995; 6(1): 17.

Notes

Nanba, H. Antitumor activity of orally administered D-fraction from maitake mushroom (*grifola frondosa*), *J Naturopathic Med* 1993; 1(4): 10–15.

27. Wang, H. et al. The oxygen radical absorbing capacity of anthocyanins, *J Agric Food Chem* 1997; 45: 304–9.

28. Batkin, S. et al. Antimetastatic effect of bromelain with or without its proteolytic and anticoagulant activity, *J Cancer Res Clin Oncol* 1988; 114: 507–8.

29. Takeshita, M. et al. Antitumour effects of RBS (rice bran saccharide) on ENNG-induced carcinogenesis, *Biotherapy* 1992; 4: 139–45.

30. Weed, Susan S. *Breast Cancer? Breast Health!*, Ash Tree Publishing (USA), 1996.

31. Reddy, B. S. et al. Effect of Japanese seaweed extracts on the mutagenicity of 7, 12-dimethylbenz(a)anthracene, a breast carcinogen, and of 3, 2'-dimethyl-4-aminobiphenyl, a colon and breast carcinogen, *Mutat Res* 1984; 127: 113–18.

Liu, J. N. et al. B cell stimulating activity of seaweed extracts, *Int J Immunopharmacol* 1997; 19: 135–42.

Teas, J. et al. Dietary seaweed (Lamianria) and mammary carcinogenesis in rats, *Cancer Res* 1984; 44: 2758–61.

32. Akiyama, T. et al. Use and specificity of genistein as inhibitor of protein-tyrosine kinases, *Methods in Enzymology*, 1991; 201: 362–70.

Kim, H. et al. Mechanisms of action of the soy isoflavone genistein: emerging role for its effects via transforming growth factor B signaling pathways, *Am J Clin Nutr* 1998; 68: 1418S–25S (suppl).

33. Challem, J. and Dolby, V. *The Health Benefits of Soy*, Keats (USA), 1996.

34. Lee, H. P. et al. Dietary effects on breast cancer risk in Singapore, *Lancet* 18 May 1991; 337: 1197–200.

35. Lin, Y. L. et al. Composition of polyphenols in fresh tea leaves and associations of their oxygen-radical absorbing capacity with antiproliferative actions in fibroblast cells, *J Agric Food Chem* 1996; 44: 1387–94.

36. Sharma, O. P. Antioxidant activity of curcumin and related compounds, *Biochem Pharmacol* 1976; 25: 1811–12.

Ammon, H. P. et al. Pharmacology of Curcuma longa, *Planta Med* 1991; 57: 1–7.

Nagabhusham, M. and Bhide, S. V. Curcumin as an inhibitor of cancer, *J Am Coll Nutr* 1992; 11(2): 192–8.

37. Verma, S. P. et al. Curcumin and genistein, plant natural products, show synergistic inhibitory effects on the growth of human breast cancer MCF-7 cells induced by estrogenic pesticides, *Biochem Biophys Res Commun* 1997; 233: 692–6.

Verma, S. P. et al. The inhibition of the estrogenic effects of pesticides and environmental chemicals by curcumin and isoflavonoids, *Environ Health Perspect* 1998; 106: 807–12.

38. Conge, G. A. et al. Comparative effects of a diet enriched in live or heated

yoghurt on the immune system of the mouse, *Reprod Nutr Dev* (French) 1980; 20(4A): 929–38.

39. Hitchins, A. D. and McDonough, F. E. Prophylactic and therapeutic aspects of fermented milk, *Am J Clin Nutr* Apr 1989; (4): 675–84 (review).
40. Le, M. G. et al. Consumption of dairy produce and alcohol in a case-control study of breast cancer, *J Natl Cancer Inst* Sep 1986; 77(3): 633–6.

Reddy, G. V. Antitumour activity of yoghurt components, *Journal of Food Products* 1983; 46: 8–11.

Your Supplement Guide

1. Hutton Deborah, Cancer 2000, *UK Vogue* May 1998: 109.
2. Hoffer, A. and Pauling, L. Hardin Jones biostatistical analysis of mortality data for cohorts of cancer patients with a large fraction surviving at the termination of the study and a comparison of survival times of cancer patients receiving large regular oral doses of vitamin C and other nutrients with similar patients not receiving those doses, *J Ortho Med* 1990; 5: 143–54.
Summary of results: 129 patients were enrolled in the study and all received what the patients' doctors considered to be the appropriate oncology treatment. Then the group was subdivided. Thirty-one patients received no advice on diet or supplementation. The average lifespan of this group was less than six months. The remaining ninety-eight patients were given dietary advice, similar to that which is covered in this book, and were given therapeutic doses of vitamins C, E, beta-carotene and B3, along with a broad spectrum vitamin and mineral supplement. These were the results: the poor responders, nineteen people (or 20 per cent) lived an average of twenty months – still more than three times better than the group not given nutritional advice. Their cancers were probably quite advanced before embarking on treatment. The good responders, forty-seven people (or 50 per cent) lived an average of six years. Their cancers included leukaemia, lung, liver and pancreas. A second group of good responders, thirty-two people (or 30 per cent) were all female with reproductive/hormonal related cancers (breast, cervix, ovary, uterus) and this group lived ten years on average – with many still alive at the end of the study.
3. Lupulecu, A. The role of vitamins A, beta-carotene, E and C in cancer cell biology, *Int J Vitam Nutr Res* 1994; 64(1): 3–14.
4. Valentine, T. *Nexus*, April–May 1995 (reprinted from April 1994 issue *Acres*, PO Box 8800, Metairle, Louisiana 70011, USA).
5. Ministry of Agriculture, Fisheries and Food (MAFF) Government Food Survey 1994.
6. Cheraskin, E. and Ringsdorf Jr, W. M. Establishing a suggested optimum nutrition allowance (SONA). 1994 Contact: Department of Nutrition, University of Alabama, 1675 University Boulevard, Birmingham, Alabama 35294, USA.

7. Stephens, N. et al. Randomized controlled trial of vitamin E in patients with coronary disease: Cambridge Heart Antioxidant Study (CHAOS), *Lancet* 1996; 347(9004): 781–6.
8. Sigounas, G. et al. dl-α-Tocopherol induces apoptosis in erythroleukemia, prostate and breast cancer cells, *Nutrition and Cancer* 1997; 28(1): 30–5.
9. Bendich, A. et al. Potential health economic benefits of vitamin supplementation, *West J Med* 1997; 166(5): 306–12.
10. Rock, C. L. et al. Nutrient intakes from foods and dietary supplements in women at risk for breast cancer recurrence, *Nutrition and Cancer* 1997; 29(2): 133–9.

Vitamins

1. Longnecker, M. P. et al. Intake of foods and supplements rich in beta-carotene and vitamin A in relation to risk of breast cancer, *Am J Epidemiol* 1997; 145(11): S28.
2. Misra, N. C. et al. Intrahepatic arterial infusion of combination of mitomicin C and 5-fluorouracil in treatment of primary and metastatic liver carcinoma, *Cancer* 1977; 39: 1425–9.
3. Sketris, L. S. et al. Effects of vitamin C on the excretion of Methotrexate, *Cancer Treatment Reports* 1984; 68(2).
4. Johnston, C. S. et al. Vitamin C elevates red blood cell glutathione in healthy adults, *Am J Clin Nutr* 1993; 58(1): 103–5.

   Johnston, C. S. The antihistamine action of ascorbic acid, *Subcell Biochem* 1996; 25: 189–213.
5. Block, G. et al. Vitamin C and cancer prevention: the epidemiologic evidence, *Am J Clin Nutr* 1991; 53: 270S–82S (review).
6. Vojdani, A. and Namatalla, G. Enhancement of human Natural Killer cytotoxic activity by vitamin C in pure and augmented formulations, *J of Nutr & Env Med* 1997; 7:187–95.
7. Cameron, E. and Pauling, L. Supplemental ascorbate in the supportive treatment of cancer: prolongation of survival times in terminal human cancer, *Proc Natl Acad Sci USA* 1976; 73: 3685–9.

   Cameron, E. and Pauling, L. Supplemental ascorbate in the supportive treatment of cancer: re-evaluation of prolongation of survival times in terminal human cancer, *Proc Natl Acad Sci USA* 1978; 75: 4538–42.

   Cameron, E. and Pauling, L. Ascorbic acid as a therapeutic agent in cancer, *J Internat Acad Prev Med* 1978; 5(1): 8–29.
8. Austin, Steve and Hitchcock, Cathy. *Breast Cancer*, Prima (USA), 1994: 142–6.
9. Murata, A. et al. Prolongation of survival times of terminal cancer patients by administration of large doses of ascorbate, *Int J Vit Nutr Res* 1982; Suppl 23: 103–14.

10. Burras, R. R. et al. Vitamin D receptors in breast cancer cells, *Breast Cancer Res Treat* 1994; 31: 191–202.

    Burras et al. Modulation of vitamin D receptor level in human breast cancer cells, *Proc Annu Meet Am Assoc Cancer Res* 1993; 34: A1501.

11. Welsh, J. Induction of apoptosis in breast cancer cells in response to vitamin D and antiestrogens, *Biochem Cell Biol* 1994; 72: 537–45.

12. Vitamin D: A new perspective, *Lancet*, 16 May 1987: 1122–23.

13. Nolan, E. et al. Dissociation of vitamin D3 and anti-estrogen mediated growth regulation in MCF-7 breast cancer cells, *Mol Cell Biochem* 1998; 188: 13–20.

14. Rozen, F. et al. Antiproliferative action of vitamin D-related compounds and insulin-like growth factor binding protein accumulation, *J Natl Cancer Inst* 1997; 89(9): 652–6.

15. Wald, N. J. et al. Plasma retinol, beta-carotene and vitamin E levels in relation to the future risk of breast cancer, *Br J Cancer* 1984; 49: 321–4.

    Negri, E. et al. Intake of selected micronutrients and the risk of breast cancer, *Int J Cancer* 1996; 65: 140–4.

    Freudenheim et al. Premenopausal breast cancer risk and intake of vegetables, fruit and related nutrients, *J Natl Cancer Inst* 1996; 88: 340–8.

16. Charpentier, A. et al. RRR a tocopherol succinate enhances TGF-b1, -b2, and -b3 TGF-bR-II expression by human MDA-MD-435 breast cancer cells, *Nutrition and Cancer* 1996; 26c: 237–50.

17. Turley, J. M. et al. Vitamin E succinate induces fat-mediated apoptosis in estrogen receptor negative human breast cancer cells, *Cancer Research* 1997; 57: 881–90.

18. Nesaretnam, K. et al. Tocotrienols inhibit the growth of human breast cancer cells irrespective of estrogen receptor status, *Lipids* 1998; 33: 461–9.

19. Shklar, G. et al. Vitamin E inhibits experimental carcinogenesis and tumour angiogenesis, *Oral Oncology, European J Cancer* 1996 32B: 114–19.

20. Kimmick, G. G. et al. Vitamin E and breast cancer: a review, *Nutrition and Cancer* 1997; 27: 109–17.

    Knekt, P. et al. Serum vitamin E level and risk of female cancers, *Int J Epidemiol* 1988; 172–81.

    Dimitrov, N. V. et al. Some aspects of vitamin E related to humans and breast cancer prevention, *Adv Exp Med Biol* 1994; 364: 119–27.

    Goodman, Sandra. *Nutrition and Cancer: State of the Art*, Green Library (UK), 1995.

21. Myers, C. E. et al. Adriamycin: the role of lipid peroxidation in cardiac toxicity and tumour response, *Science* 1977; 197: 165–7.

    Van Vleet JF. Effects of selenium-vitamin E on adriamycin induced cardiomyopathy in rabbits, *J Vet Res* 1978; 39: 997–1010.

22. Wood, L. A. Possible prevention of adriamycin induced alopecia by tocopherol (letter), *NEJM* 1985; 312: 16.

23. Daniel, R. and Goodman, S. *Cancer and Nutrition*, Bristol Cancer Help Centre, October 1996: 9.

Minerals

1. Newmark, H. Teens' low-calcium diets may increase breast cancer risk, *Oncology News Intl* 1993; 2(11): 2.
2. Stadel, V. W. Dietary iodine and the risk of breast, endometrial and ovarian cancer, *Lancet* 1976; 1: 7965: 890–1.
3. Myers, Gianni and Simone. Oxidative destruction of membranes by Doxorubicin-iron complex, *Biochemistry* 1982; 21: 1707–13.
4. Stevens, R. et al. Body iron stores and the risk of cancer, *New Engl J Med* 1988; 319: 1047–52.
5. Gutteridge, J. M. C. and Halliwell, B. The measurement and mechanism of lipid peroxidation in biological systems, *Trends Biochem Sci* 1990; 15: 129–35.
6. Baldew, G. S. et al. The mechanism of interaction between cisplatin and selenite, *Bio Pharm* 1991; 141 (10): 1429–37.
7. Frost, P. et al. The effects of zinc deficiency on the immune response, *Proc Clin Biol Res* 1977; 14: 143.

Other Useful Supplements

1. Goldin, B. and Gorbach, S. L. Alterations in fecal microflora enzymes related to diet, age, lactobacillus supplements and dimethylthydrazine, *Cancer* 1977; 40: 2421–6.
   Diamond, W. John et al. *An Alternative Medicine, Definitive Guide to Cancer*, Future Medicines Publishers Inc (USA), 1997.
2. Zhang, Z. L. et al. Hepatoprotective effects of astragalus root, *J Ethnopharmacol* 1990; 30: 145–9.
3. Wang, J. et al. Enhancing effects of anti-tumour polysaccharide from astragalus or radix hedysarum on C3 clevage production of macrophages in mice, *Jpn J Pharmacol* 1989; 51: 432–4.
   Chu, D. T. et al. Immunotherapy with Chinese medicinal herbs. II. Reversal of cyclophosphamide-induced immune suppression by administration of fractionated astragalus membranaceus in vivo, *J Clin Lab Immunol*. 1988; 25: 125–9.
4. Folkers, K. et al. Survival of cancer patients on therapy with coenzyme Q10, *Biochem Biophys Res Comm* 1993: 192: 241–51.
   Jolliet, P. et al. Plasma coenzyme Q10 concentrations in breast cancer: prognosis and therapeutic consequences, *Int J Clin Pharmacol Ther*. 1998; 36: 506–9.
5. Lockwood, K. et al. Partial and complete regression of breast cancer in patients

in relation to dosage of coenzyme Q10, *Biochem Biophys Res Commun* 30 March 1994; 199(3): 1504–8.

Lockwood, K. et al. Apparent partial remission of breast cancer in patients supplemented with nutritional antioxidants, essential fatty acids and coenzyme Q10, *Mol Aspects Medicine* 1994; 15: s231–s240 (suppl).

6. Lockwood, K. et al. Progress on therapy of breast cancer with vitamin Q10 and the regression of metastases, *Biochem Biophys Res Comm* July 1995: 212: 172–7.
7. Combs, A. B. et al. Reduction in coenzyme Q10 of the acute toxicity of adriamycin in mice, *Res Commun Chem Pathol Pharmacol* 1977; 18: 565.

Judy, W. V. et al. Coenzyme Q10 reduction of adriamycin cardiotoxicity. In: Folkers, K. and Yamamura, Y. (eds). *Biochemical and Clinical Aspects of Coenzyme Q,* Elsevier Science Publ, Amsterdam, 1984, vol. 4: 231–41.
8. Luettig, B. et al. Macrophage activation by the polysaccharide arabinogalactan isolated from plant cell cultures of echinacea purpurea, *J Ntl Cancer Inst.* 1989; 81(9): 669–75.

Burger, R. A. et al. Echinacea-induced cytokine production by human macrophages, *Int J Immunopharmacol.* 1997; 19: 371-9.
9. Man-Fan, W. J. et al. Omega-3 fatty acids and cancer metastasis in humans, *World Review of Nutrition and Dietetics* 1991; 66: 477–87.
10. Stoll, B. A. et al. Essential fatty acids, insulin resistance, and breast cancer risk, *Nutr Cancer* 1998; 31(1): 72–7.
11. Lau, B. H. S. et al. Allium sativum (garlic) and cancer prevention, *Nutrition Research* 1990; 10: 937–48.
12. Wilmore, D. W. et al. Role of glutamine in immunologic responses, *Nutrition* 1998: 14: 7–8, 618–26.
13. Yoshida, S. et al. Effects of glutamine supplements and radiochemotherapy on systemic immune and gut barrier function in patients with advanced esopageal cancer, *Ann Surg* 1998; 227(4): 485–91.

Anderson, P. M. et al. Oral glutamine reduces the duration and severity of stomatitis after cytotoxic cancer chemotherapy, *Cancer* 1998; 83(7): 1433–9.
14. Souba, W. W. et al. Glutamine and cancer, *Ann Surg* 1993; 218(6): 715–28.

Austgen, T. R. et al. The effects of glutamine-enriched total parenteral nutrition on tumor growth and host tissues, *Ann Surg* 1992; 215(2): 107–13.
15. Organ, C. H. et al. Glutamine, cancer and its therapy, *Am J Surg* 1996; 172(5): 418–24.
16. Klimberg, V. S. et al. Glutamine suppresses PGE2 synthesis and breast cancer growth, *J Surg Res* 1996; 63(1): 293–7.
17. Ziegler, T. R. et al. Clinical and metabolic efficacy of glutamine-supplemented parenteral nutrition after bone marrow transplantation. A randomized, double-blind, controlled study, *Ann Intern Med* 1992; 116: 821–8.
18. Rouse, K. et al. Glutamine enhances selectivity of chemotherapy through changes in glutathione metabolism, *Ann Surg* 1995; 221(4): 420–6.

19. Rubio, I. T. et al. Effect of glutamine on methotrexate efficacy and toxicity, *Ann Surg* 1998; 227(5): 772–8, discussion 778–80.
20. Passwater, Richard A. *Lipoic Acid: The Metabolic Antioxidant*, Keats (USA), 1995.
21. Levy, J. et al. Lycopene is a more potent inhibitor of human cancer cell proliferation than either alpha-carotene or beta-carotene, *Nutr Cancer* 1995; 24: 257–66.
22. Dorgan et al. Relationships of serum carotenoids, retinol, alpha-tocopherol and selenium with breast cancer risk: results from a prospective study in Columbia, Missouri (USA), *Cancer Causes and Controls* 1998; 9: 89–97.
23. So, F. V. et al. Inhibition of proliferation of estrogen reception-positive MCF-7 human breast cancer cells by flavonoids in the presence and absence of excess estrogen, *Cancer Lett* 1997; 112(2): 127–33.

    Rodgers, E. H. et al. The effects of the flavonoids, quercitin, myricetin and epicatechin on the growth and enzyme activities of MCF-7 human breast cancer cells, *Chem Biol Interact* 1998; 116(3): 213–28.

    Stavric, B. Quercitin in our diet: from potent mutagen to probably anticarcinogen, *Clin Biochem* 1994; 27: 247–8.
24. Humfrey, C. D. et al. Phytoestrogens and human health effects: weighing up the current evidence, *Nat Toxins* 1998; 6: 51–9.
25. Stoll, B. A. et al. Eating to beat breast cancer: potential role for soy supplements, *Ann Oncol* 1997; 8(3): 223–5.

Lifestyle Choices

1. Thurne, I. et al. Physical activity and the risk of breast cancer, *N Engl J Med* 1997; 336: 1269–75.
2. Bernstein, L. et al. Physical exercise and reduced risk of breast cancer in young women, *J Natl Cancer Inst* 1994; 86(18): 1403–8.
3. Gammon, M. D. et al. Recreational and occupational physical activities and risk of breast cancer, *J Natl Cancer Inst* 1998; 90(2): 100–17.
4. Alessio, H. M. et al. Exercise-induced oxidative stress before and after vitamin C supplementation, *Int J Sport Nutr* 1997; 7(1): 1–9.
5. Huang, Z. et al. Dual effects of weight and weight gain on breast cancer risk, *JAMA* 1997; 278: 1407–11.

    Bruning, P. F. et al. Body measurements, estrogen availability and the risk of human breast cancer: a case-control study, *Int J Cancer* 1992; 51: 14–19.

    Kumar, N. B. et al. Timing of weight gain and breast cancer risk, *Cancer* 1995; 76(2): 243–9.

    Stoll, B. A. Teenage obesity in relation to breast cancer risk, *Int J Obes Relat Metab Disord* 1998; 22(11): 1035–40.
6. Verma, S. P. et al. Effects of soy-derived isoflavonoids on the induced growth

of MCF-7 cells by estrogenic environmental chemicals, *Nutr Cancer* 1998; 30: 232–9.

7. Brinton, L. A. et al. Oral Contraceptives and breast cancer risk among young women, *J Natl Cancer Inst* 1995; 87: 827–35.

   Romieu, I. et al. Oral contraceptives and breast cancer. Review and meta-analysis, *Cancer* 1990; 2253–63.

8. Le Fanu, James. Are these doctors risking your life?, *Daily Telegraph*, 21 June 1996.

9. Breast cancer and hormone replacement therapy: a collaborative reanalysis of data from 51 epidemiological studies involving 52,705 women with breast cancer and 108,411 women without breast cancer, *Lancet*, 11 October 1997.

10. Department of Health, Statistics Division 1E, Prescription Cost Analysis system.

11. Felson, D. T. et al. The effects of postmenopausal estrogen therapy on bone density in elderly women, *N Engl J Med* 1993; 329: 1141–16.

Your Basic Nutrition Plan

1. Messina, M. To recommend or not to recommend soy foods, *Journal of the American Dietetic Association* November 1994; 94(11): 1253–4.

2. Adapted from Bender, A. E. and Bender, D. A. *Food Tables*, Oxford University Press, 1986 (reprinted 1997).

3. Adapted from McCance and Widdowson's *The Composition of Foods* (5th edition), Royal Society of Chemistry, Ministry of Agriculture, Fisheries and Food.

Harmonizing Hormones

1. Kaaks, R. Nutrition, hormones and breast cancer: is insulin the missing link?, *Cancer Causes Control* 1996; 7(6): 605–25.

   Stoll, B. A. Macronutrient supplements may reduce breast cancer risk: how, when and which?, *Eur J Clin Nutr* 1997; 51(9): 573–7.

   Stoll, B. A. Nutrition and breast cancer risk: can an effect via insulin resistance be demonstrated?, *Breast Cancer Res Treat* 1996; 38(3): 239–46.

2. Stoll, B. A. et al. Impaired ovulation and breast cancer risk, *Eur J Cancer* 1997; 33(10): 1532–5.

3. Coulam, C. B. et al. Chronic annovulation may increase postmenopausal breast cancer risk, *J Am Med Assn* 1983; 249: 445.

4. Chang, K. J. et al. Influences of percutaneous administration of estradiol and progesterone on human breast epithelial cell cycle in vivo, *Fertility and Sterility* 1995; 63: 785–91.

5. Cowan, L. D. et al. Breast cancer incidence in women with a history of progesterone deficiency, *Am J of Epidemiol.* 1981; 114(2): 209–17.

6. Lecture by Dr John Lee at the Woman to Woman conference, London, 27 September 1998.

   Shi-Zong, Bu et al. Progesterone induces apoptosis and up-regulation of p53 expression in human ovarian carcinoma cell lines, *Am Cancer Society* 1997: 1944–50.

   Kandouz, M. et al. Antagonism between estradiol and progestin on Bcl-2 expression in breast cancer cells, *Int J Cancer* 1996; 68: 120–5.

7. Lee, John R. *Natural Progesterone: The multiple roles of a remarkable hormone*, John Carpenter Publishing, Oxford, 1996.

8. Well Woman's International Network, Autumn 1998 Newsletter, Le Brecque, Alderney, Channel Islands GY9 3TJ.

9. Hrushesky, W. J. M. Breast cancer, timing of surgery and the menstrual cycle: call for a prospective trial, *J of Women's Health* 1996; 5: 555–66.

10. Bergvist, L. et al. The risk of breast cancer after estrogen and estrogen-progestin replacement, *N Engl J Med* 1989; 321: 293–7.

11. Gambrell, R. D. et al. Decreased incidence of breast cancer in postmenopausal estrogen-progesterone users, *Obstet Gynecol* 1983; 62: 435–43.

    Leis, H. P. Endocrine prophylaxis of breast cancer with cyclic estrogen and progesterone, *Intern Surg* 1966; 45: 496–503.

12. McMichael-Phillips, D. F. et al. Effects of soy-protein supplementation on epithelial proliferation in the histologically normal human breast, *Am J Clin Nutr* 1998; 68 (suppl): 1431S–6S.

13. Inoh, A. et al. Protective effects of progesterone and tamoxifen in estrogen-induced mammary carcinogenesis in ovarectimized W/u rats, *Jpn J Cancer Res* 1985; 76: 699–704.

14. Langer, S. E. and Scheer, J. F. *Solved the Riddle of Illness*, Keats (USA), reprinted 1995.

15. Shering, S. G. et al. Thyroid disorders and breast cancer, *Eur J Cancer Prev.* 1996; 5: 504–6.

    Smyth, P. P. Thyroid disease and breast cancer, *J Endocrinol Invest.* 1993; 16: 396–401.

    Smyth, P. P. A direct relationship between thyroid enlargement and breast cancer, *J Clin Endocrinol Metab* 1996; 81: 937–41.

    Smyth, P. P. The thyroid and breast cancer: a significant association?, *Ann Med* 1997; 29: 189–91 (editorial).

16. Hoffman, D. A. et al. Breast cancer in hypothyroid women using thyroid supplements, *JAMA* 1984; 251: 616–19.

17. Strain, J. J. et al. Thyroid hormones and selenium status in breast cancer, *Nutr Cancer* 1997; 27: 48–52.

18. Lock, M. Contested meaning of the menopause, *Lancet* 1991; 337: 1270–72.

19. Adlercreutz, H. et al. Dietary phyto-oestrogens and the menopause in Japan, *Lancet*, 16 May 1992; 339: 1233.

20. Eden, J. A. et al. The effects of isoflavones on menopausal symptoms, *Abstract* 1996, Royal Hospital for Women, New South Wales.
21. Murkies, A. L. et al. Postmenopausal hot flushes decreased by dietary flour supplementation: effects of soya and wheat, *Am J Clin Nutr* 1998; 68 (suppl): 1533S.
22. Lee, John R. *What your doctor may not tell you about the menopause*, Warner Books (USA), 1996.
23. Gallaher et al. The effects of soy isoflavone intake on bone metabolism in post-menopausal women, September 1996: 21. Erdman et al. Short term effect of soybean isoflavones on bone in postmenopausal women, September 1996: 21. Blair, H. C. Action of genistein and other protein tyrosine kinase inhibitors in preventing osteoporosis, September 1996: 19. Arimand et al. A soy protein containing diet prevents bone loss due to ovarian hormone deficiency, September 1996: 19, *Abstract Book of Second International Symposium on the Role of Soy in Preventing and Treating Chronic Disease.*
24. Agnusdei, D. et al. A double-blind, placebo-controlled trial of ipriflavone for prevention of postmenopausal spinal bone loss, *Calcif Tissue Int* 1997; 61(?): 142–7.
25. Kenton Leslie. *Passage to Power*, Ebury Press, 1995.
26. Samman, S. et al. Minor dietary factors in relation to coronary heart disease – flavonoids, isoflavonoids and boron, *J Clin Biochem Nutr* 1996; 20: 173–80.

    Anthony et al. Effects of soy isoflavones on atherosclerosis: potential mechanism, September 1996: 26, *Abstract Book of Second International Symposium on the Role of Soy in Preventing and Treating Chronic Disease.*

    Potter, S. M. et al. Soy protein and isoflavons: their effects on blood lipids and bone density in postmenopausal women, *Am J Clin Nutr* 1998; 68: 1375S–9S.

Healthy Digestion

1. *Food Magazine* 43, 1998.
2. Xia, Xu et al. Bioavailability of soybean isoflavones depends upon gut microflora in women, *J Nutr* 1995; 125: 2307–15.
3. Adlercreutz, H. Evolution, nutrition, intestinal microflora and prevention of cancer: a hypothesis, *Proceedings of the Society for Experimental Biology and Medicine* 1998; 217: 241–6.

Detox Your System

1. South African Division of the International Association of Dental Research.

Notes

Reducing Your Stress Load

1. Levy, S. et al. Correlation of stress factors with sustained depression of natural killer cell activity and prognosis in patients with breast cancer, *J Clin Oncol* 1992; 10: 1292–8.
2. Chen, C. C. et al. Adverse life events and breast cancer: case controlled study, *British Med J* 1995; 311: 1527–30.
3. Fentiman, I. et al. Stress and relapse in breast cancer, *BMJ* 1989; 289: 291–3.
   Barraclough, J. et al. Life events and breast cancer prognosis, *BMJ* 1992; 304: 1078–81.
4. Leinster, S. J. The mind matters: the impact of psychology on surgery, *J R Coll Surg Edinb* 1994; 39: 144–9.
5. Degner, L. F. et al. Decision making during serious illness: what role do patients really want to play?, *J Clin Epidemiol* 1992; 45: 944–50.
   Leinster, S. J. et al. Treatment decision making in women newly diagnosed with breast cancer, *Cancer Nurs* 1996; 19(1): 8–19.
6. Leinster, S. J. et al. The information needs of women newly diagnosed with breast cancer, *J Adv Nurs* 1995; 22(1): 134–41.
7. Luker, K. A. et al. Meaning of illness for women with breast cancer, *J Adv Nurs* 1996: 23(6): 1194–201.

Your Medical Treatment Choices

1. *Daily Telegraph*, 29 April 1998.
2. *Sunday Times Magazine*, 1 June 1997.
3. Commons Select Committee on Health Report, 1998.

Investigative Scans

1. Hirshaut, Y. and Pressman, P. I., *Breast Cancer*, Bantam (USA), 1992.

Surgery

1. Baum, Michael et al. *Breast Cancer*, Oxford, 1994.
2. Fentiman, I. S. et al. Timing of surgery during menstrual cycle and survival of premenopausal women with operable breast cancer, *Lancet* 1991; 337: 1261–14.
3. Baum, Michael et al. *Breast Cancer*, Oxford, 1994.
4. Fentiman, I. S. et al. Effect of menstrual phase on surgical treatment of breast cancer. *Lancet* 1994; 344: 402 (letter).
5. Johnson, J. W. et al. Sensory information, instruction in coping strategy and recovery from surgery, *Research in Nursing and Health* 1978; 1: 4–17.

Webb, C. Teaching for recovery from surgery. In: Wilson-Barnett, J. (ed), *Patient Teaching*, Churchill Livingstone, Edinburgh, 1983, p. 34.

Radiotherapy

1. Hirshaut, Y. and Pressman, P. I. *Breast Cancer*, Bantam (USA), 1992.
2. Ibid.
3. Okunieff, P. Interactions between ascorbic acid and the radiation of bone marrow, skin and tumor, *Am J Clin Nutr* 1991; 54: 1281S–3S.
   Kagerud, A. et al. Tocopherol in tumour irradiation, *Anticancer Res* 1981; 1: 35–8.
4. Quillin, Patrick. *Beating cancer with nutrition*, Nutrition Times Press (USA), 1994.
5. De Froment, P. Unsaponifiable substance from alfalfa for pharmaceuticals and cosmetic use, *French Patent* 1974; 2: 187, 328.

Hormone Treatment

1. Cassidy, A. et al. Biological effects of a diet protein rich in isoflavones on the menstrual cycle of premenopausal women, *Am J Clin Nutr* 1994; 60: 333–40.
2. Austin, Steve and Hitchcock, Cathy. *Breast Cancer*, Prima (USA), 1994.
3. Magriples, U. et al. High-grade endometrial cancer in tamoxifen-treated breast cancer patients, *J Clin Oncol* 1993; 11: 485–90.
4. Graedon, J. and Graedon, T., *Deadly Drug Interactions*, St Martin's Press (USA), 1995.
5. Scottish Cancer Trials Breast Group and ICRF Breast Unit, Guy's Hospital, London. Adjuvant ovarian ablation versus CMF chemotherapy in premenopausal women with pathological stage II breast carcinomas: the Scottish trial, *Lancet* 1993; 341: 1293–41.

Chemotherapy

1. Hirshaut, Y. and Pressman, P. I. *Breast Cancer*, Bantam (USA), 1992.
2. Pauling, Linus. *How to live longer and feel better*, W. H. Freeman & Co (USA), 1986, p. 180.
3. Simone, Charles B. *Breast Health*, Avery (USA), 1995.
4. Simone, Charles B. *Cancer and Nutrition*, Avery (USA), 1994.
5. Myers, C. E. et al. Adriamycin: the role of lipid peroxidation in cardiac toxicity and tumour response, *Science* 1977; 197: 165–7.
   Van Fleet, J. F. Effects of selenium-vitamin E on adriamycin induced cardiomyopathy in rabbits, *J Vet Res* 1978; 39: 997–1010.

Wang, Y. M. et al. Effects of vitamin E against adriamycin-induced toxicity in rabbits, *Cancer Res* 1980; 40: 1022–7.

Milei, J. et al. Amelioration of adriamycin-induced toxicity in rabbits by prenylamine and vitamins A and E, *Am Heart J* 1986; 111: 95.

6. Szczepanska, I. et al. Inhibition of leukocyte migration by cancer chemotherapeutic agents and its prevention by free radical scavengers and thiols, *Eur J Hematol* 1988; 40: 69–74.

Waxman, S. et al. The enhancement of 5-FU antimetabolic activity by leucovorin, menadione, and alpha-tocopherol, *Eur J Cancer Clin Oncol* 1982; 18(7): 685–92.

Watrach, A. M. et al. Inhibition of human breast cancer cells, *Cancer Letters* 1984; 25: 41–7.

7. Wood, L. A. Possible prevention of adriamycin induced alopecia by tocopherol (letter), *NEJM* 1985; 312: 16.

8. Block, G. Vitamin C and cancer prevention: the epidemiological evidence, *Amer J Clin Nutr* 1991: 53: 270S–82S.

Taper, H. S. et al. Non-toxic sensitization of cancer chemotherapy by combined vitamin C and K3 pretreatment in mouse tumor resistant to oncovin, *Anticancer Res* 1992; 12: 1651–4.

9. Taper, H. S. et al. Non-toxic potentiation of cancer chemotherapy by combined C and K3 vitamin pre-treatment, *Int J Cancer* 1987; 40: 575–9.

De Loecker, W. et al. Effects of sodium ascorbate (vitamin C) and 2-methyl-1,4-naphthoquinone (vitamin K3) treatment on human tumor cell growth in vitro. II. Synergism with combined chemotherapy action, *Anticancer Res* 1993; 13: 103–6.

10. Combs, A. B. et al. Reduction in coenzyme Q10 of the acute toxicity of adriamycin in mice, *Res Commun Chem Pathol Pharmacol* 1977; 18: 565.

Judy, W. V. et al. Coenzyme Q10 reduction of adriamycin cardiotoxicity. In: Folkers, K. and Yamamura, Y. (eds), *Biochemical and Clinical Aspects of Coenzyme Q*, Elsevier Science Publ., Amsterdam, 1984 vol. 4: 231–41.

11. Burns, C. P. and Spector, A. A. Effects of lipids on cancer therapy, *Nutr Rev.* 1990; 48(6): 233–40.

12. Chen, G. et al. Potentiation of the anti-tumour activity of cisplatin in mice by 3-aminobenzamide and nicotinamide, *Cancer Chemother Pharmacol* 1988; 22: 303–7.

13. Ohkawa, K. et al. The effects of co-administration of selenium and cis-platin on cis-platin induced toxicity and antitumour activity, *Br J Cancer* 1988; 58: 38–41.

14. Israel, L. et al. Vitamin A augmentation of the effects of chemotherapy in metastatic breast cancers after menopause. Randomized trial in 100 patients, *Annales de Médecine Interne* 1985; 136(7): 551–4.

15. Ciaccio, M. et al. Vitamin A preserves the cytotoxic activity of adriamycin

while counteracting its peroxidative effects in human leukemic cells in vitro, *Biochem Mol Bio* 1994; 34: 329–35.

16. Nagai, Y. et al. Vitamin A, a useful biochemical modulator capable of preventing intestinal damage during methotrexate treatment, *Pharmacol Toxicol* 1993; 73: 69–74.

17. Rouse, K. et al. Glutamine enhances selectivity of chemotherapy through changes in glutathione metabolism, *Ann Surg* 1995; 221(4): 420–6.

18. Goringe, A. P. et al. Glutamine and vitamin E in the treatment of hepatic veno-occlusive disease following high-dose chemotherapy, *Bone Marrow Transplant* 1998; 21: 829–32.

19. Rubio, I. T. et al. Effect of glutamine on methotrexate efficacy and toxicity, *Ann Surg* 1998; 227(5): 772–8; discussion 778–80.

20. Zhang, Z. L. et al. Hepatoprotective effects of astragalus root, *J Ethnopharmacol* 1990; 30: 145–9.

21. Wang, J. et al. Enhancing effects of anti-tumour polysaccharide from astragalus or radix hedysarum on C3 clevage production of macrophages in mice, *Jpn J Pharmacol* 1989; 51: 432–4.

22. Chu, D. T. et al. Immunotherapy with Chinese medicinal herbs. II. Reversal of cyclophosphamide-induced immune suppression by administration of fractionated astragalus membranaceus in vivo, *J Clin Lab Immunol* 1988; 25: 125–9.

23. Moss, R. W. *Questioning Chemotherapy*, Equinox Press (USA), 1995.

24. Darlington, Dr G. and Gamlin, L. *Diet and Arthritis*, Vermilion Press: 293.

25. Golomb, F. M. Agents used in cancer chemotherapy, *Am J Surg* 1963; 105: 579–90.

26. Sketris, I. S. and Farmer, P. S. Effects of vitamin C on the excretion of Methotrexate, *Cancer Treat Rep* 1984; 68(2) 446–7 (letter).

27. Miller, L. G. Herbal medicinals: selected clinical considerations focussing on known or potential drug-herb interactions, *Arch Intern Med* 1998; 158: 2200–11.

28. Ibid.

Bibliography

Abstract Book of Second International Symposium on the Role of Soy in Preventing and Treating Chronic Disease, September 1996

Anthony et al. Effects of soy isoflavones on atherosclerosis: potential mechanism: 26

Arimand et al. A soy protein containing diet prevents bone loss due to ovarian hormone deficiency: 19

Blair, H. C. Action of genistein and other protein tyrosine kinase inhibitors in preventing osteoporosis: 19

Erdman et al. Short term effect of soybean isoflavones on bone in postmenopausal women: 21

Gallaher et al. The effects of soy isoflavone intake on bone metabolism in post-menopausal women: 21

Adlercreutz, H. et al. Determination of urinary lignan and phytoestrogen metabolites, potential antioestrogens and anticarcinogens in urine of women on various habitual diets, *J Steroid Biochem* 1986; 25: 791–7

Adlercreutz, H. et al. Dietary phyto-oestrogens and the menopause in Japan, *Lancet* 16 May 1992; 339: 1233

Adlercreutz, H. et al. Soybean phytoestrogen intake and cancer risk, *J Nutr* 1995; 125: 757S–70S

Adlercreutz, H. Evolution, nutrition, intestinal microflora and prevention of cancer: a hypothesis, *Proc Soc Experim Biol Med* 1998; 217: 241–6

Agarwal, K. C. Therapeutic actions of garlic constituents, *Med Res Rev* 1996; 16: 111–24

Agnusdei, D. et al. A double-blind, placebo-controlled trial of ipriflavone for prevention of postmenopausal spinal bone loss, *Calcif Tissue Int* 1997; 61(2): 142–7

Akiyama, T. et al. Use and specificity of genistein as inhibitor of protein-tyrosine kinases, *Methods in Enzymology* 1991; 201: 362–70

Alessio, H. M. et al. Exercise-induced oxidative stress before and after vitamin C supplementation, *Int J Sport Nutr* 1997; 7(1): 1–9

Ammon, H. P. et al. Pharmacology of Curcuma longa, *Planta Med* 1991; 57: 1–7

Anderson, P. M. et al. Oral glutamine reduces the duration and severity of stomatitis after cytotoxic cancer chemotherapy, *Cancer* 1998; 83(7): 1433–9

Arnold, S. F. et al. Synergistic activation of estrogen receptor with combinations of environmental chemicals, *Science* 1996; 272: 1489–92

Austgen, T. R. et al. The effects of glutamine-enriched total parenteral nutrition on tumor growth and host tissues, *Ann Surg* 1992; 215(2): 107–13

Austin, Steve and Hitchcock, Cathy. *Breast Cancer*, Prima (Rocklin, CA, USA), 1994

Baldew, G. S. et al. The mechanism of interaction between cisplatin and selenite, *Bio Pharm* 1991; 141(10): 1429–37

Banerjee, S. et al. Influence of certain essential oils on carcinogen metabolizing enzymes and acid-soluble sulfhydryls in mouse livers, *Nutr Cancer* 1994; 21: 263–9

Barbosa, J. C. et al. The relationship among adiposity, diet and hormone concentrations in vegetarian and non-vegetarian postmenopausal women, *Am J Clin Nutr* 1990; 51(5): 798–803

Barnes, S. et al. Chemical modification of isoflavones in soyafoods during cooking and processing, *Am J Clin Nutr* 1998; 68: 1486S–91S (suppl)

Barnes, S. et al. Soybeans inhibit mammary tumours in models of breast cancer, *Prog Clin Biol Res* 1990; 347: 239–53

Barraclough, J. et al. Life events and breast cancer prognosis, *BMJ* 1992; 304: 1078–81

Batkin, S. et al. Antimetastatic effect of bromelain with or without its proteolytic and anticoagulant activity, *J Cancer Res Clin Oncol* 1988; 114: 507–8

Baum, Michael et al. *Breast Cancer*, Oxford, 1994

Baxevanis, C. N. et al. Elevated prostaglandin E2 production by monocytes is responsible for the depressed levels of natural killer and lymphokine-activated killer cell function in patients with breast cancer, *Cancer* 1993; 72: 491–501

Bendich, A. et al. Potential health economic benefits of vitamin supplementation, *West J Med* 1997; 166(5): 306–12

Bergvist, L. et al. The risk of breast cancer after estrogen and estrogen progestin replacement, *N Engl J Med* 1989; 321: 293–7

Bernstein, L. et al. Physical exercise and reduced risk of breast cancer in young women, *J Natl Cancer Inst* 1994; 86(18): 1403–8

Bingham, S. A. et al. Phyto-oestrogens: where are we now? *Br J Nutr* 1998; 79: 393–406

Block, G. Epidemiologic evidence regarding vitamin C and cancer, *Am J Clin Nutr* 1991; 54(6): 1310S–14S

Block, G. et al. Vitamin C and cancer prevention: the epidemiologic evidence, *Am J Clin Nutr* 1991; 53: 270S–82S (review)

Block, G. and Reinli, K. Phytoestrogen content of foods – a compendium of literature values, *Nutrition and Cancer* 1996; 26(2): 123–48

Borgeson, D. E. et al. Effects of dietary fish oil on human mammary carcinoma and on lipid-metabolizing enzymes, *Lipids* 1989; 24: 290–5

Bougnoux, P. et al. Alpha-linolenic acid content of adipose breast tissue: a host determinant of the risk of early metastasis in breast cancer, *Br J Cancer* August 1994; 70(2): 330–4

Bibliography

Boyd, N. F. Ontario Cancer Treatment and Research Foundation in Toronto, *Canadian Diet and Breast Cancer Prevention Study Group*

Boyd, N. F. et al. Effects of a low-fat, high carbohydrate diet on plasma sex hormones in premenopausal women: results from a randomized trial, *Breast Cancer Res Treat* 1997; 76: 127–35

Breast cancer and hormone replacement therapy: a collaborative reanalysis of data from 51 epidemiological studies involving 52,705 women with breast cancer and 108,411 women without breast cancer, *Lancet* 11 October 1997

Brinton, L. A. et al. Oral contraceptives and breast cancer risk among young women, *J Natl Cancer Inst* 1995; 87: 827-35

Brisson, J. et al. Diet, mammographic features of breast tissue, and breast cancer risk, *Am J Epidemiol* 1989; 130: 14–24

Bruning, P. F. et al. Body measurements, estrogen availability and the risk of human breast cancer: a case control study, *Int J Cancer* 1992; 51: 14–19

Burger, R. A. et al. Echinacea-induced cytokine production by human macrophages, *Int J Immunopharmacol*. 1997; 19: 371–9

Burns, C. P. and Spector, A. A. Effects of lipids on cancer therapy. *Nutr Rev* 1990; 48(6): 233–40

Burras, R. R. et al. Modulation of vitamin D receptor level in human breast cancer cells, *Proc Annu Meet Am Assoc Cancer Res* 1993; 34: A1501

Burras, R. R. et al. Vitamin D receptors in breast cancer cells, *Breast Cancer Res Treat* 1994; 31: 191–202

Cameron, E. Cancer Nutriprevention Project, Linus Pauling Institute of Science and Medicine 10 June 1987

Cameron, E. and Pauling, L. Supplemental ascorbate in the supportive treatment of cancer: prolongation of survival times in terminal human cancer, *Proc Natl Acad Sci USA* 1976; 73: 3685–9

Cameron, E. and Pauling, L. Supplemental ascorbate in the supportive treatment of cancer: re-evaluation of prolongation of survival times in terminal human cancer, *Proc Natl Acad Sci USA* 1978; 75: 4538–42

Cameron, E. and Pauling, L. Ascorbic acid as a therapeutic agent in cancer, *J Internat Acad Prev Med* 1978; 5(1): 8–29

Cao, G. et al. Increases in human plasma antioxidant capacity after consumption of controlled diets high in fruit and vegetables, *Am J Clin Nutr* 1998; 68: 1081–7

Cao. G. et al. Serum antioxidant capacity is increased by consumption of strawberries, spinach, red wine in elderly women, *J Nutr* 1998; 128(12): 2383–90

Cassidy, A. et al. Biological effects of a diet of protein rich in isoflavones on the menstrual cycle of premenopausal women, *Am J Clin Nutr* 1994; 60: 333–40

Cavalieri, E. L. et al. Molecular origin of cancer: Catechol estrogen-3,4 quinones as endogenous tumour initiators, *Proc Natl Acad Sci* 1997; 94: 10937–42

Challem, J. *Nutrition Science News* August 1997; 2(8) www.nutritionscience-news.com

Challem, J. and Dolby, V. *The Health Benefits of Soy*, Keats, New Canaan (CT, USA), 1996

Chang, K. J. et al. Influences of percutaneous administration of estradiol and progesterone on human breast epithelial cell cycle in vivo, *Fertility and Sterility* 1995; 63: 785–91

Charpentier, A. et al. RRR a tocopherol succinate enhances TGF-bl, -b2, and -b3 TGF-br-II expression by human MDA-MD-435 breast cancer cells, *Nutrition and Cancer* 1996; 26c: 237–50

Chen, C. C. et al. Adverse life events and breast cancer: case controlled study, *British Med J* 1995; 311: 1527–30

Chen, G. et al. Potentiation of the anti-tumour activity of cisplatin in mice by 3-aminobenzamide and nicotinamide, *Cancer Chemother Pharmacol* 1988; 22: 303–7

Chen, J. et al. Antioxidant status and cancer mortality in China, *Int J Epidem* 1992; 21: 625–34

Cheraskin, E. and Ringsdorf, W. M. Jr. *Establishing a suggested optimum nutrition allowance (SONA)*, 1994. Contact: Department of Nutrition, University of Alabama, 1675 University Boulevard, Birmingham, Alabama 35294, USA

Chihara, G. et al. Antitumor and metastasis inhibitory activities of lentinan as an immunomodulator: an overview, *Cancer Detect Prev* 1987; 1: 423–43 (suppl)

Chu, D. T. et al. Immunotherapy with Chinese medicinal herbs. II. Reversal of cyclophosphamide-induced immune suppression by administration of fractionated astragalus membranaceus in vivo, *J Clin Lab Immunol* 1988; 25: 125–9

Ciaccio, M. et al. Vitamin A preserves the cytotoxic activity of adriamycin while counteracting its peroxidative effects in human leukemic cells in vitro, *Biochem Mol Bio* 1994; 34: 329–35

Cobleigh, M. A. et al. Hormone replacement therapy and high S-phase in breast cancer, *JAMA* 1999; 28: 528–30

Cohen, L. A. et al. Dietary fat and mammary cancer. 1. Promoting effects of different dietary fats on n-nitrosomethylurea-induced rat mammary tumourgenesis, *J Natl Cancer Inst* 1986; 77: 33–42

Colborn, T. et al. Developmental effects of endocrine disrupting chemicals in wildlife and humans, *Environ Health Perspect* 1993; 101: 378–84

Colborn, Theo et al. *Our Stolen Future*, Little, Brown & Co (USA), 1996: 184–5

Combs, A. B. et al. Reduction in coenzyme Q10 of the acute toxicity of adriamycin in mice, *Res Commun Chem Pathol Pharmacol* 1977; 18: 565

Commons Select Committee on Health Report, 1998

Conge, G. A. et al. Comparative effects of a diet enriched in live or heated yoghurt on the immune system of the mouse, *Reprod Nutr Dev* (French) 1980; 20(4A): 929–38

Coulam, C. B. et al. Chronic annovulation may increase postmenopausal breast cancer risk, *J Am Med Assn* 1983; 249: 445

Bibliography

Cowan, L. D. et al. Breast cancer incidence in women with a history of progesterone deficiency, *Am J Epidemiol* 1981; 114(2): 209–17

Crawford, Michael and Marsh, David. *Nutrition and Evolution*, Keats, Canaan (CT, USA), 1995

Daniel, R. and Goodman, S. *Cancer and Nutrition* October 1996, Bristol Cancer Help Centre: 7–9

Daniels, Rosie, *Healing Foods*, Thorsons (UK), 1996, p. 117

Darlington, G. and Gamlin, L. *Diet and Arthritis*, Vermilion Press, p. 293

De Froment, P. Unsaponifiable substance from alfalfa for pharmaceuticals and cosmetic use, *French Patent* 1974; 2: 187, 328

Degner, L. F. et al. Decision making during serious illness: what role do patients really want to play?, *J Clin Epidemiol* 1992; 45: 944–50

De Loecker, W. et al. Effects of sodium ascorbate (vitamin C) and 2 methyl-1,4-naphthoquinone (vitamin K3) treatment on human tumor cell growth in vitro. II. Synergism with combined chemotherapy action, *Anticancer Res* 1993; 13: 103–6

Department of Health, Statistics Division 1E, Prescription Cost Analysis System

Diamond, W. John et al. *An Alternative Medicine, Definitive Guide to Cancer*, Future Medicines Publishers Inc (USA), 1997

Dimitrov, N. V. et al. Some aspects of vitamin E related to humans and breast cancer prevention, *Adv Exp Med Biol* 1994; 364: 119–27

Dorgan, J. F. et al. Relationships of serum carotenoids, retinol, alpha tocopherol and selenium with breast cancer risk: results from a prospective study in Columbia, Missouri (USA), *Cancer Causes and Controls* 1998; 9: 89–97

Downing, D. Effective Nutritional Medicine. The application of nutrition to major health problems: *A report of the British Society for Allergy and Environmental Medicine with the British Society for Nutritional Medicine* (Southampton, UK), 1995

Drasar, B. S. and Irving, D. Environmental factors and cancer of the colon and breast, *Br J Cancer* 1973; 27: 167–72 (review)

Drewnowski, A. and Rock, D. L. The influence of genetic taste markers on food acceptance, *Am J Clin Nutr* 1995; 62: 506–11

Dwivedy et al. Synthesis and characterization of estrogen 2,3- and 3,4-quinones. Comparisons of DNA aducts formed by the quinones versus horseradish peroxidase-activated catechol estrogens, *Chem Res Toxicol* 1992; 5: 828–33

Dwyer, J. T. et al. Health aspects of vegetarian diets, *Am J Clin Nutr* 1988; 48(3 suppl): 712–38 (review)

Eden, J. A. et al. The effects of isoflavones on menopausal symptoms, *Abstract* 1996, Royal Hospital for Women, New South Wales

Editorial. Low-fat diet lengthens menstrual cycle, *J Am Diet Assoc* 1993; 1501

Eisen, A. and Weber, B. L. Prophylactic mastectomy – the price of fear, *N Engl J Med* 1999; 340(2): 137–8 (editorial)

Erasmus, Udo. *Fats that Heal, Fats that Kill*, Alive Books (Canada), 1995

Fahey, J. W. et al. Broccoli sprouts: an exceptionally rich source of inducers of enzymes that protect against chemical carcinogens. *Proceedings of the National Academy of Sciences of the USA* 1997; 94: 10367–72

Felson, D. T. et al. The effects of postmenopausal estrogen therapy on bone density in elderly women, *N Engl J Med* 1993; 329: 1141–6

Fentiman, I. et al. Stress and relapse in breast cancer, *BMJ* 1989; 298: 291–3

Fentiman, I. S. et al. Timing of surgery during menstrual cycle and survival of premenopausal women with operable breast cancer, *Lancet* 1991; 337: 1261–4

Fentiman, I. S. et al. Effect of menstrual phase on surgical treatment of breast cancer, *Lancet* 1994; 344: 402 (letter)

Fenwick, G. R. and Hanley, A. B. The genus allium – part 1/2/3, *Crit Rev Food Sci Nutr* 1985; 22: 199–271, 273–377; 23: 1–73

Folkers, K. et al. Survival of cancer patients on therapy with coenzyme Q10, *Biochem Biophys Res Comm* 1993; 192: 241–51

Foster, H. D. Selenium and cancer prevention, *J Nutr* 1988; 118: 237 (letter)

Franceschi, S. et al. Intake of macronutrients and risk of breast cancer, *Lancet* 1996, 347: 1351–6

Freudenheim, J. L. et al. Premenopausal breast cancer risk and intake of vegetables, fruit and related nutrients, *J Natl Cancer Inst* 1996; 88: 340–8

Fritsche, K. L. and Johnston, P. V. Effects of dietary alpha-linolenic acid on growth, metastasis, fatty acid profile and prostaglandin production of two murine adenocarcinomas, *J Nutr* December 1990; 120(12): 1601–9

Frost, P. et al. The effects of zinc deficiency on the immune response, *Proc Clin Biol Res* 1977; 14: 143

Fürst C. J. et al. DNA pattern and dietary habits in patients with breast cancer, *Eur J Cancer* 1993; 29A(9): 1285–8

Gambrell, R. D. et al. Decreased incidence of breast cancer in postmenopausal estrogen-progesterone users, *Obstet Gynecol* 1983; 62: 435–43

Gammon, M. D. et al. Recreational and occupational physical activities and risk of breast cancer, *J Natl Cancer Inst* 1998; 90(2): 100–17

Garland, M. et al. Antioxidant micronutrients and breast cancer, *J Am Coll Nutr* 1993; 12: 400–11 (review)

Goldin, B. R. and Gorbach, S. L. Alterations in fecal microflora enzymes related to diet, age, lactobacillus supplements and dimethylhydrazine, *Cancer* 1977; 40: 2421–6

Goldin, B. R. et al. Estrogen excretion patterns and plasma levels in vegetarian and omnivorous women, *N Engl J Med* 1982; 307: 1542

Goldin, B. R. et al. Estrogen excretion patterns and plasma levels in vegetarian and omnivorous women, *N Engl J Med* 1982; 307: 1542–7

Golomb, F. M. Agents used in cancer chemotherapy, *Am J Surg* 1963; 105: 579–90

Bibliography

Gonzalez, M. J. et al. Dietary fish oil inhibits breast carcinoma growth: a function of increased lipid peroxidation, *Lipids* 1993; 28(9): 827–32

Goodman, M. T. et al. The association of diet, obesity and breast cancer in Hawaii, *Cancer Epidem Bio Prev.* 1992; 1, 269–75

Goodman, Sandra. *Nutrition and Cancer: State of the Art*, Green Library, 1995

Goodwin, J. S. and Tangrum, M. R. Battling quackery. *Arch Intern Med* 1998; 158: 2195–7

Goringe, A. P. et al. Glutamine and vitamin E in the treatment of hepatic veno-occlusive disease following high-dose chemotherapy, *Bone Marrow Transplant* 1998; 21: 829–32

Graedon, J. and Graedon, T. *Deadly Drug Interactions*, St Martin's Press (USA), 1995

Graham, S. et al. Diet in the epidemiology of breast cancer, *Am J Epidemiol* 1982; 116: 68–75

Grubbs, C. J. et al. Chemoprevention of chemically-induced mammary carcinogenesis by indole-3-carbinol, *Anticancer Research* 1995; 15: 709–16

Guthrie, N. et al. Inhibition of mammary cancer by citrus flavonoids, *Adv Exp Med Biol* 1998; 439: 227–36

Gutteridge, J. M. and Halliwell, B. The measurement and mechanism of lipid peroxidation in biological systems, *Trends Biochem Sci* 1990; 15: 129–35

Hankin, J. H. et al, Diet and breast cancer: a review, *Am J Clin Nutr* 1978; 31: 200–205

Harding, C. et al. Dietary soy supplementation is estrogenic in menopausal women, *Am J Clin Nutr* 1998; 68: 1531–3S (suppl)

Hawrylewicz, E. J. Fat-protein interaction defined 2-generation studies, Dietary Fat and Cancer. In: Ip, C. et al. (eds), *Progress in Clinical and Biological Research*, Alan R. Liss Inc (New York, USA), 1986; 222: 4033–4

Hawrylewicz, E. J. et al. Dietary soybean isolate and methionine supplementation affect mammary tumour progression in rats, *J Nutr*, October 1991; 121(10): 1693–8

Hawrylewicz, E. J. et al. Soy and experimental cancer: animal studies, *J Nutr*, March 1995; 125: 698–708 (suppl 3)

Helzisouer, K. J. et al. Association between glutathione S-transferase M1, P1, and T1 genetic polymorphisms and breast cancer, *J Natl Cancer Inst* 1998; 90(7): 512–18

Hems, G. and Stuart, A. Breast cancer rates in populations of single women, *Br J Cancer* 1975; 31(1): 118–23

Hin-Peng, L. Diet and breast cancer: an epidemiologist's perspective. *Crit Rev Oncol Hematol* 1998; 28: 115–19

Hirshaut, Yasher and Pressman, Peter I. *Breast Cancer*, Bantam (New York, USA), 1992

Hitchins, A. D. and McDonough, F. E. Prophylactic and therapeutic aspects of fermented milk, *Am J Clin Nutr* April 1989; 4: 675–84 (review)

Hoffer, Abram and Pauling, Linus. Hardin Jones biostatistical analysis of mortality data for cohorts of cancer patients with a large fraction surviving at the termination of the study and a comparison of survival times of cancer patients receiving large regular oral doses of vitamin C and other nutrients with similar patients not receiving those doses, *J Ortho Med* 1990; 5: 143–54

Hoffman, D. A. et al. Breast cancer in hypothyroid women using thyroid supplements, *JAMA* 1984; 251: 616–19

Holm, L. E. et al. Treatment failure and dietary habits in women with breast cancer, *J Natl Cancer Inst* 1993; 85(1): 32–6

Homberger, F. et al. Inhibition of murine subcutaneous and intravenous benzo(rst)pentaphene carcinogenesis by sweet orange oils and d-limonene, *Oncology* 1971; 25: 1–20

Horrobin, D. F. and Seely, S. Diet and breast cancer: the possible connection with sugar consumption, *Med Hypotheses* 1983; 11(3): 319–27

Howard, V. Synergistic effects of chemical mixtures – can we rely on traditional toxicity?, *The Ecologist* 1997; 27(5): 192–5

Howe, G. R. et al. Dietary factors and risk of breast cancer: combined analysis of 12 case-control studies, *J Natl Cancer Inst* 1990; 82(7): 561–9

Hoyer, A. P. et al. Organochlorine exposure and risk of breast cancer, *Lancet* 1998; 352: 1816–20

Hrushesky, W. J. M. Breast cancer, timing of surgery and the menstrual cycle: call for a prospective trial, *J of Women's Health* 1996; 5: 555–66

Huang, H. H. et al. Effects of protein diet on release of prolactin and ovarian steroids in female rats, *Nutr Rpts Int* 1982; 26, 807–20

Huang, Z. et al. Dual effects of weight and weight gain on breast cancer risk, *JAMA* 1997; 278: 1407–11

Hughes, C. Phytochemical mimicry of reproductive hormones and modulation of herbivore fertility by phytoestrogens, *Environm Health Persp* 1988; 78: 171–5

Humfrey, C. D. et al. Phytoestrogens and human health effects: weighing up the current evidence, *Nat Toxins* 1998; 6: 51–9

Ingrams, D. et al. Case-control study of phyto-oestrogens and breast cancer, *Lancet* 1997; 350: 990–4

Inoh, A. et al. Protective effects of progesterone and tamoxifen in estrogen-induced mammary carcinogenesis in ovarectimized W/u rats, *Jpn J Cancer Res* 1985; 76: 699–704

Institute of Food Research, Norwich, press release 12 June 1998. www.ifrn.bbsr.ac.uk

Ip, C. et al. Mammary cancer prevention by regular garlic and selenium enriched garlic, *Nutr Cancer* 1992; 17: 279–86

Ip, C. and Lisk, D. J. Bioactive selenium from Brazil nut for cancer prevention and selenoenzyme maintenance, *Nutr Cancer* 1994; 21: 203–12

Bibliography

Ip, C. and Lisk, D. J. Efficacy of cancer prevention by high-selenium garlic is primarily dependent on the actions of selenium, *Carcinogenesis* 1995; 16: 2649–52

Israel, L. et al. Vitamin A augmentation of the effects of chemotherapy in metastatic breast cancers after menopause. Randomized trial in 100 patients, *Annales de Médecine Interne* 1985; 136(7): 551–4

Johnson, J. W. et al. Sensory information, instruction in coping strategy and recovery from surgery, *Research in Nursing and Health* 1978; 1: 4–17

Johnston, C. S. The antihistamine action of ascorbic acid, *Subcell Biochem* 1996; 25: 189–213

Johnston, C. S. et al. Vitamin C elevates red blood cell glutathione in healthy adults, *Am J Clin Nutr* 1993; 58(1): 103–5

Jolliet, P. et al. Plasma coenzyme Q10 concentrations in breast cancer: prognosis and therapeutic consequences, *Int J Clin Pharmacol Ther* 1998; 36: 506–9

Judy, W. V. et al. Coenzyme Q10 reduction of adriamycin cardiotoxicity. In: Folkers, K. and Yamamura, Y. (eds), *Biochemical and Clinical Aspects of Coenzyme Q*, Elsevier Science Publ, Amsterdam, 1984, vol. 4K: 231–41

Jumaan, A. O. et al. Beta-carotene intake and risk of postmenopausal breast cancer, *Epidemiology* 1999; 10: 49–53

Kaaks, R. Nutrition, hormones and breast cancer: is insulin the missing link?, *Cancer Causes Control* 1996; 7(6): 605–25

Kagawa, Y. Impact of Westernization on the nutrition of Japan: Changes in physique, *Cancer* 1978; 7: 205

Kagerud, A. et al. Tocopherol in tumour irradiation, *Anticancer Res* 1981; 1: 35–8

Kaizer, L. et al. Fish consumption and breast cancer risk: an ecological study, *Nutr Cancer* 1989; 12: 61–8

Kandouz, M. et al. Antagonism between estradiol and progestin on Bcl-2 expression in breast cancer cells, *Int J Cancer* 1996; 68: 120–5

Katsouyanni, K. et al. Diet and breast cancer: a case-control study in Greece, *Int J Cancer* 1986; 38: 815–20

Kaufmann, M. (ed.), *Breast Diseases*, Springer-Verlag, Berlin, 1990, pp. 79–96

Kazer, R. R. Insulin resistance, insulin-like growth factor I and breast cancer: a hypothesis, *Int J Cancer* 1995; 62: 403–6

Kelsey, K. T. and Wiencke, J. K. Growing pains for the environmental genetics of breast cancer: observations on a study of the glutathione-S-transferases, *J Natl Cancer Inst* 1998; 90(7): 484–5 (editorial)

Kennedy, A. and Little, J. B. Effects of protease inhibitors on radiation transformation in vitro, *Cancer Res* 1981; 41(6): 2103–8

Kennedy, A. R. The evidence for soybean products as cancer preventive agents, *J Nutr* 1995; 125: 733S–43S

Kenton, Leslie, *Passage to Power*, Ebury Press, London, 1995

Keys, A. et al. The diet and 15-year death rate in the seven countries study, *Am J Epidemiol* 1986; 124: 903–15

Kim, H. et al. Mechanisms of action of the soy isoflavone genistein: emerging role for its effects via transforming growth factor β signaling pathways, *Am J Clin Nutr* 1998; 68: 1418S–25S (suppl)

Kim, J. H. et al. The use of high dose vitamins as an adjunct to conventional cancer treatment, *Cancer and Nutrition* 1998: 205–12

Kimmick, G. G. et al. Vitamin E and breast cancer: a review, *Nutrition and Cancer* 1997; 27: 109–17

Kinne, D. Management of male breast cancer, *Oncology* March 1991: 45–8

Klimberg, V. S. et al. Glutamine suppresses PGE2 synthesis and breast cancer growth, *J Surg Res* 1996; 63(1): 293–7

Knekt, P. et al. Serum vitamin E level and risk of female cancers, *Int J Epidemiol* 1988; 172–81

Knight, D. C. et al. A review of the clinical effects of phytoestrogens. *Obstet Gynecol* 1996; 87: 897–904

Kohlmeier, L. Future of dietary exposure assessment, *Am J Clin Nutr* 1995; 61: 702S–9S (suppl)

Kroman, N. et al. Should women be advised against pregnancy after breast-cancer treatment?, *Lancet* 1997; 350: 319–22

Kumar, N. B. et al. Timing of weight gain and breast cancer risk, *Cancer* 1995; 76(2): 243–9

Kunstmann, J. M. et al. Decline in semen quality among fertile men in Paris during the past 20 years, *N Engl J Med* 1995; 332: 281–5

Kurzer, M. S. et al. Dietary phytoestrogens, *Annu Rev Nutr* 1997; 17: 353–81

Lamartiniere, C. A. et al. Genistein studies in rats: potential for breast cancer prevention and reproductive and developmental toxicity, *Am J Clin Nutr* 1998; 68: 1400S–5S (suppl)

Lancet Editorial. Vitamin D: A new perspective. 16 May 1987: 1122–3.

Langer, S. E. and Scheer, J. F. *Solved the Riddle of Illness*. Keats, New Canaan (CT, USA), 1994

Lau, B. H. et al. Allium sativum (garlic) and cancer prevention, *Nutrition Research* 1990; 10: 937–48

Lau, B. H. et al. Garlic compounds modulate macrophage and T-lymphocyte functions, *Mol Biother* 1991; 3: 103–7

La Vacchia, C. et al. Dietary factors and the risk of breast cancer, *Nutr Cancer* 1987; 10: 205–14

Le, M. G. et al. Consumption of dairy produce and alcohol in a case-control study of breast cancer, *J Natl Cancer Inst* September 1986; 77(3): 633–6

Lee, H. P. et al. Dietary effects on breast cancer risk in Singapore, *Lancet* 1991; 337: 1197–1200

Lee, J. R. *Natural Progesterone: The multiple roles of a remarkable hormone*. John Carpenter Publishing, Oxford, 1996

Bibliography

Lee, John R. *What your doctor may not tell you about the menopause.* Warner Books, New York, 1996

Le Fanu, James. Are these doctors risking your life? *Daily Telegraph*, 21 June 1996

Leinster, S. J. The mind matters: the impact of psychology on surgery, *J R Coll Surg Edinb* 1994; 39: 144–9

Leinster, S. J. et al. The information needs of women newly diagnosed with breast cancer, *J Adv Nurs* 1995; 22(1): 134–41

Leinster, S. J. et al. Treatment decision making in women newly diagnosed with breast cancer, *Cancer Nurs* 1996; 19(1): 8–19

Leis, H. P. Endocrine prophylaxis of breast cancer with cyclic estrogen and progesterone, *Intern Surg* 1966; 45: 496–503

Levy, J. et al. Lycopene is a more potent inhibitor of human cancer cell proliferation than either alpha-carotene or beta-carotene, *Nutr Cancer* 1995; 24: 257–66

Levy, S. et al. Correlation of stress factors with sustained depression of natural killer cell activity and prognosis in patients with breast cancer, *J Clin Oncol* 1992; 10: 1292–8

Lin, R. S. et al. Epidemiological findings in male breast cancer, *Proc Am Assoc Cancer Res* 1980; 21: 72

Lin, Y. L. et al. Composition of polyphenols in fresh tea leaves and associations of their oxygen-radical absorbing capacity with antiproliferative actions in fibroblast cells, *J Agric Food Chem* 1996; 44: 1387–94

Liu, J. N. et al. B-cell stimulating activity of seaweed extracts, *Int J Immunopharmacol* 1997; 19: 135–42

Lock, M. Contested meaning of the menopause, *Lancet* 1991; 337: 1270–72

Lockwood, K. et al. Partial and complete regression of breast cancer in patients in relation to dosage of coenzyme Q10, *Biochem Biophys Res Commun* 30 March 1994; 199(3): 1504–8

Lockwood, K. et al. Apparent partial remission of breast cancer in patients supplemented with nutritional antioxidants, essential fatty acids and coenzyme Q10, *Mol Aspects Medicine* 1994; 15: s231–s240 (suppl)

Lockwood, K. et al. Progress on therapy of breast cancer with vitamin Q10 and the regression of metastases, *Biochem Biophys Res Comm* 1995; 212: 172–7

Longnecker, M. P. et al. Alcoholic beverage consumption in relation to risk of breast cancer: Meta-analysis and review, *Cancer Causes Controls* 1994; 5: 73–82

Longnecker, M. P. et al. Intake of foods and supplements rich in beta-carotene and vitamin A in relation to risk of breast cancer, *Am J Epidemiol* 1997; 145(11): S28

Lowry, S. F. et al. Effects of protein malnutrition on host-tumor composition and growth, *Surgical Forum* 1977; 28: 143–5

Lubin, F. et al. Role of fat, animal protein and dietary fibre in breast cancer etiology: a case-control study, *J Natl Cancer Inst* 1986; 77: 605–12

Luettig, B. et al. Macrophage activation by the polysaccharide arabinogalactan isolated from plant cell cultures of echinacea purpurea, *J Ntl Cancer Inst* 1989; 81(9): 669–75

Luker, K. A. et al. Meaning of illness for women with breast cancer, *J Adv Nurs* 1996; 23(6): 1194–201

Lupulecu, A. The role of vitamins A, beta-carotene, E and C in cancer cell biology, *Int J Vitam Nutr Res* 1994; 64(1): 3–14

Mabuchi, K. et al. Risk factors for male breast cancer, *JNCI* 1985; 74: 371–5

Magriples, U. et al. High-grade endometrial cancer in tamoxifen-treated breast cancer patients, *J Clin Oncol* 1993; 11: 485–90

Malins, D. C. et al. The aetiology of breast cancer: characteristic alterations in hydroxyl radical-induced DNA base lesions during oncogenesis with potential for evaluating incidence risk, *Cancer* 1993; 71: 3036–43

Malins, D. C. et al. Tumour progression to the metatastic state involves structural modification in DNA markedly different from those associated with primary tumour formation. *Proceedings of the National Academy of Sciences of the USA* 1996; 93: 14047–52

Man-Fan, W. J. et al. Omega-3 fatty acids and cancer metastasis in humans, *World Review of Nutrition and Dietetics* 1991; 66: 477–87

Martin, M. E. et al. Interactions between phytoestrogens and human sex steroid binding protein, *Life Sciences* 1996; 58(5): 429–36

McMichael-Phillips, D. F. et al. Effects of soy-protein supplementation on epithelial proliferation in the histologically normal human breast, *Am J Clin Nutr* 1998; 68: 1431S–6S (suppl)

Messina, M. et al. Phyto-oestrogens and breast cancer, *Lancet* 1997; 350: 971–2

Messina, M. J. et al. Soy intake and cancer risk: A review of the in-vitro and in-vivo data, *Nutrition and Cancer* 1994; 21(2): 112–31

Michnovicz, J. J. et al. Altered estrogen metabolism and excretion in humans following consumption of indole-3-carbinol, *Nutr Cancer* 1991; 16: 59–66

Milei, J. et al. Amelioration of adriamycin-induced toxicity in rabbits by prenylamine and vitamins A and E, *Am Heart J* 1986; 111: 95

Miller, L. G. Herbal medicinals: selected clinical considerations focussing on known or potential drug-herb interactions, *Arch Intern Med* 1998; 158: 2200–11

Mills, P. K. et al. Animal products consumption and subsequent fatal breast cancer risk among Seventh-day Adventists, *Am J Epidemiol* 1988; 127: 440–53

Mills, P. K. et al. Dietary habits and breast cancer incidence among Seventh-day Adventists, *Cancer* 1989; 64: 582–90

Ministry of Agriculture, Fisheries and Food (MAFF). *Government Food Survey* 1994

Misra, N. C. et al. Intrahepatic arterial infusion of combination of mitomicin C and 5-fluorouracil in treatment of primary and metastatic liver carcinoma, *Cancer* 1977; 39: 1425–29

Moss, R. W. *Questioning Chemotherapy*, Equinox Press (USA), 1995

Bibliography

Murata, A. et al. Prolongation of survival times of terminal cancer patients by administration of large doses of ascorbate, *Int J Vit Nutr Res* 1982; 23: 103–14 (suppl)

Murkies, A. L. et al. Postmenopausal hot flushes decreased by dietary flour supplementation: effects of soya and wheat, *Am J Clin Nutr* 1998; 68: 1533S (suppl)

Myers, C. E. et al. Adriamycin: the role of lipid peroxidation in cardiac toxicity and tumour response, *Science* 1977; 197: 165–7

Myers, Gianni and Myers, Simone. Oxidative destruction of erythrocyte ghost membranes catalyzed by doxorubicin-iron complex, *Biochemistry* 1982; 21: 1707–12

Nagabhusham, M. and Bhide, S. V. Curcumin as an inhibitor of cancer, *J Am Coll Nutr* 1992; 11(2): 192–8

Nagai, Y. et al. Vitamin A, a useful biochemical modulator capable of preventing intestinal damage during methotrexate treatment, *Pharmacol Toxicol* 1993; 73: 69–74

Nanba, H., Antitumor activity of orally administered D-fraction from maitake mushroom (grifola frondosa), *J Naturopathic Med* 1993; 1(4): 10–15

Nanba, H. Maitake mushroom: immune therapy to prevent cancer growth and metastasis, *Explore* 1995; 6(1): 17

Negri, E. et al. Intake of selected micronutrients and the risk of breast cancer, *Int J Cancer* 1996; 65: 140–4

Nesaretnam, K. et al. Tocotrienols inhibit the growth of human breast cancer cells irrespective of estrogen receptor status, *Lipids* 1998; 33: 461–9

Newmark, H. Teens' low-calcium diets may increase breast cancer risk, *Oncology News Intl* 1993; 2(11): 2

Nihoff, W. A. et al. Effects of consumption of Brussels sprouts on intestinal and lymphocytic glutathione-S-transferase in humans, *Carcinogenesis* 1995; 16(9): 2125–8

Nolan E. et al. Dissociation of vitamin D3 and anti-estrogen mediated growth regulation in MCF-7 breast cancer cells, *Mol Cell Biochem* 1998; 188: 13–20

Nordevang, E. et al. Dietary habits and mammographic patterns in patients with breast cancer, *Breast Cancer Res Treat* 1993; 26(3): 207–15

Normura, A. M. Y. et al. The effects of dietary fat in breast cancer survival among Caucasian and Japanese women in Hawaii, *Breast Cancer Res Treat* 1991; 18: S135–41

Norwegian Polar Institute June 1998

Office of National Statistics, National Cancer Registration Database

Ohkawa, K. et al. The effects of co-administration of selenium and cis-platin on cis-platin induced toxicity and antitumour activity, *Br J Cancer* 1988; 58: 38–41

Okunieff, P. Interactions between ascorbic acid and the radiation of bone marrow, skin and tumor, *Am J Clin Nutr* 1991; 54: 1281S–3S

Organ, C. H. et al. Glutamine, cancer and its therapy, *Am J Surg* 1996; 172(5): 418–24

Organic foods vs supermarket foods: element levels, *Journal of Applied Nutrition* 1993: 45(1)

Passwater, Richard A. *Cancer Prevention and Nutritional Therapies*, Keats, New Canaan (CT, USA), 1993

Pauling, Linus. *How to Live Longer and Feel Better*, W. H. Freeman & Co (New York), 1986, p. 180

Pesticides News Residues in food and water, 30 December 1995

Peterson, T. G. et al. The role of metabolism in mammary epithelial cell growth inhibition by the isoflavones genistein and biochanin A, *Carcinogenesis* 1996; 17(9): 1861–9

Peterson, T. G. et al. Metabolism of the isoflavones genistein and biochanin A in human breast cancer cell lines, *Am J Clin Nutr* 1998; 68: 1505S–11S (suppl)

Pierce, J. P. et al. Feasibility of a randomized trial of high vegetable diet to prevent breast cancer recurrence, *Nutrition and Cancer* 1997; 28(3): 282–8

Potter, S. M. et al. Soy protein and isoflavones: their effects on blood lipids and bone density in postmenopausal women, *Am J Clin Nutr* 1998; 68: 1375S–9S

Pritchard, G. A. et al. Lipids in breast carcinogenesis, *Br J Surg* 1989; 76: 1069–73

Quillin, P. *Beating cancer with Nutrition*, Nutrition Times Press (Tulsa, OK, USA), 1994: pp. 53, 112

Raloff, J. This fat may fight cancer in several ways, *Science News*, 19 March 1994

Reddy, B. S. et al. Effect of Japanese seaweed extracts on the mutagenicity of 7,12-dimethylbenz(a)anthracene, a breast carcinogen, and of 3,2'-dimethyl-4-aminobiphenyl, a colon and breast carcinogen, *Mutat Res* 1984; 127: 113–18

Reddy, G. V. Antitumour activity of yoghurt components, *Journal of Food Products* 1983; 46: 8–11

Riboli, E. et al. Identifiability of food components for cancer chemoprevention, *IARC Sci Publ* 1996; 139: 23–31

Riggs, B. L. et al. Effect of fluoride treatment on the fracture rate in post-menopausal women with osteoporosis, *N Eng J Med* 1990; 322: 802–9

Rock, C. L. et al. Nutrient intakes from foods and dietary supplements in women at risk for breast cancer recurrence, *Nutrition and Cancer* 1997; 29(2): 133–9

Rodgers, E. H. et al. The effects of the flavonoids, quercitin, myricetin and epicatechin on the growth and enzyme activities of MCF-7 human breast cancer cells, *Chem Biol Interact* 1998; 116(3): 213–28

Romieu, I. et al. Oral contraceptives and breast cancer. Review and meta-analysis, *Cancer* 1990; 2253–63

Rothkopf, M. Fuel utilization in neoplastic disease: Implications for the use of nutritional support in cancer patients, *Nutrition* 1990; 6(4): 14S–16S (suppl)

Rouse, K. et al. Glutamine enhances selectivity of chemotherapy through changes in glutathione metabolism, *Ann Surg* 1995; 221(4): 420–6

Rozen, F. et al. Antiproliferative action of vitamin D-related compounds and insulin-like growth factor binding protein accumulation, *J Natl Cancer Inst* 1997; 89(9): 652–6

Rubio, I. T. et al. Effect of glutamine on methotrexate efficacy and toxicity, *Ann Surg* 1998; 227(5): 772–8; discussion: 778–80

Safe, S. H. Xenoestrogens and breast cancer, *N Engl J Med* 1997; 337(18): 1303–4 (editorial)

Saitoh, S. et al. p53 gene mutations in breast cancers in midwestern US women: null as well as missense-type mutations are associated with poor prognosis, *Oncogene* 1994; 9: 2869–75

Samman, S. et al. Minor dietary factors in relation to coronary heart disease – flavonoids, isoflavonoids and boron, *J Clin Biochem Nutr* 1996; 20: 173–80

Santisteban, G. A. et al. Glycemic modulation of tumor tolerance in a mouse model of breast cancer, *Biochem Biophys Res Commun* 1985; 132: 1174–9

Schulphan, W. Nutritional value of crops as influenced by organic and inorganic fertilizer treatments, *Qualitas Plantarum Plant Foods for Human Nutrition* 1974; 23(4): 333–58

Scottish Cancer Trials Breast Group and ICRF Breast Unit, Guy's Hospital, London. Adjuvant ovarian ablation versus CMF chemotherapy in premenopausal women with pathological stage II breast carcinoma: the Scottish trial, *Lancet* 1993; 341: 1293–4

Seely, S. and Horrobin, D. F. Diet and breast cancer: the possible connection with sugar consumption, *Med Hypotheses* 1993; 11(3): 319–27

Sepkovic, D. W. et al. Catechol estrogen production in rat microsomes after treatment with indole-3-carbinol, ascorbigen, or β-naphthaflavone, *Steroids* 1994; 59: 318–23

Serraino, M. et al. The effects of flaxseed supplementation on early risk markers for mammary carcinogenesis, *Cancer Lett* 1991; 60: 135–42

Serraino, M. and Thompson, L. The effects of flaxseed supplementation on the initiation and promotional stages of mammary tumourgenesis, *Nutr Cancer* 1992a; 17: 153–9

Sharma, O. P. Antioxidant activity of curcumin and related compounds, *Biochem Pharmacol* 1976; 25: 1811–12

Sharpe, R. and Skakkeback, N. Are oestrogens involved in the falling sperm counts and disorders of the male reproductive tract?, *Lancet* 1993; 341: 1392–5

Shekhar et al. Environmental estrogen stimulation of growth and estrogen receptor function in preneoplastic and cancerous human breast cell lines, *J Natl Cancer Inst* 1997; 89(23); 1774–82

Shering, S. G. et al. Thyroid disorders and breast cancer, *Eur J Cancer Prev* 1996; 5: 504–6

Shi-Zong, Bu et al. Progesterone induces apoptosis and up-regulation of p53 expression in human ovarian carcinoma cell lines, *Am Cancer Society* 1997: 1944–50

Shklar, G. et al. Vitamin E inhibits experimental carcinogenesis and tumour angiogenesis, *Oral Oncology, European J Cancer* 1996; 32B: 114–19

Shun-Zhang, Y. et al. A case-controlled study of dietary and non-dietary risk factors for breast cancer in Shanghai, *Cancer Res* 1990; 50: 5017–21

Sigounas, G. et al. dl-a-Tocopherol induces apoptosis in erythroleukemia, prostate and breast cancer cells, *Nutrition and Cancer* 1997; 28(1): 30–5

Sigounas, G. et al. S-allylmercaptocysteine inhibits cell proliferation and reduces the viability of erythroleukemia, breast and prostate cancer cell lines, *Nutr Cancer* 1997; 27: 186–91

Simone, Charles B. *Breast Health*, Avery (USA), 1995

Simone, Charles B. *Cancer and Nutrition*, Avery (USA), 1994

Sketris, I. S. et al. Effects of vitamin C on the excretion of Methotrexate, *Cancer Treat Rep* 1984; 68(2): 446–7 (letter)

Smith-Barbaro, P. et al. Carcinogen binding to various types of dietary fibre, *J Natl Cancer Inst* 1981; 67(2): 495–7

Smyth, P. P. Thyroid disease and breast cancer, *J Endocrinol Invest* 1993; 16: 396–401

Smyth, P. P. A direct relationship between thyroid enlargement and breast cancer, *J Clin Endocrinol Metab* 1996; 81: 937–41

Smyth, P. P. The thyroid and breast cancer: a significant association?, *Ann Med* 1997; 29: 189–91 (editorial)

So, F. V. et al. Inhibition of human breast cancer cell proliferation and delay of mammary tumourgenesis by citrus juices, *Nutr Cancer* 1996; 26(2): 167–81

So, F. V. et al. Inhibition of proliferation of estrogen reception-positive MCF-7 human breast cancer cells by flavonoids in the presence and absence of excess estrogen, *Cancer Lett* 1997; 112(2): 127–33

Souba, W. W. et al. Glutamine and cancer, *Ann Surg* 1993; 218(6): 715–28

Sowers, M. F. et al. A prospective study of bone mineral content and fracture in communities with different fluoride exposure, *Am J Epidemiol* 1991; 134: 649–60

Stadel, V. W. Dietary iodine and the risk of breast, endometrial and ovarian cancer, *Lancet* 1976; 1: 7965: 890–1

Stavric, B. Antimutagens and anticarcinogens in food, *Food Chem Oxicol* 1994; 32: 79–90

Stavric, B. Role of chemopreventers in human diet, *Can Biochem* 1994; 27: 319–32

Stavric, B. Quercitin in our diet: from potent mutagen to probably anticarcinogen, *Clin Biochem* 1994; 27: 245–8

Stephens, N. et al. Randomized controlled trial of vitamin E in patients with coronary disease: Cambridge Heart Antioxidant Study (CHAOS), *Lancet* 1996; 347(9004): 781–6

Stevens, R. et al. Body iron stores and the risk of cancer, *New Engl J Med* 1988; 319: 1047–52

Bibliography

Stoll, B. A. Diet and exercise regimens to improve breast carcinoma prognosis, *Cancer* 1996; 78(12): 2465–70

Stoll, B. A. Nutrition and breast cancer risk: can an effect via insulin resistance be demonstrated?, *Breast Cancer Res Treat* 1996; 38: 239–46

Stoll, B. A. Breast cancer: further metabolic-endocrine risk markers?, *Br J Cancer* 1997; 76(12): 1652–4

Stoll, B. A. Macronutrient supplements may reduce breast cancer risk: how, when and which?, *Eur J Clin Nutr* 1997; 51(9): 573–7

Stoll, B. A. et al. Eating to beat breast cancer: potential role for soy supplements, *Ann Oncol* 1997; 8(3): 223–5

Stoll, B. A. et al. Essential fatty acids, insulin resistance, and breast cancer risk, *Nutr Cancer* 1998; 31(1): 72–7

Stoll, B. A. Teenage obesity in relation to breast cancer risk, *Int J Obes Relat Metab Disord* 1998; 22(11): 1035–40

Strain, J. J. et al. Thyroid hormones and selenium status in breast cancer, *Nutr Cancer* 1997; 27: 48–52

Sunday Times Magazine. Cancer, Special Report, 1 June 1997

Surh, Y. J. et al. Chemoprotective properties of some pungent ingredients present in red pepper and ginger, *Mutat Res* 1998; 402: 259–67

Szczepanska, I. et al. Inhibition of leukocyte migration by cancer chemotherapeutic agents and its prevention by free radical scavengers and thiols, *Eur J Hematol* 1988; 40: 69–74

Takata, T. et al. Specific inhibitory effect of dietary eicosapentaenoic acid on N-nitroso-N-methylurea-induced mammary carcinogenesis in female Sprague-Dawley rats, *Carcinogenesis* November 1990; 11(1): 2012–9

Takeshita, M. et al. Antitumour effects of RBS (rice bran saccharide) on ENNG-induced carcinogenesis, *Biotherapy* 1992; 4: 139–45

Talamini, R. et al. Selected medical conditions and risk of breast cancer, *J Cancer* 1997; 75(11): 1699–703

Taper, H. S. et al. Non-toxic potentiation of cancer chemotherapy by combined C and K3 vitamin pre-treatment, *Int J Cancer* 1987; 40: 575–9

Taper, H. S. et al. Non-toxic sensitization of cancer chemotherapy by combined vitamin C and K3 pretreatment in mouse tumor resistant to oncovin, *Anticancer Res* 1992; 12: 1651–4

Teas, J. et al. Dietary seaweed (Lamianria) and mammary carcinogenesis in rats, *Cancer Res* 1984; 44: 2758–61

Thompson, L. U. et al. Flaxseed and its lignan and oil components reduce mammary tumour growth at a late stage of carcinogenesis, *Carcinogenesis* 1996; 17: 1373–6

Thompson, L. U. et al. Antitumorigenic effect of a mammalian lignan precursor from flaxseed, *Nutr Cancer* 1996; 26: 159–65

Thurne, I. et al. Physical activity and the risk of breast cancer, *N Engl J Med* 1997; 336: 1269–75

Tinsley, I. J. et al. Influence of dietary fatty acids on the incidence of mammary tumours in the C3H mouse, *Cancer Res* 1981; 41: 1460–5

Toniolo, P. et al. Calorie-providing nutrients and risk of breast cancer, *JNCI* 1989; 81: 278–86

Toniolo, P. et al. Consumption of meat, animal products, protein and fat and risk of breast cancer – a prospective cohort study in New York, *Epidemiology* 1994; 5: 391–7

Turley, J. M. et al. Vitamin E succinate induces fat-mediated apoptosis in estrogen receptor negative human breast cancer cells, *Cancer Research* 1997; 57: 881–90

Unnikrishnan, M. C. et al. Cytotoxicity of extracts of spices to cultured cells, *Nutr Cancer* 1988; 11: 251–7

Ursin, G. et al. Use of oral contraceptives and risk of breast cancer in young women, *Breast Cancer Res Treat* 1998; 50: 175–84

Valentine, T. The hidden hazards of microwave cooking, *Nexus* April/May 1995 (reprinted from April 1994 issue *Acres*, PO Box 8800, Metairle, Louisiana 70011, USA)

Van Vleet, J. F. Effects of selenium-vitamin E on adriamycin induced cardio-myopathy in rabbits, *J Vest Res* 1978; 39: 997–1010

Verma, S. P. et al. Curcumin and genistein, plant natural products, show synergistic inhibitory effects on the growth of human breast cancer MCF-7 cells induced by estrogenic pesticides, *Biochem Biophys Res Commun* 1997; 233: 692–6

Verma, S. P. et al. The inhibition of the estrogenic effects of pesticides and environmental chemicals by curcumin and isoflavonoids, *Environ Health Perspect* 1998; 106: 807–12

Verma, S. P. et al. Effects of soy-derived isoflavonoids on the induced growth of MCF-7 cells by estrogenic environmental chemicals, *Nutr Cancer* 1998; 30: 232–9

Verhagen, H. et al. Reduction of oxidative DNA-damage in humans by Brussels sprouts, *Carcinogenesis* 1995; 16(4): 969–70

Verhoeven, D. T. et al. A review of mechanisms underlying anticarcinogenicity by brassica vegetables, *Chem Biol Interact* 1997; 103(2): 79–129

Verma, S. P. et al. Effects of soy-derived isoflavonoids on the induced growth of MCF-7 cells by estrogenic environmental chemicals, *Nutr Cancer* 1998; 30: 232–9

Vessey, M. P. Effects of endogenous and exogenous hormones on breast cancer: epidemiology, *Verh Dtch Ges Pathol* 1997; 81: 493–501

Vojdani, A. and Namatalla, G. Enhancement of human Natural Killer cytotoxic activity by vitamin C in pure and augmented formulations, *J of Nutr & Env Med* 1997; 7: 187–95

Von Fournier, D. et al. Natural growth rate of primary breast cancer and its metastases. In: Kubli, F. et al. (eds), *Breast Diseases*, Springer-Verlag (Berlin), 1990: pp. 79–96

Bibliography

Wald, N. J. et al. Plasma retinol, beta-carotene and vitamin E levels in relation to the future risk of breast cancer, *Br J Cancer* 1984; 49: 321–4

Wang, C. et al. Lignans and flavonoids inhibit aromatase enzyme in human preadiposites, *J Steroid Biochem Mol Biol* 1994; 50: 205–12

Wang, D. Y. et al. Serum hormone levels in British and rural Chinese females, *Breast Cancer Res Treat* 1991; 18: S41–5

Wang, H. et al. The oxygen radical absorbing capacity of anthocyanins, *J Agric Food Chem* 1997; 45: 304–9

Wang, J. et al. Enhancing effects of anti-tumour polysaccharide from astragalus or radix hedysarum on C3 clevage production of macrophages in mice, *Jpn J Pharmacol* 1989; 51: 432–4

Wang, T. T. et al. Molecular effects of genistein on estrogen receptor mediated pathways, *Carcinogenesis* 1996; 17(2): 271–5

Wang, Y. M. et al. Effects of vitamin E against adriamycin-induced toxicity in rabbits, *Cancer Res* 1980; 40: 1022–7

Watrach, A. M. et al. Inhibition of human breast cancer cells, *Cancer Letters* 1984; 25: 41–7

Wattenberg, L. W. et al. Inhibition of polycyclic aromatic hydrocarbon induced neoplasia by naturally occurring indoles, *Cancer Res* 1978; 38: 1410–13

Waxman, S. et al. The enhancement of 5-FU antimetabolic activity by leucovorin, menadione, and alpha-tocopherol, *Eur J Cancer Clin Oncol* 1982; 18(7): 685–92

Webb, C. Teaching for recovery from surgery. In: Wilson-Barnett, J. (ed.), *Patient Teaching*, Churchill Livingstone (Edinburgh), 1983: p. 34

Weed, Susan S. *Breast Cancer? Breast Health!*, Ash Tree Publishing (USA), 1996

Well Woman's International Network, Autumn 1998 Newsletter. Le Brecque, Alderney, Channel Islands GY9 3TJ, UK

Welsch, C. W. Dietary fat, calories and mammary gland tumourgenesis, *Adv Exp Med Biol* 1992; 322: 203–22

Welsch, C. W. Caffeine and the development of the normal and neoplastic mammary gland, *Proc Soc Exp Biol Med* 1994; 207(1): 1–12

Welsch, C. W. et al. Suppression of growth by dietary fish oil of human breast carcinomas maintained in three different strains of immune-deficient mice, *Nutr Cancer* 1993; 20: 119–27

Welsh, J. Induction of apoptosis in breast cancer cells in response to vitamin D and antiestrogens, *Biochem Cell Biol* 1994; 72: 537–45

Westin, J. et al. The Israel breast cancer anomaly, *Acad Sci* 1990; 609: 269–79

White, E. et al. Breast cancer among young US women in relation to oral contraceptive use, *J Natl Cancer Inst* 1994; 86: 505–14

Willett, W. C. et al. Dietary fat and fibre in relation to risk of breast cancer, *JAMA* 1992; 268: 2037–44

Wilmore, D. W. et al. Role of glutamine in immunologic responses, *Nutrition* 1998; 14; 7–8, 618–26

Wolff, M. S. et al. Blood levels of organochlorine residues and risk of breast cancer, *J Natl Cancer Inst* 1993; 85: 648–52

Wood, A. J. Tamoxifen in the treatment of breast cancer, *Drug Therapy* 1998; 339(22): 1609–18

Wood, L. A. Possible prevention of adriamycin induced alopecia by tocopherol, *N Engl J Med* 1985; 312: 16 (letter)

Woods, M. N. et al. Low fat, high fibre diet and serum estrone sulphate in premenopausal women, *Am J Clin Nutr* 1989; 49: 1179–93

World Cancer Research Fund and American Institute for Cancer Research, *Food, Nutrition and the Prevention of Cancer: A Global Perspective*, 1998

Wynder, E. L. et al. Diet and breast cancer in causation and therapy, *Cancer* 1986; 58: 1804–13

Xia Xu, et al. Bioavailability of soybean isoflavones depends upon gut microflora in women, *J Nutr* 1995; 125: 2307–15

Yam, D. Insulin–cancer relationships: possible dietary implication. *Med Hypotheses* 1992; 38(2): 111–17

Yoshida, S. et al. Effects of glutamine supplements and radiochemotherapy on systemic immune and gut barrier function in patients with advanced esophageal cancer, *Ann Surg* 1998; 227(4): 485–91

Zarid, D. et al. Diet, alcohol consumption and reproductive factors in a case-control study of breast cancer in Moscow, *Int J Cancer* 1991; 48: 493–501

Zava, D. T. and Duwe, G. Estrogenic and antiproliferative properties of genistein and other flavonoids in human breast cancer cells in vitro, *Nutr Cancer* 1997; 27(1): 31–40

Zava, D. T. et al. Estrogen and progestin bioactivity of foods, herbs and spices, *Proceedings of the Society for Experimental Biology and Medicine* 1998; 217: 369–78

Zhang, Z. L. et al. Hepatoprotective effects of astragalus root, *J Ethnopharmacol* 1990; 30: 145–9

Zheng, W. et al. Well-done meat intake and the risk of breast cancer, *J Natl Cancer Inst* 1998; 90(22); 1724–9

Ziegler, T. R. et al. Clinical and metabolic efficacy of glutamine supplemented parenteral nutrition after bone marrow transplantation. A randomized, double-blind, controlled study, *Ann Intern Med* 1992; 116: 821–8

Recipe Index

General Index

General Index

General Index

General Index

insecticides 28, 60, 107, 187
insomnia 262
insulin 58–9, 75, 77, 168, 245, 246, 248
insulin resistance 73, 247
interferon 14, 143, 150
interleukin 14, 143
International Agency for Research on
Cancer 13
invasive ductal carcinoma 43
iodine 147, 168, 258, 260
ipriflavone 264
iron 73, 131, 155, 162, 168–9, 232, 264,
348
irritability 26
irritable bowel syndrome 28, 154, 268, 298
isoflavones 77, 101, 117, 119, 137, 141,
147, 149, 181–2, 212, 263
isothiocyanates 137, 138
Israel 110, 198

James, Professor Philip 6
Japan 109, 258
Japanese diet 84, 87, 116, 203
Japanese women 12, 64, 65, 67, 87–8, 103,
147, 191, 261
Johns Hopkins University 251
Journal of the Royal College of Surgery 293
juices 15, 132–3, 205–6, 247, 271, 317

kaempferol 137
kafir 150
kava 299
Kellogg, Dr John Harvey 115
kidneys
kidney damage 157
kidney stones 12, 162
and vitamin C 162
King's College Hospital, London 254, 290
Klinefelter's syndrome 48
'Knitbone' 318
Kobe Pharmaceutical University, Japan 143
Kombucha 136

L-glutamine 155, 177–9, 233, 234, 248,
275, 287, 340, 341
Lactobacilli species 173, 340
lactose 150
laetrile 138
Lancet 190, 254, 261
laxatives 268
LDL cholesterol levels 265, 266, 325
lead 131, 167, 172, 287, 288
leben 150
lecithin 148, 347

Lee, Dr John 21, 251–2, 256, 266
*Natural Progesterone: The Multiple Roles of
a Remarkable Hormone* 251
legumes 138, 141
Leinster, Sam 293
lemon juice 286, 341
lentils 72, 146, 209
Leucovorin 161, 342
Levin, Ronald 151
libido 262
licorice 142, 248
lignans 76, 77, 101, 117, 142, 143, 146,
173, 209, 268, 279
limonene 140
Lindane 108–9
linoleic acid 83
linseeds 117, 119, 142, 216–17, 233, 263,
268
recommended amounts 226
lipid peroxidation 165, 209
lipoic acid 179, 233, 234, 248, 349
liver
and chemopreventive foods 14
and coffee 126
detoxification 178
forms glucuronides 268
improving liver health 286–7
processes spent oestrogens 268
protecting from chemotherapy damage
341–2
and ultrasound 309
liver damage 157
liver detoxifiers 206
liver infections 48
lobules 33, 34
carcinoma 43
Lockwood, Knud 158
lumpectomy 308, 310
as an option 4, 303, 305
lycopene 101, 149, 180, 233, 234, 349
lymph flow, improving 196
lymph glands *see* lymph nodes
lymph nodes
acting as filters 33
calcifications 39
clearance 4, 19
lumps 34
spread of breast cancer into 89
surgery 34, 304, 310, 316
and the TNM system 55–6
lymph system 283–5, 310
lymph vessels 33
lymphatic system 33–4
lymphoedema 34, 315–16, 318–19, 320

426

General Index

General Index

General Index